CASE MANAGEMENT FOR THE HEALTH, HUMAN, AND VOCATIONAL REHABILITATION SERVICES

FIRST EDITION

Edited by

Keith B. Wilson
Southern Illinois University Carbondale

Carrie L. Acklin
University of Wisconsin, Stout

Si-Yi Chao
Southern Illinois University Carbondale

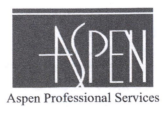

Aspen Professional Services

2018

PUBLISHED BY
Aspen Professional Services
63 Duffers Drive
Linn Creek, MO 65052

Case Management for the Health, Human, and Vocational Rehabilitation
Services
[Edited by] Keith B. Wilson
              Carrie L. Acklin
              Si-Yi Chao

Includes bibliographical references
ISBN 978-0-9853389-8-5

TABLE OF CONTENTS

PART II: CASE MANAGEMENT IN ACTION:
NAVIGATING VARIOUS CASE MANAGEMENT SERVICE
SETTINGS

Acknowledgements

There are many people that we would like to thank that made this edition of the book possible. First, we would like to formally acknowledge the work and dedication of all the contributing authors who committed both time and creatively to this project. For many, we asked things as editors that might not be considered normal when contributing to such a book. We say thanks for your outstanding contributions. Secondly, we would like to thank our families, friends and colleagues for their support in facilitating the completion of our most ambitious book project. We hope that our readers will get as much as we did in producing this first edition.

Editors:
Keith B. Wilson
Carrie L. Acklin
Si-Yi (Jessica) Chao

EDITORS AND CONTRIBUTORS

EDITORS

CARRIE L. ACKLIN, PHD, is an Assistant Professor and Director of Rehabilitation and Criminal Justice at the University of Wisconsin-Stout. Dr. Acklin earned her PhD in rehabilitation from Southern Illinois University, Carbondale. Her professional background includes working with individuals who have substance use and mental health disorders. In her five years of professional experience, Dr. Acklin has worked as both a case manager and a therapist. She has worked in several treatment settings that include outpatient, intensive outpatient, partial hospitalization, residential, hospital-based, and community-based care. Dr. Acklin's research focuses on culturally competent care for individuals of underrepresented groups, people living with HIV, and increasing consumer engagement in services.

SI-YI CHAO, M.S., is a doctoral student in rehabilitation counseling and administration program in the Rehabilitation Institute of Southern Illinois University Carbondale. She has work for 10 years as a licensed physical therapist in the hospital where she provided physical therapy, rehabilitation counseling, and case management for people with neurological impairments, chronic pain, cancer, people living with HIV/AIDS, and people with work injuries. Part of her responsibilities was to supervise new employees and conduct internship training programs. She received her bachelor's degree in physical therapy at China Medical University and master's degree in rehabilitation counseling at the Changhua University of Education in Taiwan. Ms. Chao has served people who used intensive care, inpatient or outpatient services through the holistic model. She provided treatment programs, required information, and integrated resources of medical, psychological, vocational, academic, and social aspects based on the needs of customers. Additionally, she created a community-based rehabilitation program funded by Taiwan's government. This program administered evaluation, treatment plans, education of health promotion, psychological adaptation, coping strategies, advocacy, and resource integration for customers. Moreover, she provided outreach services to nursing facilities, community organizations, and schools for physical and mental health promotion. Ms. Chao's research interests include life care planning for people with disabilities, community-based rehabilitation applications, quality of life promotion, life care management, supervisor education training, and multicultural competences of human service professionals. She received the Dorothy Dykema Endowed Scholarship and the National Association of Rehabilitation Leadership Award presented by the Rehabilitation Institute at Southern Illinois University Carbondale.

KEITH B. WILSON, PHD, CRC, ABDA, NCC, LPC (PA), LCPC (IL), is a Professor in the Rehabilitation Institute at Southern Illinois University Carbondale (SIUC). He served as administrator and faculty member at The Pennsylvania State University (Penn State) for 15 years and Dean of the College of Education and Human Services at SIUC. During his tenure at Penn State University, he was also the owner and Director of Counseling, Consultation and Psychotherapy, and Services (CCPS) in State College, PA. He received his B.A., M. Ed., and PhD degrees from Wilberforce University, Kent State University, and The Ohio State University, respectively. As a professor, he routinely teaches undergraduate, masters, and doctoral level students. Dr. Wilson has approximately 100 scholarly publications (e.g., journal articles, book, and book chapters) and an estimated 170 presentations at the local, state, national, and international levels. His research interests are primarily centered around two areas: 1. Cross-cultural/multicultural issues among persons with disabilities and 2. Privilege based on phenotype (e.g., skin color, gender) in the United States. His current research is looking at improving the Multicultural Counseling Competencies to use more application approaches to cross-cultural trainings in both education and the human services.

Committed to the ideals of research, teaching, and service, he has been honored in several service, research, and lifetime achievement awards including the Researcher of the Year Award from the National Council of Rehabilitation Education, the Virgie Winston-Smith Lifetime Achievement Award, presented by the National Association of Multicultural Rehabilitation Concerns, and the James F. Garrett Distinguished Career in Rehabilitation Research Award, presented by the American Rehabilitation Counseling Association. Dr. Wilson's expertise is widely solicited by many agencies in the U.S. He was recently invited to participate in the Healthy People 2020 Law and Health Policy project as member of the Report Working Group for Disability and Health. This project is sponsored by the CDC Foundation, in collaboration with the U.S. Department of Health and Human Services' (HHS), Office of Disease prevention and Health promotion (ODPHP), the Robert Wood Johnson Foundation, and the Centers for Disease Control and prevention. Dr. Wilson has been active in

Upward Bound, Summer Opportunity Research Program (SORP), and McNair programs contributing as a workshop presenter, social, and research mentor for the past 30 years. These programs are in place to facilitate college and/or graduate school success for students from underrepresented populations. He is a Certified Rehabilitation Counselor (CRC), National Certified Counselor (NCC), Licensed Professional Counselor (LPC) in Pennsylvania, Licensed Clinical Professional Counselor (LCPC) in Illinois, and American Board of Disability Analysts (ABDA) Diplomat.

CONTRIBUTORS

SHIRLENE SMITH AUGUSTIN, PHD, D.A., is an Associate Professor and the Recruitment and admissions Coordinator in the Department of Counseling at North Carolina Agricultural & Technical State University. Dr. Smith-Augustine's research interests include international counseling, multicultural and social justice issues, school counseling, spirituality in counseling, teen pregnancy, and advising/mentorship for graduate learners.

JAMES ATHANASOU, PHD, is a Psychologist in private practice, specializing in vocation assessment of persons with an injury. He is also Associate Professor in Rehabilitation Counseling (2014-2018) at The University of Sydney. He lectures in the Master's program in Vocational Development and Applied Psychosocial and Medical aspects of Rehabilitation. In 2017, he coordinates the dissertation subject.

CHANDRA DONNELL CAREY, PHD, CRC., is an Associate Professor of Rehabilitation Counseling and currently serves as the Interim Chair of the Department of Rehabilitation and Health Services. Dr. Carey has served as an editorial board member for the Journal of Multicultural Counseling and Development and is the former President for the National Association of Multicultural Rehabilitation Concerns. She is a Certified Rehabilitation Counselor and previously held a Licensed Professional Counselor intern designation in the State of Michigan (2005-2009). She is currently the Co-Investigator on a two-year, $353,000 Minority Health Research Grant Program project sponsored by the Texas Higher Education Coordinating Board, and a four-year, $1.2 million-dollar Department of Health and Human Services, Health Resources, and Services Administration Behavioral Health Grant. Dr. Carey has contributed well over 25 refereed publications and book chapters to the literature and completed 39 national presentations over her 16-year career as a scholar. She is the recipient of 7

Research and service awards and is regarded in her discipline as one of the top multicultural researchers. Her research interests include: multicultural competency in rehabilitation counselor education and practice; multicultural clinical supervision practices; and women of color with severe mental illness and rehabilitation outcomes.

DENISE CATALANO, PHD, is an Associate Professor and Graduate Coordinator in the Department of Rehabilitation and Health Services at the University of North Texas.

MARTHA H. CHAPIN, PHD, LPC, CRC, CDMS, NCC, is a Professor and Director of the Bachelor of Science in Rehabilitation Services program at East Carolina University. She worked for 17 years as a rehabilitation counselor in private for-profit rehabilitation and for one year with the state federal rehabilitation agency handling their workers' compensation caseload. Her research interest includes employment for persons with spinal cord injuries, quality of life, and using positive psychology techniques in rehabilitation counseling. She also enjoys writing about case management techniques in practice.

RALPH M. CRYSTAL is Wallace Charles Hill Professor of Rehabilitation Counseling and Chair, Department of Early Childhood, Special Education, and Rehabilitation Counseling at the University of Kentucky (1981-Present). Previously he was Coordinator of the Rehabilitation Counseling program. He was an Assistant Professor of Rehabilitation Counseling and Research Director of a Rehabilitation Research Institute at the University of Michigan (1977-1981). His research interests are related to employment law and forensic rehabilitation. He is a Certified Rehabilitation Counselor and a Licensed Professional Counselor in the Commonwealth of Kentucky. He maintains a forensic rehabilitation practice and is on the roster of vocation experts of the U.S. Social Security Administration.

YASMIN E. GAY, MS, CCJP, LCAS, LPC, MAC, CRC, CCS, is a doctoral student at North Carolina Agricultural and Technical State University pursuing a PhD in Rehabilitation Counseling and Rehabilitation Counseling Education. She received her master's degree in Rehabilitation Counseling from Winston Salem State University and a bachelor's degree in Criminal Justice from Fayetteville State University. Yasmin has worked in the human service profession for several years in residential, outpatient, and intensive outpatient settings. She is currently an adjunct instructor with the Human Services Department at Guilford Technical Community College and independently contracts with community agencies providing clinical supervision, consultation, and counseling services. Yasmin holds credentials in Licensed Clinical Addictions Specialist (LCAS), Licensed Profession Counselor (LPC), Master Addiction Counselor (MAC), Certified Rehabilitation Counselor (CRC), Certified Clinical Supervisor (CCS), and Certified Criminal Justice Addictions Professional (CCJP). Yasmin's research interests include substance abuse, clinical supervision, and wellness.

BRYAN O. GERE, PHD, is an Assistant Professor in the Psychology and Counseling program at Alabama A&M University, Normal (Huntsville), AL. His research interests include efficiency in vocational rehabilitation service delivery, innovative service delivery, and fiscal management in state vocational rehabilitation agencies and community rehabilitation programs.

JASON E. GINES, PHD, is the Director of Inclusion and Diversity Engagement in the College of Information Sciences and Technology at Pennsylvania State University (University Park). He obtained the PhD in Counselor Education & Supervision with a specialized focus in Rehabilitation Counseling from Penn State University. He earned two Master's degrees in Counselor Education and Divinity from Penn State and Vanderbilt University, respectively.

MICHAEL T. HARTLEY, PHD, is an Associate Professor in the Counseling Program at the University of Arizona. Much of his scholarship on ethics has targeted distributive justice issues and his scholarship on ethical obligations has focused on the importance of promoting resilience and advocating against ableism or the preference of able-bodiedness. Dr. Hartley was the primary investigator of grants to promote resilience among military veterans with spinal cord injuries and youth with disabilities during the school-to-work transition. Recently, his research on ethical issues in rehabilitation counseling practice were used to guide recent revisions to the 2017 Commission on Rehabilitation Counselor Code of Ethics (CRCC) and a taskforce he served on. Dr. Hartley is knowledgeable about the profession and professional practice of rehabilitation counseling, and is committed to defining and better preparing rehabilitation counselors to work ethically and effectively with persons with disabilities.

JULIE C. HILL, M.ED., NCC, is a doctoral candidate in Counselor Education and Supervision at the University of Arkansas. Her research interests include psychosocial adaptation to chronic illness and disability and career implications of chronic illness. She has conducted several national presentations and authored or co-authored book chapters and articles in peer-reviewed rehabilitation journals.

SARA P. JOHNSTON, PHD, is an Assistant Professor and program director for the Clinical Rehabilitation Counseling program in the Department of Clinical Counseling and Mental Health at Texas Tech University Health Sciences Center. Dr. Johnston has over 10 years' experience in the counseling field, primarily in the areas of tobacco cessation counseling and supported community living counseling for individuals with psychiatric and cognitive disabilities. Dr. Johnston was also employed as ADA Wisconsin Project Coordinator. Dr. Johnston's research interests include ethics and ethical practice, global health and disability issues, health and wellness promotion for individuals with disabilities, and ADA accommodations under the Americans with Disabilities Act. Dr. Johnston currently serves as president for the Rehabilitation Counselor and Educators Association, and is past-president of the National Association of Disability Benefits Specialists. She also served as a member of the Commission on Rehabilitation Counselor Certification 2017 Code of Ethics Revision Task Force.

AMBER KHAN, is a Nationally Certified Counselor and a Licensed Professional Counselor Associate. In 2008, she graduated with a Bachelor's degree in Psychology from the University of North Carolina at Greensboro. In 2012, Amber earned a Master's degree in School Counseling at North Carolina Agricultural and Technical State University. Currently, she is a second-year doctoral student in the Rehabilitation Counseling and Rehabilitation Counselor Education program at North Carolina Agricultural and Technical State University. Amber is an active member of the American Counseling Association and the North Carolina School Counselors Association. She has 15 years of advocacy and community service work experience. Serving on various non-profit boards, one of her goals is to continue to bridge the gaps of communication between the several organizations and institutions that she is affiliated with in the Central North Carolina region.

LYNN KOCH, PH.D, CRC, is a Professor in the Rehabilitation Counseling Program at the University of Arkansas. Her current research interests include the psychosocial and vocational aspects of emerging disabilities, the treatment of people with disabilities in the workplace, and the persistence of students with disabilities in higher education. She has authored or co-authored more than 100 publications on these and related topics. In 2017, she co-authored a textbook entitled Rehabilitation

Counseling and Emerging Disabilities: Medical, Psychosocial, and Vocational Aspects that was published by Springer Publishing Company. As a former state vocational rehabilitation counselor, Dr. Koch has a unique understanding of the psychosocial and workplace experiences of people with disabilities. Because of this professional background, her research and teaching emphasize consumer perspectives regarding how to remove barriers to education, employment, and community integration so that individuals with disabilities can enjoy all the rights and privileges of the rest of American society.

SHAKEERRAH D. LAWRENCE, LPC, PVE, is a second-year doctoral student in Rehabilitation Counselor Education at North Carolina Agricultural and Technical State University. She possesses master's degrees in Rehabilitation Counseling and Adult Education. Her professional experience includes working as a Vocational Evaluator, professional Counselor, and a Vocational Expert. Her research interests are rehabilitation counselor wellness, spirituality in counseling, and the mental health needs of diverse populations.

SHALINI MATHEW, is a second-year doctoral student at North Carolina Agricultural and Technical State University pursuing her Ph.D. in Rehabilitation Counseling and Counseling Education. She received her first master's degree in Behavior Science and a bachelor's degree in Family and Community Science from Mahatma Gandhi University, India. She also received a second master's degree in School Counseling from Martin Luther Christian University, India. Shalini has worked in the behavioral health profession for several years in outpatient and inpatient settings. Currently, she is a graduate assistant in the Assessment and Analytics department of the Office of Strategic Planning and Institutional Effectiveness at North Carolina Agricultural & Technical State University. Her research interests include Specific Learning Disabilities, Counselor Wellness, Mindfulness, Clinical Supervision, and Challenges of International Students.

DEANA LACY MCQUITTY, PHD, CCC-SLP, is currently the Speech Program Director (Speech-Language Pathology and Audiology and Speech/Communication Concentrations) and Assistant Professor in the Department of Administration and Instructional Services in the College of Education at North Carolina Agricultural and Technical State University. She received her Master's in Science in Communication Sciences and Disorders from Southern Connecticut State University in New Haven, Connecticut, and her Doctorate in Speech Language Pathology from Nova Southeastern University in Fort Lauderdale, Florida. She has worked for over 17 years as a speech language pathologist and as an academician. She has provided skilled speech language pathology in a variety of settings including early intervention, school-based speech language pathology, skilled nursing facilities and medical based speech language pathology. She has taught an array of courses that expand across the lifespan including Development of Speech Language in Children, Neuroanatomy in Communication Sciences and Disorders, Language Disorders, Early Intervention in Infants and Toddlers, Clinical Practicum in Developmental Disorders, Clinical Practicum in Acquired Adult Disorders and Diagnostics in Communication Sciences and Disorders.

VANESSA M. PERRY, PHD, CRC, is an Assistant Professor of Practice in the Counseling Program at University of Arizona. As an American Red Cross Disaster Mental Health Volunteer, she responded to the aftermath of the 2014 tornadoes in North Carolina. Dr. Perry has been a rehabilitation counselor, disability rights advocate, social service support to military families, clinical mental health counselor, and clinical supervisor. Most recently, she provided outreach and counseling services to homeless veterans via a mobile clinic. Her research interests include the clinical supervision experience of Spanish-English bilingual supervisees.

JENNIFER DASHIELL-SHOFFNER, has been an educator at North Carolina Agricultural and Technical State University for 14 years. She possesses master's degrees in Industrial/Organizational Psychology and Rehabilitation Counseling, and is currently pursuing a doctorate in Rehabilitation Counselor Education. She has taught numerous courses in psychology and counseling and is knowledgeable in other areas such as public health, autism spectrum disorder, and gerontology. She has presented at several conferences and served as a research assistant on projects that have been associated with both the community health and counseling fields.

ALAYNA THOMAS, received her Bachelor's Degree in Psychology from the University of North Carolina at Greensboro in 2012. Alayna continued her education and pursued her Masters in Rehabilitation Counseling at North Carolina Agricultural and Technical State University. Currently, Alayna is a doctoral student in the Rehabilitation Counseling and Counselor Education program at North Carolina Agricultural and Technical State University and anticipates graduating in May 2019. Alayna is a Certified Rehabilitation Counselor who has work experience in the public and non-profit sectors working with individuals and families. As a client centered counselor, her greatest passion is assisting clients in finding healthy perceptions of themselves and strengthening their relationships, so they can know themselves as peaceful, complete, whole, and safe.

TYRA TURNER WHITTAKER, PHD, LPC, CRC, is currently a Professor of Counseling and the Coordinator of the PhD in Rehabilitation Counseling and Rehabilitation Counselor Education Program at North Carolina A&T State University. She has received over 13 million in grant funds to meet the needs of racial and ethnic minorities with disabilities and addictive behaviors. Additionally, she assisted in the development of the PhD in Rehabilitation Counseling and Rehabilitation Counselor Education with an emphasis on Trauma and Trauma Informed Care. She has also served as the Co-Principal Investigator on grants to establish certificate programs in Vocational Evaluation, Work Adjustment, Rehabilitation Psychology, and Behavioral Medicine. She has worked with the university's counseling center to obtain grant funding in substance abuse prevention. She has numerous presentations and publications in rehabilitation and multicultural counseling and has served on numerous professional boards including the Arkansas Board of Examiners in Counseling, Commission on Rehabilitation Counseling Certification (CRCC), National Council on Rehabilitation Education (NCRE), and the Council for Accreditation of Counseling and Related Educational Programs (CACREP).

INTRODUCTION TO BOOK

PART I: CASE MANAGEMENT FUNDAMENTALS

Most of what is presented in the first part of this book is foundational. It describes what case management tools are utilized across many areas of expertise in the human, allied health, and rehabilitation services. Included are one or two chapters that readers might consider unique and helpful for professional development (e.g., *Documentation Evolution: Electronic Health Records*).

With the changing diversity of the United States, it has become increasingly salient that service providers expand their toolbox of service delivery to maintain standards of care for all clients. Thus, it is our belief that high quality and competent services begin with effective case management covering a wide-range of services. As with many service delivery modes, case management services occur across many specializations including health care, behavioral health, allied health, and vocational rehabilitation services.

While the processes in many delivery systems are admittedly different, there is an overwhelming similarity of processes that must occur to deliver high quality and competent service delivery for those serving health, human, and vocational rehabilitation services in the United States. The aim of this book is to inform best practices across several areas of specializations to:

➢ show a connection between delivery systems to provide better services to clients and families, and

➢ include the latest trends related to serving underrepresented groups to facilitate better outcomes for all client populations.

Part I of this book covers fundamental, yet critical, case management functions across several areas including the intake interview, counselling skills, medical and psychosocial aspects, ethics, possible employment barriers, multicultural and family considerations, referral options, substance use disorders, and electronic health records.

The order of chapters is based upon our belief that counseling skills are paramount to providing effective services to our clients. Thus, communication skills and multicultural considerations anchor the books with foundational content to assist students in serving all populations they may encounter in the future. These and other chapters will generally provide:

1. Empirical data to support best practices in case management services, and

2. A standardized process, focusing on the commonalities of case management services across several human and health care service areas.

Because of the writing style of this book, instructors of both undergraduate and graduate education can tailor content to facilitate learning objectives for many audiences.

PART II: CASE MANAGEMENT IN ACTION: NAVIGATING VARIOUS CASE MANAGEMENT SERVICE SETTINGS

Most of what is presented in Part II of this book is foundational for unique areas of practice that occur in social work, psychology, counselor education, and rehabilitation services. We attempt to differentiate between several areas of expertise to provide a more in-depth examination of skills used in these areas (*e.g., Case Management in Forensic Environments, Case Management, Mental Health, Substance Abuse*). Additionally, because of the interconnectedness, once students understand the foundational information covered in Part I of the book, Part II will introduce students to areas and expertise needed to work in environments and, by extension, work with different case management populations to facilitate better services.

PART I: CASE MANAGEMENT FUNDAMENTALS

CHAPTER 1

COUNSELING SKILLS NEEDED IN CASE MANAGEMENT

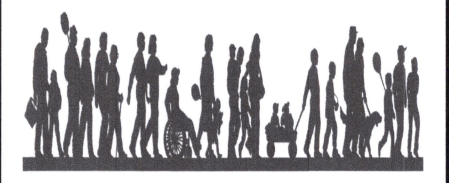

JASON E. GINES

CHANDRA DONNELL CAREY

KEITH B. WILSON

ABSTRACT

When people seeking case management services are not satisfied with the services, they tend to not come back to the human or allied health agency. Not understanding, but applying basic counseling skills across many contexts, account for many reasons why seekers of case management services are not satisfied with the services they receive. As a human being (e.g., European American, African American, gay, female) means that you are part of the diversity equation. How people communicate and have civil discourse within institutions in the United States has become a pervasive and perplexing problem for our society. Across many segments of society (e.g. education, government, and allied health services), a seminal question is being considered; how do we talk about difficult topics without devolving into highly polarized positions? Yes, case managers and other human and allied health professionals are front and center to the ever-changing face of civil discourse. This chapter will explore basic counseling skills, validation, and how to apply general counseling aids in a systematic way to positively impact clients in the case management context. The ability to recognize that both case managers and clients are cultural beings is important in understanding validation. The intersection of basic counseling skills and the application of a decision-making process are explored further in a case study with discussion questions that highlight key points in each area of a model for decision-making and better communication.

CHAPTER HIGHLIGHTS

➢ Basic Counseling Skills in Case Management;

➢ Communication that Leads to Validation;

➢ Decision Making in Context.

LEARNING OBJECTIVES

At the conclusion of the chapter, students will be able to:

➢ Describe the concept of active listening;

➢ Understand definitions of validation;

➢ Identify multiple factors that influence and interrupt validation;

➢ Understand how to apply active listening and validation to make decisions for clients;

3

➢ Understand how consistently validating clients can improve case management outcomes.

DISCUSSION QUESTIONS

1. What are the basic counseling skills that can bridge gaps with clients? How can counseling skills be applied in context for all our clients?

2. What are the necessary conditions for validating the lives and experiences of clients? Is validating clients' lives and experiences necessary for each encounter? Why or Why not?

3. What is the process of making informed decisions? How does the decision-making process ensure validation of clients' lives and experiences?

INTRODUCTION

Although this chapter is contextualized in general case management environments, ALL principles introduced can be generalized outside of the case management environment for application. Before any formal information is gathered from a client for an intake interview or first appointment with a case manager, nonverbal interactions with agency representatives are internalized as either hostile, polite, or indifferent. More pointedly, communication starts the second a client enters the office and stops at the front desk and declares, my name is Jason E. Gines and I am here to see Counselor Jane Doe. The nonverbal behavior may signal to a client that your agency may not want to assist them secure services.

A verbal counterproductive encounter is more obvious. We are all diverse beings and are subject to the slights of people who may have a negative perception of our personhood (e.g., gender, sexual orientation). This is an inescapable truth. However, groups who are minorities in the United States (U.S.), based on the context of the U.S., may be more prone to experience counterproductive interactions with human service and allied health providers than others. While we are all considered diverse, there are groups with phenotypical differences in personhood and language that may be prone to experience increased levels of counterproductive behaviors when interacting with the human and allied health services in the U.S. We can trace clients who are dissatisfied with case management services to errors in behaviors by the provider that facilitates a disconnect with the receiver of services.

Case Management, in the United States context, will need to embrace new processes that promote validation in order to stem the tide of polarization in the human and allied health professions. This polarization is taking place within tremendous shifts in racial and ethnic demographics. The U.S. Census Bureau projects that over the next 20-30 years, "more than half of all Americans are projected to belong to a minority group…by 2060, nearly one in five of the nation's total population is projected to be foreign born."[1] It is safe to say that we are living in a time that case management workloads will contain people from more places, with different experiences, than at any other time in our history. In many places in the U.S., this demographic transformation is here and human service providers are already servicing this diverse populace.

Another reason to increase our counseling skills is simple, our professional ethics dictate that we place a priority on helping clients who are "diverse." Let's learn some tools to get ready for the rapidly increasing diversity and to become more ethical. Finally, we believe that understanding what validation is and is not, will enhance positive outcomes for ALL seeking our expertise as case managers.

PRE- COUNSELING ENCOUNTERS

Have you ever had the experience of leaving a verbal encounter with a person and feeling diminished in some aspect of your identity (e.g., ability, sexual orientation, race, etc.)? If yes, what were the follow-up actions you took to determine if you were *correctly* reading the verbal exchange correctly? Whose counsel did you seek? What details did you share with your confidant about who was in the verbal encounter? How did you come to a sense of meaning about the feelings of diminishment, or not? Finally, how did the verbal encounter impact the next time you interacted with that person? This chapter will offer ways to understand and navigate counterproductive moments of verbal exchanges in case management between and among individuals.

One of the first concepts we will review, that is critical to successful navigation of these complex moments is the process of *active listening*. Active listening is arguably the cornerstone of any communicative interaction and it is important to start here. We will also define and provide examples for validating clients on multiple levels of their identity. In addition, a decision-making process will empower you with the ability to apply basic counseling skills to consistently increase opportunities to validate clients in ways that lead to more successful outcomes. Let's begin our journey to better basic counseling and decision-making skills in case management.

ACTIVE LISTENING

Exactly, what is active listening? Across most training programs (e.g., social work, psychology, nursing, counseling), students are taught a series of skills that will assist with their connection to and understanding of client issues. These skills, referred to as microskills, are facilitative in helping case managers to listen effectively and to attend empathically to the concerns of the individuals they are working with. These microskills help to foster the positive relationship needed to empower the client to reach successful outcomes. Many educational programs train students to use listening skills. However, cognitively understanding what a skill is and applying the micro skill is difficult depending upon the context.

There is a hierarchy of skills developed by Ivey and Ivey.[2] These skills move from some of the initial, most critical skills (e.g., active listening, questioning, paraphrasing, etc.) to more complex skills that assist the case manager to reflect meaning and supportively challenge when required. The foundation to the entire hierarchy is ethically grounded and is a culturally responsive practice. Skill acquisition centers on active listening.

Active listening encompasses several components. One area is attending to the intracies of verbal speech (intonation, repetition of words, etc.). What words did the client use? Which words were emphasized? What words were repeated to show significance? Another area of active listening is paying attention to non-verbal behavior (that which might belie the words being spoken). For instance, a client may state that they are excited about a new opportunity, but look away when expressing this thought or have a slumped and or tight body posture when saying so. These particular nonverbals might be commuicating something important from the clients stand point.

Lastly, it is important in active listening to acknowledge or confront the contextual meaning to the words used (what meaning is there that can provide more information about what the client is stating). For instance, when inquiring if a client agrees to a plan of action, if they respond, "I suppose," then you may want to supportively challenge how he or she understands the plan moving forward. Gaining mastery of active listening will help decidedly with the case manager's ability to validate clients, to provide the client with an opportunity to provide greater context to their story, and to allow the case manager space to fully attend to the client in a holistic and affirming way. Let's move to a case study where we will apply some of the prior outlined active listening skills.

CASE STUDY
Ms. MARTEEN

Ms. Marteen is mixed race/ethnicity (Latinx and African-American), aged 52, and resides on the outskirts of town with minimal to no access to transportation. Ms. Marteen grew up in the Deep South, and has recently relocated north to a small college town near Caitlyn Manning's alma mater. She has always wanted to provide a better life for her daughters, and has tried to establish herself in the community.

Ms. Marteen's previous experience with the local health agency is when she tried to seek mental health services for her youngest daughter. She got involved with a local college program that provided free transportation to and from mental health appointments. The experience left her with a positive view of local health care services.

Ms. Marteen has two daughters, one who recently gave birth to a little girl. Ms. Marteen's grand-daughter recently developed asthma, and it has been determined that the cause is high levels of pollution that surround her home. She is the primary caretaker of her grand-daughter, even though she has recently been diagnosed with extremely high blood pressure and diabetes.

Caitlyn Manning is also mixed race (White and Asian), aged 25, and has been in case management for one year. Caitlyn Manning was raised, attended undergraduate and graduate school, and currently resides in a predominantly White environment. Caitlyn attended a top ten counselor education program with an emphasis on multicultural education and social justice. While in college, Caitlyn got involved with several organizations focused on providing mental health care to underserved populations near her campus. Based on this work, she produced a Master's thesis on working with minority populations with mental health issues.

Outside of her formal service roles, Caitlyn has had minimal contact with cultures outside of her own, and largely considers herself to be most familiar and comfortable in, and with, "White culture" in her personal life. Ms. Marteen has been working with Caitlyn for two months at the time of the exchange below. Caitlyn's supervisor is a White male, aged 61, and is one year away from retirement.

The following interaction is presented to better examine active listening.

CAITLYN MANNING: Ms. Marteen! How are you today? I'm glad to hear you are doing well. I just wanted to follow up with you to see if you were ever able to complete that application for the transportation form I sent you. I know how hard it can be for you to get to your appointments without your own car.

Caitlyn immediately makes assumptions about Ms. Marteen's level of ease getting to appointments, instead of utilizing active listening to see what is going on with Ms. Marteen.

MS. MARTEEN: No child, honestly, I haven't even had a chance to look at that mess. You keep sending me all this stuff every week. (sigh) My grandbaby is sick in the hospital and *everyone is focused on helping her get better.* I am not really worried about *my screenings* right now. (long pause) I know they are important though.

Ms. Marteen expresses her truth to Caitlyn, and is communicating that several things have her currently frustrated. Ms. Marteen is also providing viable reasons why she has not been able to fill out paperwork or attend her screenings.

CAITLYN MANNING: My sympathies to you Ms. Marteen. Maybe I could stop by next week and we can fill out the forms together. Don't worry about those missed appointments, you have a lot going on, I can reschedule them for you in a couple of weeks. Does that sound good?

Caitlyn offers "sympathies," but immediately goes into offering a solution before fully acknowledging all that Ms. Marteen has just shared with her. This does not demonstrate active listening due to all the other cues that Caitlyn misses before offering a solution.

MS. MARTEEN: (long pause and then sigh) No…I'm not interested right now…how about I contact you in a couple of weeks? Thank you, good bye now.

Ms. Marteen does not feel heard by Caitlyn, and has become divested from the case management process.

CAITLYN MANNING: (call to supervisor) (exasperated) Well, I guess she just doesn't want help right now. She isn't showing up for any of the appointments I scheduled for her. She will say she needs help with resources, but when I send her the applications, like for transportation assistance and even to help with the costs of her medication, she won't fill them out. I feel that she is not making sufficient progression on her case.

The supervisor responds by saying, "I know it can be frustrating, but sometimes certain clients don't know what's good for them…hang in there, and don't get too frustrated by her lack of motivation." Caitlyn says thanks, and moves the case files to the bottom of her working pile.

Neither Caitlyn nor her supervisor try to investigate Ms. Marteen's lack of "sufficient progression." They immediately move to assumptions instead of engaging in active listening to find out what else may be happening with Ms. Marteen.

What happened here with Ms. Marteen? Let's review some of the words Ms. Marteen verbalized and emphasized (in italics): "mess", "everyone is focused…," "right now." Just examining those words and phrases, we might be able to conclude that Ms. Marteen is distracted and focused more on family than on her own case and health. There are certainly several dynamics to consider here and we will focus on that aspect of communication later in the chapter. Secondly, we can use Ms. Marteen's non-verbal expressions, such as sighs or pauses. Just before discussing her granddaughter and after responding about her own health, there were sighs and pauses. Case managers should note this non-verbal behavior and be ready to acquire additional information regarding potential stressful situations that Ms. Marteen is experiencing.

Lastly, the context behind some of the statements Ms. Marteen made, need to be considered. For instance, she admits that she knows her screenings are important, and she uses the phrase "right now" to perhaps indicate that she perhaps would be more open at an alternative timeframe. Actively listening and employing those skills to ask appropriate follow-up questions, empathically responding to the client's stated and implied concerns, and using the context of what the client is stating to guide your direction with the client, can lead to a stronger relationship with the client and promote the possibility of successful outcomes (e.g., client coming back for next visit). Let's hit the replay button and change the way that Caitlyn Manning responds to Ms. Marteen's verbal and nonverbal reactions in the case study:

CAITLYN MANNING: Ms. Marteen! How are you today? (pause for response).
Active listening involves slowing down to give a client an opportunity to be more descriptive of what is going on in his or her life.
MS. MARTEEN: Not well, (sighs) there is a lot going on right now.
CAITLYN MANNING: I'm sorry to hear that. Sounds like you are a bit troubled. Would you like to talk more about what's going on?
Here, Caitlyn uses several skills that we did not see in her initial response. First, she uses active listening by pausing, which provides Ms. Marteen the space to share. Second, she reflects Ms. Marteen's feelings (we will talk about this more in depth later). Last, she asks a close ended question to gauge if Ms. Marteen wanted to share more (again, we will talk about this more in depth later).
MS. MARTEEN: I just really can't right now, but you called me, so you must've had some business to discuss....
CAITLYN MANNING: Okay, I understand. Please know that if you would like to talk, that is something I can help you with. But, today, I wanted to follow up with you to see if you could complete that application for the transportation form I sent you. I know how hard it can be for you to get to your appointments without your own car.
MS. MARTEEN: No child, honestly, I haven't even had a chance to look at that mess. You keep sending me all this stuff every week. (sigh) My grandbaby is sick in the hospital and *everyone is focused on helping her get better.* I am not really worried about *my screenings* right now. (long pause) I know they are important though.
CAITLYN MANNING: Well, I am truly sorry to hear that. I do hope that your grandbaby is well and able to recover soon. I can imagine it is taking quite a bit of your attention right now. We can pause some of the work we have been doing, so that you can focus on what's important. How about you call within the next few weeks and perhaps we can start considering some of the resources for your case then?
Caitlyn continues using active listening, reflection of feeling, and close ended questions. In addition, Caitlyn is validating Ms. Marteen by offering to focus on "what's important." Validation is giving or providing truth to what a client is experiencing.

MS. MARTEEN: (big sigh) Yes, and thank you. That would probably be best. I just must be here for my family right now.

Ms. Marteen's response has completely changed from being disengaged in the earlier example to gratitude for how Caitlyn treated her and is responding to her.

CAITLYN MANNING: Sure, of course, focus on your granddaughter and family and I will focus on tracking additional resources for you. I'll keep what I find here in the office and we can review it at our next face-to-face. If anything shifts and you need my assistance sooner, don't hesitate to call and I look forward to hearing from you in a few weeks.

Caitlyn was better able to engage Ms. Marteen by demonstrating her concern and empathy for her situation and to pace their interaction in a way that respected the needs of the client.

The replay of the case study responses from the case manager appeared to be much more connected and beneficial to interactions both for Ms. Marteen and Caitlyn. Why? Actively listening to the client allowed the case manager to receive more client information regarding the client and provide a richer context to the communication challenges the case manager felt might be occurring. Additionally, the case manager could facilitate an enhanced interaction, which likely fostered a better working relationship between the two because of the attention paid to the client's verbal and nonverbal behaviors. Active listening skills, one of the foundational skills to all other techniques, are instrumental in fostering effective skills in case management.

BASIC LISTENING SEQUENCE

The case manager had a more successful interaction with Ms. Marteen by effectively using active listening skills. In any interaction with clients, it is critical to use your active listening skills; however, there are additional skills which can facilitate meaningful relationships with clients. The Basic Listening Sequence employs the use of several skills including questioning, paraphrasing and reflecting feeling. We will talk about each of these basic listening techniques as we reflect on the interaction with Ms. Marteen and her case manager, Caitlyn.

QUESTIONS

Almost every counseling encounter will involve some level of questioning. Questions allow the case manager to gather information from the client to either add or clarify the client is seeking services. There are two types of questions case managers employ: open-ended and closed-ended questions. Open-ended questions are those questions that are used to prompt and encourage the client to discuss their perception of events, as well as to discuss their feelings about these events. For example, open ended questions are a great way to engage with the client and to learn more about their needs or desires that will impact their success if they are granted services from the organization. Here is an example of using open-ended question with Ms. Marteen.

CAITLYN MANNING: Hello Ms. Marteen! You look to be in good spirits today.
Caitlyn is using non-verbal cues to make an assertion that Ms. Marteen is "in good spirits." Using non-verbal cues is a good skill for case managers to let clients know they are engaged in and tracking the conversation.
MS. MARTEEN: I'm okay...things are starting to settle down.
CAITLYN MANNING: I'm glad to hear that. It seemed to be a very stressful situation for a while there.
Could you tell me how you have been managing your health since the last time we talked (open ended question)?

Open-ended questions allow the client to provide an overview of a topic to the case manager. However, confiding can be difficult with some clients who are not as talkative. In instances where a client is not as talkative, closed-ended questions can be utilized to best initiate and support on-going dialogue. Closed-ended questions are also a great tool for gathering detailed information or perhaps redirecting the client during session. Let's return to Ms. Marteen.

CAITLYN MANNING: Hello Ms. Marteen! You look to be in good spirits today.
MS. MARTEEN: I'm okay...things are starting to settle down.
CAITLYN MANNING: I'm glad to hear that. It seemed to be a very stressful situation for a while there.
Could you tell me how you have been managing your health since the last time we talked? (open ended question)
MS. MARTEEN: Things have just been okay, you know with my grandbaby sick, everything just focused on her. And now, thank God, she is doing better. I have just been trying to play catch up! Everything just seemed to happen all at once. You know they say when it rains it pours. The doctors think she might have some type of heart condition and that is just sending her mama spinnin'. Do you know any services in the area for children? I'm assuming at some point my granddaughter might need some help too. She was just playing outside and collapsed! We thought we had lost her right there. But our neighbor is a nurse and her son was outside too, so he ran to get his mama. It seems like it's always good people that bad things happen too.
CAITLYN MANNING: Wow, well that is a lot. I can't imagine.
Is your granddaughter home now? (close ended question)

The case manager is preparing to move the conversation back to Ms. Marteen, but used active listening skills to validate (we will define later) Ms. Marteen's experience and to communicate she was listening. The question the case manager posed can allow a very talkative client to continue talking. But remember that you can also use closed questions to redirect the discussion.

CAITLYN MANNING: Wow, well that is a lot. I can only imagine how stressful that was for you.
Were you able to see your doctor at all during that time? (close ended question)

If implemented properly, a well-timed, well-formed, paced, and thoughtful question can enhance the relationship between the case manager and the client and help to provide a richer understanding of the client's issues. While the types of questions used can be helpful, there are other tools that a case manager can implement that will also enhance the relationship between the case manager and the client, while providing more information about the client's experiences.

Let's turn now to paraphrasing and how useful a tool that can be for the case manager.

PARAPHRASING

Paraphrasing is a tool to help the case manager clarify and summarize what the client is saying. It also allows the case manager the opportunity to be sure that they accurately understood what the client was articulating. Think to yourself about those moments in a conversation when you have made a statement and the person totally missed your point. The person who missed your point could have utilized a paraphrase to insure their understanding of your comment. Oftentimes, people assume they know the intended meaning being relayed during a conversation. However, that meaning can be impacted by multiple dynamics, (e.g., age, gender, racial/ethnic identity and sexual identity). Opting to paraphrase allows the case manager to check-in for clarity and understanding, which can bypass critical errors in communication. Paraphrasing, when launched in conjunction with active listening and thoughtful questioning, can facilitate positive moments in the case manager-client relationship.

MS. MARTEEN: No...I just didn't get 'round to it. I can't tell if I am coming or going. I can't sleep, I have nightmares, and I feel like a zombie throughout the day. I am so tense my body aches. No matter what I do, it just keeps getting worse.
CAITLYN MANNING: That must be difficult, to be in this dazed state, sleep-deprived, and stressed, with no real relief from it all.
The case manager summed up in her own words what the Ms. Marteen communicated to her in a succinct manner. This is paraphrasing in action.

REFLECTING FEELING

One final and critical microskill is *reflecting feeling*. Reflection of feeling helps to draw out the client's feelings and leads the case manager to a deeper exploration of emotion.

MS. MARTEEN: (Sigh) I just don't understand that doctor. One minute he says one thing and the next minute it seems like he's saying the opposite.

CAITLYN MANNING: You know it sounds like you feel confused and frustrated by that.

The case manager echoed Ms. Marteen's frustrations by using the words confused and frustrated to attach to the verbal [I just don't understand] and nonverbal [sigh] behaviors.

DEFINING VALIDATION

Defining validation. As with most words, multiple definitions are available that provide slightly different meanings. A formal definition of validation is to make valid; substantiate; confirm.[14] While technically correct, it does not capture the complexity of working in a rich environment where one is called upon to understand various ways a person may see themselves and the world around them. For example, Ms. Marteen may see herself as a woman, Latinx, African-American, grandmother, caretaker, or any number of other identities that may impact her interaction with Caitlyn Manning. The above definition of validation does not reflect a sense of responsibility that case managers need to validate an identity that may be important to a client on that given day.

A more relevant definition of validation is giving or providing truth to what a person is communicating to the case manager. This definition opens the door for both the case manager and the client to honor who they are and their respective stories at the time of exchange. In the revised versions of the conversation between Ms. Marteen and the case manager, a more empathic response was applied to the client when full consideration was given for why she had not been compliant with the case manager's requests. If applied correctly, validation is a tool that will facilitate mutual respect for different experiences in the case management environment.

A BRIEF EXAMPLE OF VALIDATION

A female client comes in a male case manager's office and after a short time, says: "I was just groped by a male colleague at work. I am feeling mad and violated." The case manager responds. "You feel mad and violated because a colleague touched you. Did you do something to invite such a response by your male colleague?" Question. Did the case manager validate the client? It is our experience that most will view the case manager's response as validating the client. In truth, the case manager's response is what most human service professionals are taught in counseling or communications 101 courses in graduate school. The case manager in the example is paraphrasing and responding to content and feelings. This is not a validation response on the part of the case manager. A validating response would be like: "You are tired of being taken advantage of by men. In fact, you get more frustrated because men tend not to believe you when you say you have been harassed." Validation is giving or providing truth to what a person is communicating. A final point in this example. Not only did the case manager not validate the client's experience, but his statement: "did you do something to invite such a response by your male colleague," added insult to injury by verbalizing that the negative experience by her male colleagues was something that she may have invited or brought on herself. This is what many women in the U.S. experience frequently from male colleagues.

Paraphrasing and responding to content and meaning is not considered validation. While gender was used in this example, substitute the gender with other variables (e.g., sexual orientation, a person who may have a disability, race) that might be associated with discrimination, bias, and prejudice. Most people would agree that the female client in this example suffered through a traumatic experience. As stated before, when clients do not feel they receive competent service by providers, they tend to not come back to that particular agency. The unfortunate observation is that many providers do not know that they are not validating their clients because this concept is not underscored in many graduate programs across the U.S. Bottom-line, a client can feel when statements are given, and not given truth by the provider. Active listening can be a helpful skill in adequately validating a client's experience. This is an example of what validation is and how validating another person's feelings, worldview, and perceptions works to enhance rapport with the client and human service provider.

APPLICATION OF COUNSELING AND VALIDATION SKILLS

At this point in the chapter, we have introduced ways Ms. Marteen (client) and Caitlyn Manning's (case manager) communication has been impacted by using basic counseling skills. We then introduced validation by providing a definition and example of a woman who experienced a traumatic interaction (e.g. sexual assault) by a male co-worker. We learned from this latter example that validation is giving or providing truth to what a person is communicating. Counseling skills are necessary to give a client the space to express his or her truth, while jointly working together towards a successful case outcome. While a case manager can have perfect basic counseling skills, and certainly be mindful of validating clients; the question becomes can they apply these skills consistently, in the right context, at the right time? Consistent application of basic counseling skills requires a decision-making process that can be repeated to more fully determine the best course of action, especially when working with clients from different backgrounds than your own. We will now briefly describe a decision-making model, DECIDE,[3] and apply it to our case study (Ms. Marteen and Caitlyn Manning).

DECIDE MODEL

The DECIDE model of decision making is designed to be a systematic, step-by-step, process for people working in the human and allied health professions[3]. Each letter in the DECIDE model represents one of the six steps of the entire decision-making process, and are listed below:

- ➢ D = define the problem.
- ➢ E = establish the criteria.
- ➢ C = consider all the alternatives.
- ➢ I = identify the best alternative.
- ➢ D = develop and implement a plan of action.
- ➢ E = evaluate and monitor the solution and feedback when necessary.[3]

Now that we have all of the steps listed, we will go through each step and apply the step to our case study. It is important to remember that, if applied correctly, this process *can be* generalized to all cultures and groups. The important thing to grasp here is the process of *how* we get to a decision, more so than the specific truth that emerges from our discussion. Perhaps you have heard this old axiom, "If you *give* a person a fish, they will eat for a day, but if you *teach* a person how to fish, they will eat for a lifetime." What the next part of this chapter wants to do is *teach* future and current case managers how to consistently utilize and apply basic counseling skills by using the DECIDE decision making model as a guide to bridge potential gaps between case managers and clients. For a reminder in this section, let's recall the multiple identities of Ms. Marteen and her Case Manager.

Ms. Marteen is mixed race/ethnicity (Latinx and African-American), aged 52, and resides on the outskirts of town with minimal to no access to transportation. Ms. Marteen grew up in the Deep South and has recently relocated north to a small college town near Caitlyn Manning's alma mater. She has always wanted to provide a better life for her daughters and has tried to establish herself in the community. Ms. Marteen's previous experience with the local health agency is when she tried to seek mental health services for her youngest daughter. She got involved with a local college program that provided free transportation to and from mental health appointments. The experience left her with a positive view of local health care services.

Ms. Marteen has two daughters, one recently gave birth to a little girl. Ms. Marteen's grand-daughter recently developed asthma, and it was determined that the cause is high levels of pollution that surround her home. Ms. Marteen is the primary caretaker of her grand-daughter, even though she has recently been diagnosed with extremely high blood pressure and diabetes.

Caitlyn is also mixed race (White and Asian), aged 25, and has been in case management for one year. Caitlyn was raised, attended undergraduate and graduate school, and currently resides in a predominantly White environment. She attended a top ten counselor education program with an emphasis on multicultural education and social justice. While in college, Caitlyn was involved with several organizations focused on providing mental health care to underserved populations near her campus. Based on this work, she produced a Master's thesis on working with minority populations with mental health issues. Outside of her formal service roles, Caitlyn Manning has had minimal contact with cultures outside of her own, and largely considers herself to be most familiar and comfortable in, and with, "White culture" in her personal life.

Ms. Marteen has been working with Caitlyn for two months at the time of the exchange below. Caitlyn's supervisor is a White male, aged 61, and is one year away from retirement.

DEFINE THE PROBLEM

The first step of the model is defining the problem. While defining the problem may sound simple, it can often be a difficult task to locate possible barriers that might impact client outcomes. For example, let's think about a few of the surface differences between Ms. Marteen and Caitlyn Manning (age, race, ethnicity, (dis)ability and work status). Which of these identities is the primary cause for the initial barrier in communication? Which of the identities is the reason for the initial interpretation by Caitlyn that assumes Ms. Marteen simply is not motivated to do what is required to help herself? An important part of applying basic counseling skills to this stage of the decisionmaking process is that it helps case managers determine the *right* problem to solve at the *right* time. In the active listening replay, Caitlyn did not *assume* a lack of motivation, but considered that something else may be going on when the client changed her pattern of speech and provided viable explanations for why she could not currently fill out paperwork. Active listening can lead to asking different questions that can begin to breakdown some of the barriers that may exist between the case manager and client. In addition, validation is giving or providing truth to what a person is communicating to the case manager. The

16

ability to validate a client's truth is essential to correctly define the correct problem(s) according to the most important needs of the client. When case managers are aware of differences that MAY present barriers to successful outcomes, they will apply counseling skills to accurately define the problem leading to the outcomes that address what clients actually need to be successful and have a positive experience during the case management process.

ESTABLISH THE CRITERIA

The second step of the model is establishing the criteria. Think of criteria as a set of considerations that help you determine whether something has been successful or not. In our case, what initial considerations would the Case Manager need to think about before making an assesment of Ms. Marteen's motivation to move forward in her case? For example, if the case manager does a quick assessment of potential differences, what might she consider differntly in her work with Ms. Marteen? Would Caitlyn Manning consider and factor in where Ms. Marteen resides and the potential challenges associated with living in a highly polluted neighborhood? Would Caitlyn consider a gap in language that may be a result of differences in age, race, or ethnicity? Or might Caitlyn consider a gap in familial responsibility as a reason why Ms. Marteen is prefering the health of a grandchild over her own? Each of these considerations can only be framed by the case manager's ability to move beyond "normal" client assumptions by considering how each aspect of a client's life and experiences impact their ability to fully engage the case management process. Using basic counseling skills to inform criteria, and then taking the next step of believing a client's truth are crucial to establishing the working criteria with a client.

CONSIDER ALL THE ALTERNATIVES

The third step of the model is considering all of the possible alternative solutions available to the case manager. This step is designed to be carried out in collaboration with others who may be able to provide perspectives that initially allude the case manager. Let's recall that at the end of the initial exchange and prior to any basic counseling reframes or applications of validation, Caitlyn Manning informed her supervisor that Ms. Marteen was not motivated to act in her own best interests. The supervisor did not offer possibilities for alternative solutions, rather he agreed with the Caitlyn's interpretation of the client. In a situation like this, it is important to seek alternative counsel in order to get different perspectives that may lead to a more informed plan of action that honors a client's truth. An important truth for seeking alternative solutions is that clients may not always come from people in your place of work. For example, Caitlyn could have gone to the hospital that was serving Ms. Marteen's grand-daughter to see how hospital personnel work effectively with clients with similar backgrounds. Another resource could have been civic or community organizations in Ms. Marteen's neighborhood working to ameliorate conditions for those living in a polluted community.

Case managers can utilize basic counseling skills to create useful connections to community partners that can provide important information leading to alternative plans of action that fit with a client's background and presenting needs. Case managers should not limit themselves to supervisory structures when working to create solutions for clients because critical resources may be available in clients' communities. Utilizing the vast network in a clients world can offer alternative solutions that better address a clients' needs.

IDENTIFY THE BEST ALTERNATIVE

The fourth step of the model is identifying the best alternative. Determining a high quality solution involves considering all of the criteria from step two, generating informed alternatives from step three, and then selecting the best course of action that maximizes the chance for a positive outcome for the client. In our case study, several factors were missed due to a lack of applying basic counseling skills and not validating who Ms. Marteen is, nor where she was from. With the application of basic counseling skills to set criteria, we were able to determine some key considerations that should inform consultation with others with key data that may lead to a high quality plan of action for Caitlyn Manning. Caitlyn, in consultation with others with relevant data on the client, will select the best alternative that fits the truth presented by Ms. Marteen. A case manager's ability to arrive at a high quality alternative solution that maximizes a client's chance of success is dependent on his or her ability to enter the world of the client and determine viable sources of good information.

DEVELOP AND IMPLEMENT A PLAN OF ACTION

The fifth step of the model is developing and implementing a plan of action. Let's put the important parts of this stage up front, communication and coordination. A case manager can create a perfect plan, utilize basic counseling skills with the client, but without effective communication case management plans may not be fully implemented. In addition, if a case manager does not consistently create informed considerations (i.e. Step Two: Establishing the Criteria), then coordination efforts may not fit a client's needs. For example, once Ms. Marteen was hesitant about coming in to complete paperwork, Caitlyn Manning could have sought alternative ways to approach the case by first establishing the critera by which success would be determined. Using basic counseling skills, the Case Manager works with Ms. Marteen and others to find the highest quality solution. For Ms. Marteen, any solution that would not account for her caretaker status, transporation issues, and commitment to the health and well being of her family would not fufill a quality outcome for the client because these are essential elements of a successful outcome for her. The individual planning phase of this model considers communication and coordination to be of utmost importance after considering all of the factors that impact the client. Effective case managers will shift their modes of communication (e.g. in-person, telephone, home visit) to fit the needs of the client, and coordinate efforts according to the needs of the client.

EVALUATE AND MONITOR THE SOLUTION

The sixth step of the model is evaluating and monitoring the selected solution. Case managers will have several layers of supervision for their caseloads. While supervision is very important, the ability to have a separate process to evaluate high quality solutions informed by what a client brings to the office, is equally valuable. Each step of the plan of action developed by case managers should have a way to be evaluated for effectiveness. For example, if a plan of action for Ms. Marteen was to provide babysitting services while she completed paperwork, then an evaluation would look at whether or not her compliance with completing documents was impacted by the provided service. Case managers will comply with all normal supervision provided in the structure of their workplace, but normal supervision should not prevent them from creating their own system of evaluation for interventions made from informed considerations.

CONCLUSION

Case managers are more effective when utilizing basic counseling skills, validation, and informed decision-making processes. In the context of the U. S., increasing numbers of minority populations has created the need for case management professionals to expand their skillset to serve ALL clients. This chapter has introduced some important basic considerations for how to approach work in the current context. For example, Active listening skills provide the foundation for understanding a client, and their needs, instead of making assumptions based on preconceived notions of case managers. Additional counseling skills (i.e., open and closed ended questions, paraphrasing, and reflection of feeling) provide further tools to understanding the client's world to better validate them by giving or providing truth to what a client is communicating to the case manager. Again, validation is giving or providing truth to what a person is communicating to the case manager, believing them, which is critical to the process of meeting clients where they are.

Basic counseling skills inform the DECIDE[3] decision-making process to consistently create solutions for the client that honors their lives and experiences. We believe that utilizing basic counseling and validation skills to inform the decision making for a diverse caseload will best position the case manager to have more successful outcomes for all clients with similar and different backgrounds.

REFERENCES

[1]Colby, S. L., & Ortman, J. M. (2014). Projections of the size and composition of the U.S. population: 2014 to 2060. Current Population Reports, P25-1143, *U.S. Census Bureau*, Washington, DC, 1-13.

[2]Ivey, A. E., & Ivey, M. B. (2014). Intentional interviewing and counseling: Facilitating client development in a multicultural society (8th ed.). Pacific Grove, CA: Brooks/Cole.

[3]Guo, K. L. (2008). DECIDE: A decision-making model for more effective decision making by health care managers. *The Health Care Manager, 27*(2), 118-127. doi:10.1097/01.HCM.0000285046.27290.90

[4]Validation (n. d.). *Dictionary.com unabridged.* Retrieved August 19, 2017 from Dictionary.com Website http://www.dictionary.com/browse/validation?s=t

CHAPTER 2

MULTICULTURAL CONSIDERATIONS IN CASE MANAGEMENT

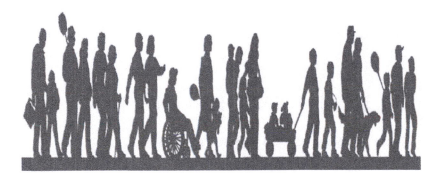

KEITH B. WILSON

ABSTRACT

As the United States becomes more diverse, the need to acquire, shape, and maintain our ability to serve all populations is more apparent now more than ever. Past research in the human, health and allied professions suggests that people who may be part of underrepresented groups (e.g., people with disabilities, women, racial & ethnic groups of color) tend to have poorer outcomes when compared to European Americans. This chapter will underscore the need for all service providers to become more competent when serving ALL populations, not only the populations that might be from underrepresented groups. Because providers of case management services can facilitate productive outcomes by applying the tools presented in this chapter, when a group that is considered marginalized (e.g., women) is used as an example to illustrating a point, please replace this group with others marginalized groups. Marginalized groups share common reasons for being marginalized. Bottom-line, the recommended tools to simplify positive outcomes are applicable to all marginalized groups, not only the group used in the example. To simulate critical thoughts, there are discussion questions to facilitate a more in-depth understanding of the need to increase our helping skills with all populations seeking case management services in the United States.

CHAPTER HIGHLIGHTS

➤ Changing Demography of the United States;

➤ Generalizing from Variables of Discrimination (VOD);

➤ Brief Overview: Multicultural Counseling Competencies (MCC).

LEARNING OBJECTIVES

➤ Identify the three levels of the Multicultural Counseling Competencies;

➤ Understanding why it is important to generalize from Variables of Discrimination (VOD);

➤ Identify reasons why it is important to apply the Multicultural Counseling Competencies;

➤ Identify the reasons why case management and case management systems are multicultural processes.

CONNECTING DIVERSITY TO THE PRACTICE OF CASE MANAGEMENT

If we are honest, many of us hold biases about identities (e.g., gender, disability, sexual orientation) that might be different from the identities that we perceive as salient in ourselves. Much of how we come to internalize these and other perceptions about others are formed in complex interactions that start with our family and other support systems (e.g., religious, educational) growing up as children. This process of influencing our behaviors as children continues well into adulthood for all of us. It also must be recognized that while serving a diverse clientele in an effective and productive way is emphasized in most of our professional ethics documentation; there are some that do not feel the need to understand themselves, let alone understand others in a way that can facilitate services to the people they are serving.

The author believes that being homophobic, for example, is not the problem. The problem is how you treat people who may have a different sexual orientation than you do. Most of us have isms (e.g., sexism, racism) and do not treat the people of that ism negatively many times. Yes, it is the belief of this author that you can have values and perceptions that are negative about certain groups without projecting your beliefs on these groups, not only as a case manager, but any person *delivering services*. The truth is that many times we cannot hold our negative perceptions away from the behaviors that will yield subpar services for people we have harmful perceptions about. As some would say, this chapter on *Multicultural Considerations in Case Management* just got real! The question is: Do you want to get better at your job in providing services to all your clients? I know for some of you the jury is still out. Smile! The journey can be fun and challenging. Connecting diversity to case management services must start with an honest assessment of ourselves and the motivation to become better professionals and people we may have authority over and or influence in our personal lives.

For years, the author has started both his graduate and undergraduate case management classes the same way. The first day, talk about current events that connect and do not connect to the class, introductions, go over the class syllabus and dismiss class. In truth, this has been the routine for almost thirty years in teaching in higher education, regardless of the classes taught. However, in his recent graduate case management class, the author decided to try something different. "How can I get students to acknowledge that many processes are inherently connected to possible diversity conflicts in not only case management, but interactions professionals might view as standard to either accessing or giving information to clients. It is unavoidable." After the usual first day established protocol utilized for close to three decades, the author decided to ask this probing question to his students. "Please raise your hand if you have had any case management experience working in the human services, allied health, or medical field? If so, can you describe one of the most difficult clients you had and the reasons that made this a challenging client for you?" While the author was not surprised, one by one, students began to disclose to the class the reasons that made these clients problematic. In short, students started to talk about some (not an exhaustive list) of the following Variables of Discrimination (VOD) that made clients very challenging to deal with during the case management process: a. Gender, and b. Race.

GENDER ROLES

One student mentioned that because of her upbringing, she was taught that women and men had different roles they should possess at home and in the vocational world. However, she also noted that her most challenging client was a male who wanted to stay home and raise the kids. As the student reported, "the interactions were made more stressful because the client had no plans to work and was happy in his role as housewife." While the student reported being professional during the interaction, she commented to the class of not approving her male client staying home and taking care of the kids.

RACE AND ETHNICITY

Another student reported that he worked in a prison with the population being primarily people of color (i.e., African American, Latino/Hispanic). In many interactions when communicating with his clients, the student reported his frustration when his clients used language that he did not understand. The use of language (slang) by its clients upset the student because he believed he should not have to keep asking his clients to interpret what they were saying to him during the session. The student was further put off because the client appeared to be frustrated when the student would not retain what was interpreted by the client in prior interactions. As seen in this illustration of most demanding clients, our philosophical differences might interfere with rapport building efforts if we are not open to modifying our behaviors to facilitate building rapport with our clients.

It is painfully apparent that the two previous examples in case management connect cultural competence with case management and other services. Additionally, it is also evident that providers of case management services must understand and deal with their own biases to facilitate services for all clients. Without going into much detail, there were several other VOD highlighted by the class for discussion. After 90 minutes of processing, I said the following to the class. "Every challenging client that you talked about was difficult because they had a VOD. Not my words, yours." After laying the foundation with the initial open-ended questions, discussions took off like a jet on a tarmac. Wow! As the instructor, I had to be able to connect the dots for the class to integrate a diversity theme throughout the rest of the class. The deliberations were so fruitful that we continued the discussions the following class period for another 90 minutes. So, what's the point? I am sure you have heard this phrase before.

24

"You can lead a horse to water, but you cannot make it drink." True. However, it is the job of the class facilitator to make the horse thirsty enough that the horse will want to drink on its own. Lay the foundation, connect the dots, and expand to a broader application of real life. Students appreciate this approach to learning. Given the changing face of the United States (U.S.) population, becoming a culturally competent case manager is a necessity to providing effective services for all clients.

GENERALIZING FROM VARIABLES OF DISCRIMINATION (VOD)

Personal attributes (e.g., gender, race, ethnicity, disability status) by either nature or nurture that one might get discriminated against are called Variables of Discrimination, otherwise known as VOD. To decrease redundancy in examples using a particular VOD, it is recommended to substitute other VODs when applying interventions and tools because these tools (e.g., not being demeaning to clients) can be used to increase positive outcomes and to advocate for ALL marginalized and non-marginalized groups seeking case management services. Thus, examples used in writings, workshops and speeches, advocate for substituting one VOD with others in your mind because of the appropriate generalizations that can be made across groups.[13, 14] This author embraces the same philosophy because of the utility to decrease cognitive dissonance when receivers of a message might get defensive because of a VOD used in an example to illustrate a point. Additionally, it is redundant to keep listing what groups apply to what example(s). While many groups who are marginalized may have different experiences, tools and interventions used to increase productive outcomes in case management, the interventions can be applied to all clients.

CHANGING DEMOGRAPHICS

Because discrimination comes in many forms (e.g., race, ethnicity, socioeconomic status, geographical location, sexual orientation, and age),[14] it is recommended that human and allied health care providers be attuned to how biases may be manifested by the actions of people serving a particular clientele. With the everchanging demographics in the U.S., the population of individuals who are diverse based on disability status, race, gender, for example, will show up in increasing numbers to human and allied health providers. In many places in the U.S. (e.g., California & Florida), this demographic transformation can more readily be seen. Thus, increasing the opportunities for service providers to engage in interventions that will facilitate services for groups other than European Americans.[4] Additionally, it has already been reported that both domestic underrepresented groups and immigrants may have problems accessing many arms of the social and allied health systems (e.g., mental health; substance abuse; rehabilitation; education) when compared to people who are European American.[6] The changing complexion of the U.S. is an important observation for several reasons:

➢ Depending on what VOD (e.g., a person with a disability, socioeconomic status) a person might bring to the case management environment, individuals who are part of underrepresented groups tend to have counterproductive experiences in the human service delivery system. Thus, there is a need for providers to be able to understand and apply interventions that might facilitate a more positive outcome.

➢ Because most of us tend to have unconscious or conscious biases against groups that might not be part of our primary identities (e.g., sexual orientation), understanding the connection between the changing complexion of the U.S. and the role that unconscious or conscious bias play in receiving case management services is vital to decrease counterproductive outcomes for underrepresented groups.

➢ If we understand the concept of social justice, the application to provide the best services to all is critical.

As stated before, it is apparent that both underrepresented domestic groups and immigrants tend to have gaps in accessing human and allied health services when compared to European Americans. While the rate of accessing services may vary, it is imperative for human service providers to recognize their role in creating a counterproductive gap in the quality of services delivered for all of their clients.

While gender, race, and socioeconomic status (SES) tend to receive the lion's share of outcomes related to the shifting demographics in the U.S., people who classify as Lesbian, Gay, Bisexual, and Transgender (LGBT) encounter analogous outcomes as other underrepresented groups in the U.S. It is also important to note that people who are LGBT are increasing in numbers as well. For example, people who are considered LGBT increased from 1.5 million to 11.7 million from 2005 to 2011.[5] Without the understanding and empathy of providers, people who are part of the LGBT community are likely to experience not only discrimination, but depression because of the lack of support and validation.[9] While providers might not be able to visually see if a person is part of the LGBT community, it is important to understand that people who classify as LGBT are likely to encounter discrimination and counterproductive outcomes when seeking behavioral health and other services in the U. S. Next, let us look at ways to increase the competence to facilitate services for people who are part of the LGBT community and other groups who might be part of the underrepresented group umbrella.

BRIEF OVERVIEW: MULTICULTURAL COUNSELING COMPETENCIES (MCC)

While there are other components (i.e., application) of multicultural competencies,[13] the following is a solid foundation to begin your journey to being able to provide competent case management and other services to people who may look and behave differently than you do. We will start with the well-articulated MCC set forth by Sue[11] over twenty years ago. Examples are illustrated to lay a basis for generalizing to other groups for application. Please apply the same principles to other groups who may be considered underrepresented, marginalized, and are not considered part of the "majority" group when delivering case management services. It is important to note the word "majority" may be contextually defined. For example, in a class of elementary school teachers, one would more and likely observe more females than males. In this example, the underrepresented group might be males (regardless of race & ethnicity) because of the overwhelming number of females in this vocational area.

AWARENESS OF ATTITUDES AND BELIEFS. Awareness is the first step to positively interacting with, treating, and developing a rapport with people who are different than we are. As emphasized by Sue,[11] awareness is being conscious of one's own, and other's values and belief systems. More importantly, being aware of how these belief systems might interact with belief systems that are different from one's self. For example, not recognizing that some groups (e.g., Asians, African Americans) may teach their children to decrease eye contact when interacting with elders/people in authority. In this example, not looking authority figures directly in the eyes shows respect for the individual who is in a position of authority or power. There are countless examples of providers who view less eye contact as being less assertive and not trustworthy. In this example of awareness, less eye contact can be equated as a defect in personhood and may likely result in misinterpretation and an inaccurate diagnosis on the part of the provider. If a human service provider is not aware of how their belief system is similar, or not, from clients they are serving, it is nearly impossible to modify counterproductive behaviors that you are not aware you may possess. In many professions, not equitably serving seekers of your services is considered unethical. Thus, it is important to get feedback to become a better facilitator of services to all clients. Being aware of your, and others, attitudes and beliefs is the first step in the process of becoming a better deliverer of case management services.

KNOWLEDGE. Knowledge is the second step to becoming a more equitable deliverer of case management services. As stated by Sue [11], this level of the MCC has to do with acquiring information to provide culturally competent services to your clients. The more you know about yourself and the populations that you serve, the better you can facilitate case management services in a more informed manner. Since most case managers routinely encounter diverse populations, it is not surprising from time-to-time that case managers might have researched about why some clients may prefer several members of their immediate family present with them during a critical part of the case management process, the intake interview, for example. Not allowing family members to engage the case management process can hinder the development of rapport building, which is a key function of facilitating services for all populations. Additionally, it would be helpful to have this kind of information (knowledge) about different groups beforehand to continue a seamless flow in the delivery of case management services. While information about different populations can be gathered from an endless reservoir of sources (e.g., books, movies, associates, etc.), never forget the most direct, and possibly the best source for information about the people you serve, the clients themselves. Please do not be afraid to ask if you do not understand cultural information about the people you serve. Lastly, please use both diplomacy and directness when seeking information that can simplify your job. Although information gathering will help inform case managers how to serve their clientele, clients might be the best resource for accurate information to build trust and show that the case manager is invested in the best possible outcomes for all clients.

SKILLS. After having a good awareness and knowledge of one's self and the clientele being served, it is now time to fine tune what you know into a deliverable skill(s). Sue [11] reported that skills are the manifestations of both awareness and knowledge. However, it is important to note that having skills is not the same as application, as reported recently by Wilson [14]. Wilson [14] and his colleagues further indicated that it takes more than awareness, knowledge, and skills to yield the application of what a case manager should do when interacting with a diverse clientele. Simply stated, because a case manager might have mastered the MCC's above, this mastery will not guarantee application of skills. An example of application would be to have the awareness, knowledge, and skills of performing cardiopulmonary resuscitation (CPR). However, you decide to use the tools learned for CPR on a person with a broken leg. It is very apparent that the skills used for CPR is not associated with the high standards of care when applying the CPR skills to a person with a broken leg. [14] The context in which the skills are delivered is a key component of application. In the CPR example, the context is applying CPR to a person who needs a leg splint. Please see Wilson [14] for more information about the distinction between *behavior/action* and *application of MCC*. Even though there is a difference between *behavior/action* and the *application* principles, it is essential to develop skills to facilitate more efficient case management services for all populations, including groups that might be underrepresented based on disability status, gender, and sexual orientation.

WHAT IS A CASE MANAGER OR CASE MANAGEMENT?

A case manager and case management process involve the integration of services by facilitating, coordinating, advocating and planning for the individual and family needs through a comprehensive net of services. When a person reaches full potential, there are several winners, including the family and various reimbursement sources.[3] While a case manager may emphasize certain service outcomes (e.g., vocational, clinical mental health) depending on the environment in which case management services are rendered, the general facilitation of a broad list of services that include community and agency services are typically part of professional locations that case management services are carried out. Although there are differences in case management services based on the type of environment delivered, the general function of services will be similar in many settings.

Perhaps, many would like to think that advocating and coordinating services would be the mainstay of providing case management services to all clients. True. However, depending on the agency, center, or hospital protocols for collecting data from your clients, having a good sense of possible multicultural concerns during an intake session, for example, can not only improve rapport, but garner more success on behalf of the case manager and agency. After talking to many case managers, health care providers, and counselors over the years, one thing is clear. When clients are not satisfied with services received, they typically vote with their feet. They do not come back to the agency because of being dissatisfied with services provided. In many instances, the human service organization might not know why a client was dissatisfied with the services provided. It is also important to note that many counterproductive outcomes from people who are part of underrepresented groups (e.g., gender, low SES, race) have been influenced by bias and prejudice as reported by several authors [1, 10, 14] over the years. Thus, providing competent services includes applying interventions to multicultural elements of personhood for your clients, especially since many case management environments may have a time limit on the collection of data during an intake interview. Being able to address multicultural issues that may arise, while continuing to collect the required data can be tricky. The best case managers continue to gather data and address multicultural issues in sessions because they realize that multicultural issues might arise during any part of the case management process. Furthermore, addressing multicultural issues during the case management process is providing efficient and competent services to clients. In the end, it is the competent awareness, knowledge, and skills of the case manager to address multicultural issues when they arise with their clients. Although the case management process might be less dynamic in some places, a good case manager understands that being able to appropriately address possible cultural concerns that might not have anything to do with his or her role, can either lead to early termination or increased rapport on the part of the client. Now, let's apply the MCC to the following Case Study. The case of Richard (case manager/counselor) and Neal (client).

CASE STUDY
RICHARD AND NEAL

Richard is a European American case manager/counselor in a community mental health center where he has been employed for the past ten years. As background, Richard's father is European American and his mother is African American. While Richard is technically biracial, many think he is European American because of his physical features. Richard graduated from an accredited university and program in counselor education and was well respected by his peers and professors at the university. One professor commented when talking about Richard, "he had a difficult time in school because he had to work to earn money to attend the university to maintain his scholarship. Money did not come easily to him." Furthermore, Richard has communicated that he has been a social justice advocate for years because of his exposure to diversity issues growing up with his parents being of different races. At the request of a community referral, Neal, who is African American, is meeting with Richard for the first time for an intake interview to determine if he is eligible for services at the community mental health center. As background, Neal was raised in an upper-class home environment where he and his brothers and sisters went to private schools and vacationed twice a year in the Hamptons and places overseas. Neal's wife had a similar upbringing as his. After a bit of small talk to build rapport, Richard begins to ask questions that are outlined on the intake form for his agency. However, before Richard can complete the first question located on the intake form, Neal begins to talk about an incident that involved his eight-year-old daughter when he and his wife (African American) were looking to take their daughter from the public school she was presently enrolled into a private school in the area.

Neal indicated to Richard that "me and my wife visited three schools in the area for our daughter, Imani, who is going to the fourth-grade next year. All three schools had a predominantly European

American enrollment. We met with the principal and assistant principal at each school to talk about requirements for enrollment, tuition, the culture of the school and start date for the upcoming school year." Neal continued. "Secondly, all of the representatives of the schools were European American and mostly female." As Neal looked at Richard during the intake, he paused. Then Neal reported the following theme from him and his wife's school visits of three private schools in the area. "Each school administrator they met with said their faculty and staff would treat our daughter just like any other student in the school."

After listening to Neal and seeing the frustration on his face as he recounted the recent school visits from him and his wife, Richard said to Neal: "I am not sure what the problem is, Neal. If the school is going to treat your daughter like the other students at the three schools, this shows that the school's administrators, faculty, and staff are going to be fair to your daughter. Are you frustrated because you wish there were more African Americans in the schools for your daughter to associate with?" Neal responded, "no, that is not it, Richard." While Richard appeared a little confused about why Neal felt frustrated, Richard thought to himself. "Why do Blacks want to make everything about race?" Richard then asked Neal if he could continue with the intake interview because they only had 45 minutes remaining to complete this part of the eligibility determination process. While Neal did not feel validated by Richard and just wanted to talk about his experiences visiting the three schools, he decided to continue the intake interview for the next 45 minutes. Finally, both Richard and Neal maintained professional and friendly interactions, joking from time-to-time throughout the intake interview.

CASE STUDY
DISCUSSION QUESTIONS

1. Do you identify with any person in the case study? If so, why or why not?

2. Are there any VOD (e.g., disability status, gender) in the case study? Yes or No?

3. If yes to question 2, what are the VOD in the Case Study?

4. If there are VOD present in the case study, should these variables be addressed before, during or after the initial intake interview? Why or why not?

5. What MCC should Richard improve, if any? Why?

WAYS TO BECOME MORE MULTICULTURALLY COMPETENT

While there are many avenues to become a more competent professional when dealing with diverse populations, the ultimate decision will be the person delivering services. There is no substitute for the willingness to get better, despite your own negative enculturation (i.e., the process of being trained to survive in your own group) process towards diverse populations, to facilitate services and learn how to become less self-centered and more client-centered. As the message over the intercom during a flight reminds us, "we must first put the mask on our faces before attempting to put the mask on a loved one." It is this concept that I submit two ideas for consideration in becoming a more well-rounded deliverer of case management services to all clients.

KNOWING YOURSELF

It is virtually impossible to deliver competent services if one is not aware of their own biases and shortcomings towards others who may look and behave differently than they do. Thus, it makes it difficult, at best, to be able to predict what your actions will do to others because of ignorance. Hey, we all have some degree of ignorance and cannot be expected to know everything about every culture and population representing those cultures. This next point is critical. Knowing yourself includes knowing what other populations (people) think of you because of a VOD or not having a VOD. This point is vital because once you know how others perceive your gender (e.g., as a client or case manager), for example, you can anticipate behaviors, perceptions, and attitudes that you can counteract to deliver competence services to all of your clients. Knowing your shortcomings and doing something about your shortcomings is the key. While there is a lot more that can be said about knowing yourself, this level of understanding will get you on the road to providing effective services to your clients. The residual usually facilitate better relationships with family, friends, and co-workers as well. Knowing yourself is the first stage in this never-ending process we call professional and personal development. Only you can make a better you...

APPLYING WHAT YOU KNOW

Once you gain the necessary knowledge about yourself, knowledge about others, and you have the tools to make a difference, you must look at the application of what you know to make a difference in the lives of your clients. Now, this author will not assume that people will automatically apply what they know when it comes to the application of diversity-related knowledge and concepts. As Wilson[14] reported on several occasions, this assumption is incorrect and can lead to professionals not providing appropriate services to their clientele. Moreover, to be open and transparent, to advocate for others that are not connected in any way to a primary identity that you possess, can leave the health professional in an isolated position within their in-group. We must push through the negative enculturation (e.g., the way in which your family and friends trained you to be a part of the group as a child) we received growing up and apply these newly learned skills to the people that we serve. Applying what you know can be difficult, especially since members of our in-group influence most of us in ways that might not be positive to those that might not be in our in-group.[14]

There is indeed a gap in what we know and applying the MCC.[2,14] Most people tend to advocate for individuals that are part of their in-group. This outcome of enculturation makes it very difficult for some groups who might be considered marginalized, to receive fair and efficient services in and outside of your agency. In many instances, professionals espouse social justice principles. Nevertheless, the application of these principles on marginalized populations are far from realizing their full potential in the U.S. We are all challenged to make our world a better place that we all can be proud of.[14] While applying the MCC can be challenging at times for a plethora of reasons, this author is still optimistic that we can be just a little better in applying the MCC than we were the day before to ALL the people that we serve.

CONCLUSION

The changing demographics in the U.S. challenges us to get prepared for populations coming into service delivery systems that may have been different from past populations in their racial, sexual orientation, and gender makeup. Finding ways to connect case management to diversity can be challenging for many, especially when they may not want to hear or discuss issues related to diversity because of their preconceived negative biases about people who are different from themselves. Moreover, because of the enculturation process, some of us will not change much in the delivery of services to underrepresented populations because we believe our enculturation. Individuals with such thinking will be among us in every profession. The truth of the matter is that some of these individuals do not see that they are doing anything wrong... That being said, most of us have negative views about identities that are different from ourselves. However, our harmful and counterproductive views about other groups do not have to end with providers delivering subpar services to these populations of the clients we serve. **Millions of providers deliver excellent, consistent services to clients they have undesirable perceptions about because of the harmful enculturation experienced in their childhood.** When the behavior of these perceptions is kept in check, we can do our jobs ethically. When these behaviors of our perceptions are not kept at bay, we have the potential to not only deliver subpar services but do irreparable harm to the people that we serve. If we do not care, we all should care enough not to harm others during the process of what we are getting paid to do. Please remember that one of the most important ways to gain information about the people that you are serving is to directly ask them about their culture, for example, to facilitate service provision. While managing our negative feelings about people that are different, being able to discuss diversity issues in "mixed company" will provide a way to facilitate discussions that may lead to more self-growth to facilitate services for our clientele.

Lastly, when looking at VOD, it is crucial to apply interventions to other populations to facilitate service delivery. This idea comes from understanding that all populations will benefit from interventions that are appropriately applied to facilitate services, within the appropriate context. The tools outlined in the MCC has a broad application that can facilitate communication and understanding to many people and groups across the spectrum of services that human, allied and medical professions provide. In the end, being able to provide effective services to diverse populations means that the provider (e.g., social worker, rehabilitation counselor, psychologist, clinical mental health counselor) can provide service regardless of the official title they may hold. Good luck in your journey to becoming the best you can become as a service provider that will facilitate services for all of your clients.

REFERENCES

[1]Alvidrez, J., & Weinstein, R. S. (1999). Early teacher perceptions and later student academic achievement. *Journal of Educational Psychology*, *91*(4), 731-746.

[2]Ahmed, S. Wilson, K. B., Henriksen, R. C., & Jones, J. W. (2011). What does it mean to be a culturally-competent counselor? *Journal for Social Action in Counseling Psychology*, *3*(1)17-28.

[3]Case Management Society of America (n. d.). *What is a case manager?* Retrieved July 16, 2017 from http://www.cmsa.org/Home/CMSA/WhatisaCaseManager/tabid/224/Default.aspx

[4]Chan, F., Tarvydas, V., Blalock, K., Strauser, D., & Atkins, B. J. (2009). Unifying and elevating rehabilitation counseling through model-driven, diversity-sensitive evidence-based practice. *Rehabilitation Counseling Bulletin*, *52*(2), 114-119.

[5]Gates, G. J. (2011). How Many People are Lesbian, Gay, Bisexual and Transgender? UCLA: The Williams Institute. Retrieved from: https://escholarship.org/uc/item/09h684x2

[6]Horvitz-Lennon, M., Volya, R., Donohue, J. M., Lave, J. R., Stein, B. D., & Normand, S. T. (2014). Disparities in Quality of Care among Publicly Insured Adults with Schizophrenia in Four Large U.S. States, 2002-2008. *Health Services Research*, *49*(4), 1121-1144. doi:10.1111/1475-6773.12162

[7]Khan, M. (2016). *Black students nearly 4 times as likely to be suspended*. Retrieved from http://abcnews.go.com/US/black-students-times-suspended/story?id=39670502

[8]Kelman, B. M. (2013). *Study: Black students suspended more often than others*. Retrieved from https://www.usatoday.com/story/news/nation/2013/05/12/black-student-suspensions/2151423/

[9]King, M., Semlyen, J., Tai, S. S., Killaspy, H., Osborn, D., Popelyuk, D., & Nazareth, I. (2008). A systematic review of mental disorder, suicide, and deliberate self-harm in lesbian, gay and bisexual people. *BMC Psychiatry*, *8*(70), 1-17.

[10]Skiba, R., Michael, R., Nardo, A., & Peterson, R. (2002). The color of discipline: Sources of racial and gender disproportionality in school punishment. *The Urban Review*, *34*(4), 317-342.

[11]Sue, D., Arredondo, P., & McDavis, R. (1992). Multicultural counseling competencies and standards: A call to the profession. *Journal of Multicultural Counseling and Development*, *20*, 64-88.

[12]Validation (n. d.). *Dictionary.com unabridged*. Retrieved August 29, 2016 from Dictionary.com Website http://www.dictionary.com/browse/validation?s=t

[13]Wilson, K. B. (2010, March). *What does it mean to be a culturally-competent counselor?* Paper presented at the meeting of the American Counseling Association, Multicultural Social Justice Leadership Academy, Pittsburgh, PA.

[14]Wilson, K. B., Pitt, J. S., Raheem, M. A., Acklin, C. L., & Wilson, J. M. (2017). Multicultural counseling competencies: Why is it difficult to apply what we know…? In Leavitt, L., Wisdom, S. & Leavitt, K. (Eds.*), Cultural Awareness and Competency Development in Higher Education* (pp. 237-254). Hershey, Pennsylvania: IGI Global.

CHAPTER 3

THE INTAKE INTERVIEW

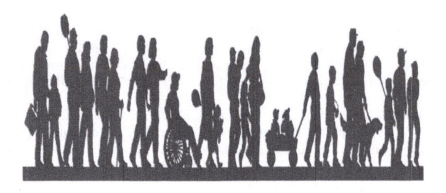

LYNN KOCH
JULIE HILL

ABSTRACT

In this chapter, the authors discuss purposes and uses of intake interviews in case management. The authors highlight the key components and structures of the intake interview and provide an overview of interviewing skills for effectively informing applicants about what to expect and gathering data for preliminary planning. They also discuss multicultural considerations in conducting culturally competent intake interviews. Additionally, the authors present unique challenges that can complicate the intake interview process and suggest techniques for responding to these challenges. Underscoring the important role of intake interviews in not only gathering information, but perhaps most importantly, in building the foundation for strong therapeutic relationships with applicants for services, the authors use the working alliance as a framework for the intake interview. Finally, the authors provide readers with an example of an intake interview report.

CHAPTER HIGHLIGHTS

➢ A comprehensive overview of skills and techniques for structuring and conducting the intake interview that have applications to practitioners working in a variety of health and human service disciplines and settings.

➢ Introduction of the working alliance as a framework for intake interviewing.

➢ An in-depth discussion of multicultural considerations for conducting culturally-responsive intake interviews.

➢ A description of unique challenges that can be present in intake interviews and techniques for responding to these challenges.

➢ Inclusion of an intake interview report to illustrate the concepts discussed in the chapter.

LEARNING OBJECTIVES

➢ Understand the purposes of the intake interview in case management.

➢ Use the working alliance as a framework for conducting intake interviews.

➢ Select techniques that can be used to effectively prepare for the intake interview.

➢ Develop skills and techniques for structuring intake interviews.

➤ Provide applicants with the necessary information they need to make informed decisions about applying for services and participating in the programming and services offered by the case manager.

➤ Identify important information to gather during the intake interview that will enable the case managers and applicants for services to make expedient eligibility decisions, determine additional assessment data that may be needed, elucidate treatment needs, and specify treatment goals.

➤ Use effective interviewing skills to gather comprehensive data from applicants for services.

➤ Consider the influence of culture on applicants' presenting problems, help-seeking behaviors, and specification of treatment services and goals.

➤ Develop multicultural awareness and culturally-responsive practices in conducting intake interviews.

➤ Recognize potential challenges that may arise in the intake interview and how to respond to these challenges.

INTRODUCTION

The intake interview, typically the first formal interaction between the practitioner and the applicant for services, has been described as a conversation that has specific purposes and a mutually agreed upon goal.[19] The goal is to identify client objectives, preferences, service needs, and desired outcomes to begin to develop a treatment plan. Other purposes include providing information to applicants about the practitioner's program, agency, or organization; establishing the groundwork for a positive working alliance; collecting information from the applicant to determine eligibility for services, identifying service needs and client goals; and determining if additional evaluations are necessary.

The intake interview is one of the first processes that will yield significant information for service recipients. It is a critical and vital first step in the coordination and delivery of medical, healthcare, behavioural, and human services. Accuracy and completeness of information gathered in the intake interview enables the practitioner and applicant to determine the next steps for treatment. This chapter is unique as it addresses (a) how to prepare for the intake interview; (b) purposes of the interview; (c) recommendations for structuring the interview; (d) effective interviewing skills to facilitate good communication between the case manager and applicant; (e) multicultural considerations, and (f) common problems and barriers that may occur during the intake interview process and how to respond to these. In the next section, the authors define the intake interview, describe its purposes, and discuss options for structuring the interview.

THE INTAKE INTERVIEW: AN OVERVIEW

Interviewing is a method of gathering information about the applicant for services to describe the individual in terms of his or her presenting problem(s), service needs, and goals of treatment. The initial interview provides both the practitioner and the applicant with a greater understanding of presenting problems and offers direction and support to the applicant in resolving the presenting problem(s).[7]

Roessler, Rubin, and Rumrill[19] underscored the importance of structuring the intake interview session with the applicant for services because it indicates to the applicant that the interviewer is professional and knowledgeable. It can also alleviate anxiety that applicants may have because they are not sure what to expect. During the intake interview, the practitioner typically takes greater control of what is discussed than may occur in future sessions because of the specific focus of the interview. Ivey, Ivey, and Zalaquet[9] offered a five-stage framework for interviewing that includes (a) building the relationship; (b) listening to the applicant's story to draw out her or his strengths; (c) setting goals; (d) re-storying (i.e., through beginning to identify potential solutions to problems), and (e) action. Along with this framework, they discuss specific communication skills that assist with each stage of the interview. This five stage approach has many benefits to applicants because it communicates to them that they are truly being heard and understood by the practitioner, helps them to realize that they have strengths they may not have previously recognized to cope with their presenting problem(s), and leaves them with hope that by working with the service provider, their situation can change and their lives can improve.

Intake interviews can be structured or semi-structured. Structured interviews are highly directive and typically follow a preset format that directs the questions to be asked and the sequence in which they are to be asked. Semi-structured interviews are more flexible, allowing the interviewer to determine questions to be asked and providing interviewees with a greater freedom to focus on issues that are important to them. Although structured interviews have sounder psychometric properties (e.g., reliability, validity), they are less conducive than semi-structured interviews to building rapport with interviewees. Semi-structured interviews are more conducive to rapport building but have been criticized for their relative subjectivity. Checklists and intake forms are often completed by the applicant either prior to or during the intake interview. These forms are used to collect basic applicant information (e.g., name, contact information, address, birth date, referral source, diagnosis, health status, reason for referral, applicant issues of concern). Obtaining information using checklists and intake forms prior to the intake interview can be time-saving and free the case manager to focus the interview more specifically on the applicant's presenting problem(s) in a more flexible and person-centered manner. Checklists and forms can also be used during the intake interview to enable the practitioner to observe and record behavioral patterns, cognitive competencies (e.g., reading, writing, comprehension), social skills, and interaction styles of the applicant. This information can be critical to the treatment planning process.

Experts in the area of interviewing in health care and human services have identified key purposes of the intake interview as (a) establishing a positive working alliance with the interviewee; (b) providing information to the applicant about the practitioner's agency, program, or organization; (c) determining eligibility for services; (d) gathering data about the applicant's presenting problem(s); (e) identifying additional evaluations that may be warranted; and (f) anticipating service needs and treatment goals. These purposes will be discussed in subsequent sections of this chapter.

In summary, the intake interview is a frequently used assessment tool by case managers to develop rapport with applicants; provide important information to the applicant about the program, agency, or organization from which they are requesting services; understand the applicant's concerns and presenting problem(s); and begin to consider implications for further evaluation, treatment, and goal-setting. The skills of the practitioner in conducting comprehensive interviews set the stage for a strong working alliance and development of a comprehensive treatment plan. In the remainder of this chapter, we explore these purposes of the intake interview in greater detail. We begin by presenting the working alliance as a framework for the intake interview as well as all future interactions between the practitioner and applicant for services.

THE WORKING ALLIANCE AS A FRAMEWORK FOR THE INTAKE INTERVIEW

Perhaps the most important purpose of the intake interview is to establish the ground work for a positive working alliance between the practitioner and applicant for services as well as among all service providers involved in the service recipient's treatment plan. Bordin[3] introduced the term "working alliance" to characterize the collaborative effort between the helping professional and the service recipient (as well as all other members of the treatment team) that is characterized by opportunities for every member of the working alliance to equally contribute to the relationship and all activities completed within this relationship.

The key components of the working alliance are bonds, goals, and tasks.[3] Bonds refer to the mutual trust, acceptance, and respect that are developed as a result of shared commitment to all activities of the working alliance. Interviewers establish these bonds by being genuine, empathic, nonjudgmental, and communicating unconditional positive regard for the applicant. Bonding occurs when applicants have the freedom to express what is of importance to them, feel understood, and validated (i.e., the case manager responds to their presenting problems, issues, and concerns with empathy and concern rather than judgment, minimization, or dismissal). Please see Chapter 1 for more information on validation. Bonds are best established when the interviewee perceives the case manager as trustworthy and is confident that the practitioner has the ability to help remediate the interviewee's presenting problem(s).[19] Please see Chapter 1 for more information on validation. Goals of the working alliance are mutually agreed upon targets for intervention.[3] Goals may include return to work, increased independence, better self-management of mental and physical health, decreased symptoms, improved functionality, and development of more effective coping skills. Tasks refer to the specific activities that will be carried out by the practitioner, the recipient of services, and all other members of the treatment team or other providers to whom the applicant is referred. These tasks must be perceived as relevant to all members, and shared responsibility for the completion of tasks must be maintained. Of utmost importance is for practitioners to keep their promises in performing agreed upon tasks and admit if they make mistakes. Doing so communicates to the applicant for services that the practitioner is reliable, responsive, trustworthy, and authentic.

The intake interview addresses all components of the working alliance because of its focus on building rapport with the applicant for services and beginning to identify treatment needs and goals as well as each partner's responsibilities for performing the tasks to achieve the goals of the alliance. A substantial base of research has demonstrated that positive working alliances are associated with positive treatment outcomes, treatment adherence, satisfaction with services, and high ratings of the working alliance. However, practitioners must keep in mind that establishing rapport and developing bonds with applicants does not always occur in one meeting. It may take time, and practitioners must ensure that all interactions with applicants and service recipients' focus on building and maintaining a relationship based on mutual trust and respect. In the next section, we discuss how to adequately prepare for conducting intake interviews that are premised on establishing the groundwork for a positive working alliance.

PREPARING FOR THE INTAKE INTERVIEW

Because the intake interview sets the stage for all future interactions between the practitioner and service recipient, the practitioner should be prepared ahead of time to establish a positive first interaction. Failure to do so can result in delays in treatment, collection of inadequate information, and possible damage to the bonding process. Roessler et al.[19] recommend that practitioners ask themselves the following questions to help guide planning for the intake interview:

> ➢ What are my goals for the interview?

> ➢ What information should be provided to the client during the intake interview?

> ➢ What information do I need to collect from the client during the intake interview?

> ➢ What is the most effective way for exchanging that information?

In preparing for the intake interview, interviewers must take into consideration the physical environment in which the interview is conducted, their mental preparation for the interview, time allotment to the interview, and whether to read preliminary forms and records prior to meeting with the applicant.

ARRANGING THE PHYSICAL ENVIRONMENT AND MENTALLY PREPARING FOR THE INTAKE INTERVIEW

The first consideration in preparation for the intake interview should be arranging and controlling the physical environment in which the interview will take place. Practitioners should ensure that the location of the interview is private and distraction free. The focus of the intake interview should be solely on the applicant, and practitioners should proactively prevent interruption by turning off cell phones and setting office phones to go straight to voicemail or, if possible, to an administrative assistant or answering service. If necessary, practitioners should have information available about who to contact in case of emergency as part of their outgoing voicemail message in case clients/patients call needing emergency assistance. Practitioners should be on time for appointments and avoid completing other tasks while the applicant is present.

When meeting with the applicant in the practitioner's office space, it is helpful to set up the office in a way that is inviting and warm. For applicants such as individuals who use wheel chairs or individuals who are blind, this also means making sure the building and the practitioner's office is accessible and does not require them to navigate an obstacle of furniture.[19] If possible, avoid having a desk between the interviewer and the applicant; instead having chairs across from each other promotes a positive, equal status interaction. As an alternative, chairs for applicants can be positioned at the side of practitioners' desks. When possible, ensure that the height of the chairs of both parties is the same to reduce any perceived power differentials between applicants and practitioners. Additionally, practitioners should remove distractions (e.g., paper work, confidential client files and records) from view so that both the applicant for services and the practitioner can exclusively focus on the intake interview.[19] Finally, practitioners can best begin to build rapport by greeting applicants in waiting areas. By greeting them and taking them to their offices, practitioners create a welcoming first impression and reduce power imbalances that can impede the development of a strong working alliance.

Because many professionals (e.g., social workers, rehabilitation counselors, nurses, crisis interventionists) work in the field, they should identify meeting places that are nearby the applicant, on a bus line for those who use public transportation, and offer private rooms for interviews. For example, they may meet with the applicant in a church office, a meeting room in a community center, an office in another community agency, or a private study room in a library. They should also ensure that these meeting places are physically accessible to individuals with disabilities and that accessible transportation is available to them.

Practitioners should also ensure that they are mentally prepared for the intake interview. During the interview, their minds should be focused on the here-and-now interaction with the applicant rather than being distracted by other tasks or client/patient concerns. To ensure that they are mentally present, practitioners may want to take a few minutes before the interview to meditate, practice breathing exercises, listen to music, or take a short walk.

ALLOTTING ADEQUATE TIME TO THE INTAKE INTERVIEW

Practitioners should avoid overwhelming themselves with back-to-back appointments. Although this may be challenging for some practitioners because of large caseloads, it can prevent making errors or unintentionally giving the impression to the applicant that the practitioner is too busy to listen to their concerns and provide them the services they need in a timely manner. Schedules should be structured so that each applicant receives adequate time and attention, while also allowing for time between meetings for reflection, case documentation, and clearing of one's mind for the next applicant or client/patient. For some, this may be ten minutes, for others this may be one hour. There is no magic number of minutes that should be allotted between meetings with clients/patients; that is a personal choice to be made by the practitioner that is also dependent on the treatment setting and types of services that are provided. If providing crisis services in a hospital setting, intake interviews may need to be delayed until applicants are stabilized and could take longer than if providing out-patient mental health maintenance services. In considering the amount of time to devote to intake interviews, practitioners want to ensure that they reduce the need to rush from appointment to appointment as well as the amount of time an applicant waits to be seen. When practitioners feel rushed, they may fail to gather or could miss important information provided by the applicant. By overscheduling interviews and not allotting sufficient time between interviews, practitioners may be late for scheduled appointments with applicants. Failure to meet with applicants on time communicates to the applicant that the practitioner may be too busy to devote sufficient attention and time to the applicant. Being late for an intake interview can result in a negative first impression, can cause applicant irritation with having to wait for the interview, and can result in frustration that interferes with establishing a positive working alliance.

READING INTAKE FORMS AND APPLICANT RECORDS BEFORE THE INTERVIEW

To read intake forms and records before the interview is a debatable issue. On one hand, information may bias the practitioner prior to even meeting the applicant. On the other hand, important information that can inform aspects of how the interview is conducted may be missed if intake forms and records are not read prior to the interview. If practitioners decide to review these records or already have information from other sources about the applicant, they should reflect on any pre-existing biases they may have about applicants and set these biases aside. All practitioners are likely to have their own philosophies regarding the amount of background information to collect about the applicant before the intake meeting. Furthermore, the setting in which a practitioner works may dictate the amount of information collected or received about an applicant. Practitioners working in private practice settings may only have the name and phone number of the applicant and basic information from the applicant about her or his reason for seeking services, whereas public agency settings may have more detailed information about an applicant collected on intake forms or gathered from previous agency records. This information may include assessment reports, school records, health history, and diagnostic information. Emergency and crisis intervention settings may have no information about patients or clients who present for treatment.

It may useful to review objective information such as diagnosis before meeting the applicant for the first time. Review of medical information may be especially important when meeting with individuals who have a diagnosis with which the practitioner might be unfamiliar or only vaguely familiar. Preliminary research about these conditions can then be conducted using resources such as websites for the Centers for Disease Control and Prevention, the National Organization of Rare Disorders, and the National Institute of Health. Individuals with rare disorders and conditions that are not well understood should not be put in the position of spending the bulk of the intake take interview educating the practitioner about their condition.[12] Practitioners should disclose if they do not have experience working with individuals with the specific condition of these applicants but have done some preliminary research and will continue to educate themselves about the condition. By doing so, they communicate to these applicants that they are invested in learning more so that they can best assist them to achieve their treatment goals.

PURPOSES OF THE INTAKE INTERVIEW

Adequate preparation for the intake interview serves to increase the likelihood that the practitioner will be able to comprehensively dispense and gather information essential to planning in a manner that focuses on actively listening to the applicant's story. It also illustrates professionalism and a focused, empathic approach to interviewing. In the next sections we describe the purposes of the intake interview, beginning with educating applicants about the practitioner's role and agency, program, or organization so applicants can make informed decisions about whether to pursue the services provided by the practitioner.

PROVIDING INFORMATION ABOUT THE AGENCY, PROGRAM, OR ORGANIZATION

To make informed decisions about participating in the activities of the agency, program, or organization represented by the practitioner, the applicant for services needs sufficient information about programmatic aspects such as eligibility criteria, agency mission, clientele served, qualifications and scope of practice of the case manager, privacy and limits of confidentiality, services offered, and the roles and functions of the case manager and client in the working alliance. This information should be provided both orally and in writing to applicants. In reviewing codes of ethics for practitioners from various disciplines (e.g., nursing, counseling, social work), the authors identified information that these codes specify as necessary to be disclosed at the outset of the professional relationship. This information includes: (a) the qualifications, credentials, and relevant professional experience of the practitioner; (b) the purpose of services, limits of services, potential risks and benefits of services, costs of services, reasonable alternatives, and frequency and length of services; (c) confidentiality, preservation of service recipients' records, policies regarding releases of information, and exceptions to protecting information obtained from service recipients (i.e., to prevent imminent and foreseeable harm to the applicant or other individuals); (d) contingencies for continuation of services upon the extended absence, incapacitation, or death of the service provider; (e) risks and limitations associated with electronic communication and provision of services via electronic media; and (f) legal issues affecting services.

Information should be communicated in a manner that is consistent with the applicant's level of understanding. The practitioner should invite and answer any questions the applicant may have about the information provided to ensure understanding. Sometimes the sheer breadth of this information can be overwhelming and may even discourage applicants from returning for a second appointment. Therefore, this information may need to be reiterated or expanded upon during subsequent sessions with the practitioner. If the applicant's primary language differs from the primary language used by the practitioner, arrangements should be made for a qualified interpreter or translator to facilitate communication in the intake interview and subsequent sessions.

Practitioners should also keep in mind that most Americans have poor health literacy skills (i.e., the ability to acquire and comprehend basic information about their health and the services offered by different health care and human service providers so that they can make informed decisions about their health and their need for services.)[18] Several strategies recommended by the Office of Disease Prevention and Health Promotion[18] can be implemented by the practitioner to improve applicants' understanding of the information:

➢ Use plain language and avoid using professional jargon and acronyms.

➢ Communicate in a culturally appropriate manner.

➢ Emphasize the most important points first.

➢ Break down information into manageable chunks.

➢ Observe applicants' nonverbal behaviors (e.g., facial expressions) that may indicate confusion or feeling overwhelmed with information. Then, ask the applicant directly if they are confused or overwhelmed so that the practitioner can adjust his or her communication and ensure applicant understanding of information.

➢ In addition to providing information verbally, provide information in written plain language (e.g., client handbooks, brochures, CDs) so that applicants can review and process the information on their own time.

➢ After providing information in writing, inform applicants that they can contact you if they have questions or that the practitioner can clarify information in the next sessions with applicants.

➢ Use the "teach back" method (i.e., the applicant repeats information back to the practitioner to ensure accurate understanding or to clarify misunderstood information).

➢ Before the intake interview, suggest that applicants bring a family member, friend, or advocate to the interview to take notes and provide applicants with emotional support.

Providing applicants with the information discussed above should enable them to make informed decisions about whether to pursue services. If the applicant chooses to pursue services from the practitioner, the focus of the interview shifts to determining eligibility for services.

DETERMINING ELIGIBILITY FOR SERVICES

Because (a) many agencies and programs have certain criteria that must be met for the applicant to be determined eligible to receive services, and (b) diagnoses must often be made to justify the payment for services by second parties such as insurance companies, establishing eligibility for services is a key focus of the intake interview. Practitioners must keep in mind that some applicants may have been on lengthy waiting lists or have experienced long delays in determining programmatic eligibility for other services (e.g., Social Security benefits). To ensure expediency, applicants should be sufficiently informed about documentation that should be brought to the interview. The language used in eligibility statements is also important to clarify with applicants. For example, in agencies that require diagnoses for receipt of services, some individuals may actually meet this requirement but do not yet have a formal diagnosis or lack awareness of the condition(s) for which they have been diagnosed. They may identify as having health problems or a chronic illness but may not identify with the language used in eligibility determination criteria. For example, some organizations (e.g., state vocational rehabilitation agencies) require that individuals have a disability in order to be eligible for services. In these cases, the practitioner must be cautious not to prematurely determine that an applicant is ineligible for services because she or he says "I don't have a disability" and to follow up with the applicant by asking questions such as "do you have any health issues that interfere with your ability to do home chores?" "In what ways does your chronic illness cause problems at work?" and "How do your health issues interfere with your daily activities?"[12]

Because a primary characteristic of strong working alliances is active client/patient involvement, applicants should participate in collecting records, especially if their involvement speeds up the process of eligibility determination. For example, they can be advised to contact their medical and health care providers to request that they respond immediately to forthcoming requests for information. Alternatively, they can bring signed release of information forms to their providers and follow-up with them in the next couple of days to ensure that the information was sent to the practitioner.

If an individual requests services that are not provided by the service provider's agency, program, or organization or is determined ineligible for services, it is paramount that these individuals are referred to the appropriate community organization that provides services needed by the applicant. In these cases, it is best to contact or have the applicant contact that organization during the appointment with the practitioner. Doing so underscores the importance of having strong working alliances, not only with applicants, but also with other community service providers. Such professional relationships can be beneficial to service recipients in expediently accessing the services they need. Practitioners should also ensure that applicants have directions and addresses of referral sources as well as information about bus routes and accessible transportation services to get to appointments with referrals. It is desirable, and in some cases (i.e., in crisis situations), it may be necessary for the practitioner to follow up with applicants to ensure that they receive the services they need.

Determining eligibility for services is a process that should actively involve applicants for services. Rather than the service provider being the sole decision maker (which creates a power imbalance and negates the principles of the working alliance), both parties should jointly explore how best to support eligibility decisions and to expedite the eligibility determination process. During this process, the case manager and applicant for services also collaboratively begin to identify potential service needs and treatment goals. A detail discussion of these foci of the intake interview follows.

IDENTIFYING SERVICE NEEDS AND TREATMENT GOALS

The intake interview involves a process of collecting, synthesizing, and interpreting medical, psychological, educational, cultural, and vocational information that provides direction to the practitioner and applicant for identifying service needs and preferred treatment outcomes.[12] It assists practitioners and applicants with understanding applicants' reasons for applying for services, preferences, strengths, and barriers to achieving desired goals. Understanding these issues enables the service provider and applicant to set achievable treatment goals and determine the type of assistance that will be needed to experience positive treatment outcomes. Skilled interviewers have expertise in determining what sources of data will best enable them to develop comprehensive, client/patient-centered treatment plans that reflect the applicant's preferences.

Although the data collected in the intake interview will vary dependent upon treatment setting and scope of practice of the professional conducting the interview, the following are examples of information that may be gathered:

➢ Applicant's presenting problem(s): detailed description of the problem; perceived source of the problem; antecedents and consequences; current or previous diagnoses received; medications; substance use; services currently or previously received to treat the problem; treatment providers; perceived effectiveness of services; unmet treatment needs; barriers to intrapersonal and interpersonal functioning, employment, and daily living created by the presenting problem(s);

➢ Personal and family history: marital status, number of dependents, primary source of income, perceived social supports, living arrangements, housing, governmental assistance received;

➢ Education and employment history: highest grade completed, current employment status, most recent job, previous jobs, reasons for leaving positions, job satisfaction and satisfactoriness in various positions, transferrable job skills;

➤ Observations: physical appearance of the client including hygiene, dress, cleanliness, and any signs of physical discomfort; applicants' affect; nonverbal reactions to statements made by the practitioner including changes in facial expressions, tone of voice, posture, or eye contact;

➤ Service preferences: desired services, preferred service providers, personal treatment goals;

➤ Next steps: records to be obtained for eligibility determination and preliminary identification of service needs, additional evaluations to be conducted, next appointment with case manager, tasks to be completed by case manager and client before next appointment.

In recording intake information to be included in the applicant's case file, practitioners should keep in mind that in most settings where case management services are provided, applicants have a right to review their records and, in many settings, have direct access to electronic records. Therefore, practitioners should avoid writing anything that they would not want the applicant to read. By doing so, they can prevent potential harm to the applicant or misunderstandings that could undermine the working alliance. If potentially harmful or easily misunderstood information (e.g., psychological evaluation reports) is included in the applicant's case file, practitioners should make provisions to assist applicants in understanding the information and provide counseling if any of the information is distressful. For example, the case manager and applicant can meet with a psychologist to discuss the results of a psychological evaluation, ask questions, and discuss information that the applicant finds distressful (e.g., terminology and labels used in psychological evaluation reports).

In some instances, the applicant's presenting problem may not be the largest barrier to achieving his or her treatment goals. Co-occurring illnesses (i.e., chronic health conditions that may contribute to or complicate the applicant's presenting problem, substance use disorders [SUDs], or mental health conditions) may not be voluntarily reported by the applicant so the practitioner may have to sensitively screen for comorbidities if these are suspected. In fact, because the rate of SUDs among people with chronic illnesses, mental health conditions, and disabilities is so high, many experts in addictions have recommended screening for SUDs with all applicants for services.[15] The Substance Abuse and Health Services Administration has organized a listing of screening instruments for SUDs.

In gathering assessment data during the intake interview, practitioners should be sensitive to each applicant's level of comfort in providing requested information. The applicant's comfort level can be increased by explaining that the purpose of asking for personal information is to assist the practitioner and applicant to proceed with determining eligibility for services and understand the applicant's presenting problem(s) so that appropriate planning is initiated. Also, keep in mind that applicants may simultaneously be receiving a variety of other services such as health care, housing assistance, rehabilitation, and mental health treatment. Practitioners should not misinterpret any frustration these individuals exhibit in the interview as being uncooperative or resistant. Rather, they should understand that applicants' frustration may stem from repeatedly answering the same questions. Additionally, practitioners should avoid soliciting information that is not relevant to treatment planning. Practitioners who query applicants about irrelevant information can be perceived as "information voyeurs" or "grand inquisitors."[19] As an example, an applicant for career counseling experiences discomfort in her intake interview when she is asked multiple questions by the career counselor about the details of her relationship with her spouse. She does not see the relevance of these questions to her need for career counseling and questions whether to return for a subsequent appointment with this career counselor or to search for a different career counselor. In any event, service providers should respect applicants' rights to choose what information to share and what information to withhold. As clients/patients get to know the practitioner better and increase their comfort level over time, they may then share additional information.

Collecting comprehensive information in the intake interview enables the practitioner and applicant for services to begin to identify changing goals and service priorities consistent with the applicant's preferences. In gathering information about potential services and treatment goals, it may be determined that additional information is necessary to aid in decision-making. We discuss considerations in obtaining additional evaluations and identifying appropriate providers to conduct these evaluations in the next section.

DETERMINING THE NEED FOR ADDITIONAL EVALUATIONS

Information gathered in the intake interview indicates additional documentation and specialist evaluations that will be necessary to develop a better understanding of the applicant's strengths and limitations, service needs, and achievable treatment goals.[14] Practitioners should be astute in obtaining adequate information in the intake interview to determine specific specialist evaluations that may be necessary. In some cases, they may want to consult with other practitioners within their organization to determine the most appropriate referrals for these evaluations. If additional evaluations are necessary, these evaluations should be conducted in a timely manner to prevent delays in eligibility determination. Applicants should be provided with specific details of what each evaluation entails (e.g., what will happen, how long the evaluation will take, procedures that will be used, directions to the evaluator's office) so that they can decide whether to participate in the evaluation. It is best if appointments for these evaluations are scheduled during or directly after the intake interview in the presence of the applicant. Immediate scheduling of evaluations demonstrates that the practitioner is committed to making eligibility determinations as quickly as possible. When making referrals for diagnostic evaluations (e.g., psychiatric evaluations, neuropsychological evaluations, comprehensive medical exams, medical specialist evaluations, vocational evaluations), practitioners should ask specific referral questions in referral letters or forms that will assist with identifying client service needs and establishing treatment goals. Before making referrals, applicants should be asked if they have ever had the evaluation that is being considered. Keep in mind that it will be necessary to clearly explain what that evaluation entails to prevent duplicative evaluations that are not only cost-ineffective, but more importantly, an unnecessary and potentially stressful use of the applicant's time. Because practitioners often have large caseloads to manage, making requests that applicants periodically contact them to determine if all necessary records have been received can expedite the eligibility determination process. Again, doing this helps to establish a strong working alliance because it directly involves the applicant in carrying out the tasks necessary to determine eligibility. Finally, when making referrals to other providers for additional evaluations, arrangements should be made for qualified interpreters or translators to attend appointments with individuals who do not speak the primary language used by the referral source. In these cases, interpreters and translators must have training and expertise in the terminology (e.g., medical, legal, psychological) used by the evaluator.

The focus of this section has been on how practitioners can use the intake interview to determine if additional evaluations are necessary to assist with making eligibility decisions, identifying service needs, and facilitating treatment goal planning. In the next section, we highlight key interviewing skills that aid in collecting comprehensive information and establishing the foundation for a positive working alliance that emphasizes equality between the practitioner and the applicant for services.

INTERVIEWING SKILLS FOR ESTABLISHING A POSITIVE WORKING ALLIANCE

Central to the working alliance is the recognition that before anything can be accomplished with an applicant for services, therapeutic or otherwise, the practitioner and applicant must build rapport with one another. The applicant must be able to trust and respect the practitioner before any real work or change can occur. Young[24] emphasized what he calls invitational skills in the building of a relationship between the practitioner and client/patient. These invitational skills are defined as "the basic means by which the helper invites the [client/patient] into a ... relationship"[p. 38] and are broken down into nonverbal skills and opening skills. Nonverbal skills include appropriate eye contact, body position, attentive silence, voice tone, gestures and facial expressions, physical distance, and touching. Eye contact should be direct with occasional breaks. However, practitioners should also be respectful of cultural variations in what is considered appropriate eye contact and physical distance. They should not always attribute lack of eye contact from the applicant to factors such as depression, social anxiety, or personality characteristics. Likewise, they should be attuned to how their own eye contact, especially if it violates cultural norms, could be viewed by the applicant as disrespectful or invasive. Observing applicants' nonverbal reactions (e.g., leaning away from the practitioner, moving their chair) can alert practitioners that they may be violating applicants' personal/cultural boundaries regarding physical distance. The practitioner's body position should be open and, when possible, mirror the client's own body position. By facing the client/patient directly, putting both feet on the floor, and leaning forward slightly, the practitioner is signaling to the client that he or she is ready to listen. If an interpreter or translator accompanies the applicant to the interview, the case manager should look at and direct all questions and responses to the applicant, not the interpreter or translator. It is disrespectful and a violation of cultural etiquette to direct questions to interpreters or translators.

Silence from the practitioner, especially after asking an open-ended question that requires reflection in order to answer, allows the time and space to think and respond at the applicant's own pace. Voice tone should be professional, gentle, calming, and at the appropriate volume that matches or reflects the tone of the client/patient. Practitioners should be aware of their facial expressions such as raising of the eyebrows, smiling, grimacing, or frowning and the message that these facial expressions might convey to the client/patient. Touching between the practitioner and applicant should be used with caution and limited to touch that is initiated by the applicant. Although it may seem natural to touch the shoulder of a client as a gesture of comfort, touch can be misinterpreted, and the appropriateness of touch can vary depending on the age, gender, and cultural background of an applicant. Touch should be used generally in terms of a handshake to open and/or close a meeting, but should never be forced on a client. Practitioners should also keep in mind cultural interpretations of touch (i.e., a firm hand shake may be interpreted as aggression in some cultures[23] and it may cause pain for some individuals with chronic health conditions and disabilities).

Opening skills include door openers, minimal encouragers (such as nodding the head, saying "mmhmm"), open-ended questions, and closed-ended questions. Door openers can be questions such as "how are you?" or "what brings you in today"? Open questions and statements such as "tell me about your condition" or "how does your rheumatoid arthritis affect your daily functioning?" allow the client to share stories or experiences that answer the question. Closed-ended questions can typically be answered with a "yes" or "no" or a short answer. These questions can be important in the information-seeking phase of the intake interview. Examples of closed questions include "What is your birthdate?" or "How long has it been since the onset of your symptoms?" By using these skills together in a way that is appropriate for the applicant, the practitioner can begin to establish a positive and trusting relationship with the applicant, and this relationship can foster the identification of the applicant's presenting problem, treatment goals, and a plan of action.

Observation skills are also important during the intake interview. While much can be learned from the applicant's history and verbal information she or he shares, additional information can be gained from simple observational skills. As we have noted in previous sections, the practitioner should observe the physical appearance of the client, noting hygiene, dress, cleanliness, and affect in the intake interaction. Any changes in subsequent visits should be noted. The applicant should be observed throughout the interview for nonverbal reactions to statements or questions posed by the practitioner including changes in facial expressions, tone of voice, posture, or eye contact.

SKILLS FOR CLARIFYING THE GOALS OF THE INTAKE INTERVIEW

Savickas[20] recommended beginning each meeting with a client/patient with the phrase, "How can I be useful to you?" He recommended use of the word "useful" over the word "helpful" because "[clients/patients] are not helpless. They are there to use … services." It is important to ask applicants what they want to accomplish during the interview, as well as the overall reason for coming to see the practitioner. Responses to these questions allow the practitioner to estimate the number of times they will need to meet, referrals, if any, which need to be made for additional services not provided by the practitioner, and to begin to consider how to best serve the applicant. At the same time, Roessler et al.[19] recommended that practitioners be transparent with clients/patients in describing the purpose of the intake interview, how the meeting will be structured, what will occur during the meeting, and how the meeting will be concluded. Doing so can (a) reassure applicants that they are not wasting their valuable time with yet another service provider who will simply require them to go through a lot of unnecessary bureaucratic red tape before services are initiated and (b) ease their uncertainty and anxiety about what to expect.[13]

SKILLS FOR ACTIVELY LISTENING TO THE APPLICANT'S STORY

In many circumstances, the individuals that are seen by practitioners are asked objective facts, but are rarely asked to tell their story. By asking applicants to tell their stories in relation to their goals for seeing the practitioner, the practitioner has the privilege of hopefully getting to know the applicant more intimately, which will ultimately lead to positive bonding between the two parties. Among the previously mentioned techniques, those that encourage applicants to tell their stories include minimal encouragers, facilitative body language, and open-ended questions and statements such as "Tell me more about..." "Describe examples of..." "What is a typical day like for you at work?" Paraphrasing what the applicant says (e.g., "What I hear you saying....," "Let me make sure I clearly understand you") indicates to applicants that the practitioner is sincerely interested in what they have to say and invites applicants to correct the practitioner if necessary.

SKILLS FOR GATHERING INFORMATION

Once applicants have had the opportunity to tell their stories, there may still be some information that is needed by the practitioner that was not given during the telling of their story. When this occurs, practitioners may need to ask the objective, close-ended questions such as age, birthdate, level of education, specific symptoms experienced, barriers to achieving desired goals, date of onset of issues, diagnosis, income, and previous services received. Throughout the intake interview, the practitioner should take the opportunity to paraphrase and summarize what the applicant has said and ask if the information was heard and interpreted correctly by the practitioner. Summarization is useful before moving onto the next topic. For example, the practitioner may state, "Before we move on to discussing your work history, I want to make sure I have a good understanding of the symptoms of your major depressive disorder that are most troubling to you. These appear to be........" It is also important, as we will discuss later, to summarize the interview near the conclusion of the meeting before determining next steps to be taken. After all summarizations, the practitioner should check with applicants to ensure that the practitioner's summarizations are consistent with what the applicant intended to express.

SKILLS FOR SETTING GOALS, IDENTIFYING TASKS, AND CONCLUDING THE INTERVIEW

At the beginning of the intake interview, the practitioner asks the reason for the applicant's visit and what she or he hopes to accomplish through meeting with the practitioner. At the end of the session, after summarizing what was discussed during the first session, the practitioner and applicant should work together to set goals to accomplish. Summarization of the session serves as a reminder to both the practitioner and applicant of the purpose of the meeting. It also enables the partners in the alliance to determine in future sessions when the time has come to terminate the relationship and/or close the case. Once the goals of the client/patient are met, then he or she will no longer need assistance from the practitioner, unless a new presenting problem develops. To keep the client focused on the goals and working towards those goals between meetings, the practitioner can assign homework to complete before the next meeting. The homework should be specific to the goals of the client. Homework may involve the client filling out a certain number of job applications, having a difficult conversation with a loved one, or attending a support group. After the intake interview, homework assignments may include gathering information for purposes of eligibility determination, keeping a diary of symptoms, or listing coping skills that the applicant uses to deal with stress. By assigning homework and expecting the client/patient to complete it, the power and responsibility for growth and change is placed in the hands of the client/patient and not the practitioner.

At the very end of the intake interview, the practitioner and applicant for services should determine specific tasks to be completed and who will complete them before the next appointment. These tasks should be mutually agreed upon, recorded in the intake interview report, and written down for the applicant. Then the next appointment should be scheduled, usually within a reasonable time period, but the time between meetings is highly dependent on the practitioner's schedule. However, best practices indicate that subsequent appointments should not be delayed for lengthy time periods.

Novice practitioners may let intake interviews go on much longer than is necessary because they fear that they may miss something important and may lack the experience of compassionately redirecting applicants who are very talkative. These practitioners should keep in mind that interviewing requires intensive listening, and at some point, the interviewer may develop fatigue that interferes with disseminating and gathering important information for decision-making and planning. Allowing interviews to go on longer than necessary can also put them behind in their appointments with other service recipients. Interviewing techniques such as redirection can be helpful in this respect. Redirection is a technique for informing applicants that they only have a limited amount of time left so they should focus on getting all the information they need to determine eligibility for services and decide on their next steps. Applicants should, in these cases, also be reassured that the service provider is invested in exploring their issues more in depth in subsequent meetings. Indeed, all practitioners should be aware of the potential for interviewer fatigue as well as time management issues in conducting intake interviews. When it is not possible to complete the entire interview in one session, subsequent appointments can be made to complete the interview. In emergency situations, practitioners such as nurses, social workers, clinical rehabilitation counselors, and/or mental health counselors must provide crisis intervention, suicide prevention, or other services first to stabilize individuals in physical or mental health crises before interviews can be conducted. Comments at the end of interviews such as "It was a pleasure to meet you, and I look forward to our next session" can help to facilitate bonding between the practitioner and applicant.

MULTICULTURAL CONSIDERATIONS AND COMPETENCIES

All individuals are multicultural beings with various identities that shape their worldviews and how others perceive and treat them. In this respect, all interactions with applicants can be viewed as requiring multicultural awareness, attitudes, and skills. Practitioners are required by their professional codes of ethics as well as their certifying and licensing bodies to be competent and comfortable with working with clients who have different values, beliefs, cultural practices, and identities than their own. In this section, we discuss the importance of multicultural attitudes, knowledge, skills, and application.

ATTITUDES

One of the biggest mistakes made by practitioners in working with clients/patients who are culturally different from them stems from gender role, gender identity, racial, ethnic, and disability stereotyping. Stereotyping pigeon holes individuals into preconceived notions or societal expectations that will ultimately do harm to the service recipient and impede the development of a positive and trusting relationship between the practitioner and individual applying for services. To avoid both stereotyping and imposing the practitioner's values on the service recipient, it is important for practitioners to first engage in thoughtful reflection and take inventory of their own cultural background, experiences, and potential biases about race, sex, ethnicity, religious beliefs, sexual orientation, gender identity, disability, and age. Additionally, practitioners must recognize that they too are multicultural beings with multiple identities, and self-inventories should include consideration of those aspects of their identities that are associated with power and privilege as well as those that are associated with disadvantage and oppression. This is the first step in continuously striving to understand themselves as racial and cultural beings and actively pursuing a non-racist identity.[1] Self-awareness alerts practitioners to when they may be stereotyping or imposing their own cultural values on the applicant. Awareness of one's own cultural background and biases and the ability to set aside these biases better enables practitioners to (a) honor and respect the cultural values, beliefs and practices of all applicants; (b) avoid imposition of their own cultural values, beliefs, and practices on service recipients; (c) improve their adeptness at establishing bonds with service recipients; and (d) incorporate cultural considerations into the intake interview and future treatment planning.

KNOWLEDGE

Practitioners should strive to stay in accordance with the mandates regarding multicultural competencies set forth by their professional codes of ethics. If practitioners are uncomfortable serving certain clients/patients from different backgrounds than their own, then it is incumbent on them to seek supervision and training to increase their knowledge and improve their cultural competencies. Remember that it is always better to ask a question of the applicant about his or her culture and beliefs rather than relying on assumptions. In the same vein as stereotyping, practitioners should avoid making generalizations about individuals with specific cultural identities and backgrounds, recognizing the intersectionality of multiple cultural identities that most people experience and how these identities shape individual beliefs, values, and worldviews in unique ways. For example, a practitioner may have two clients who share the same ethnicity, but the practitioner should be aware that each person is an individual and may not share the same beliefs, values, cultural identities just because they share the same ethnicity.

Practitioners should also be knowledgeable about varying cultural beliefs about help-seeking, sharing private information with individuals outside of the family, independence, interdependence, and gender-role expectations. These beliefs can all influence how the applicant participates in the intake interview, expectations about the role of the practitioner, information that is shared with the practitioner, and treatment goals. Additionally, because of well-documented health care and human service disparities experienced by females and individuals from racial and ethnic minority groups, it is completely understandable that these individuals may have preconceived suspicions about working with a practitioner who does not share their cultural values, experiences, and beliefs. Ivey et al.[9] recommended that the practitioner intentionally brings up these differences in the intake interview and discuss the applicant's level of comfort working with a practitioner who is culturally different from the applicant. If the applicant prefers to work with a practitioner who is more culturally similar, this preference should be honored. However, circumstances may exist that prevent these referrals from being possible. For example, the practitioner may be the only service provider in a particular community who represents the agency or organization from which the individual is pursing services. Limited choices of practitioners are especially an issue in rural areas. In such instances, the practitioner may explore the availability of a practitioner who shares more cultural similarities with the applicant working in another location to provide services on an itinerant basis, or the practitioner may have to explore with the applicant how to provide services in a manner that is culturally competent and helpful.

It is also critical that practitioners recognize that many individuals from marginalized cultural groups (e.g., women, African Americans, Muslims, transgender individuals, people with disabilities) have daily experiences with racism and microaggressions. Microaggressions are "the everyday verbal, nonverbal, and environmental slights, snubs, or insults, whether intentional or unintentional, which communicate hostile, derogatory, or negative messages to target persons based solely upon their marginalized group membership."[22, para. 2] Service providers should be conscientious not to invalidate these experiences. Rather, they should respond with empathy and recognition of the unfortunate reality that racism and microaggressions still prevail in contemporary society. For example, when applicants discuss experiences with microaggressions and discrimination, practitioners can respond with nonverbal expressions (e.g., of anger, despair) that mirror those of applicants for services and with statements such as "I feel both sad and angry to hear how you are being treated, and I am

very concerned about how this affects you, and what we can do about it."
Practitioners should then take active steps to remediate disparities in their own
agencies or organizations and partner with service recipients to advocate for
broader social changes. Most importantly, advocacy efforts aimed at changing
the cultural climates (e.g., school, work, neighborhoods, communities) in which
individuals experience disparities should be identified as key services in
treatment plans.

SKILLS

When interviewing individuals whose cultural backgrounds and identities
are different from those of the practitioner, Ivey et al.[9] recommended
acknowledging these differences up front, asking applicants if they have any
concerns or misgivings about working with the practitioner, addressing these
concerns by determining if the applicant would prefer to work with a
practitioner who shares more cultural similarities, or discussing ways the
practitioner can work with the applicant in a manner that bridges their cultural
differences. As an example, a male Mexican American adolescent is referred to
a school-based mental health counselor because he has developed a poor
attendance record, his grades are dropping, and his teachers are concerned
because he has also become withdrawn and sullen. In the intake interview, the
mental health counselor learns from the applicant that he has been enduring
bullying and ethnic slurs almost every day at his predominately Anglo-
American middle school. He has not told any of his teachers who are also
predominately Anglo-American because he fears that they will not do anything
or the bullying would get worse if he reports it. The mental health counselor,
who is a 34-year old Anglo-American female, acknowledges up front her
similarities to both the students who are bullying the adolescent and his
teachers. She then invites the adolescent to discuss with her whether these
similarities present concerns or misgivings for him.

Researchers have clearly established that individuals from underrepresented
groups experience disparities in both healthcare and human services. These
disparities include lack of access to healthcare and housing, rehabilitation,
social services, undertreatment and receipt of fewer services, and negative
health and treatment outcomes. When applicants discuss their feelings about
these disparities, their responses should not be attributed to personal
characteristics (e.g., paranoia, anger problems, difficulties getting along with
others, being overly sensitive) and should be acknowledged, validated, and
thoroughly explored with applicants in terms of what they would like to see
change. Furthermore, when individuals appear angry as they discuss social
injustices, their anger should also be validated by the practitioner rather than
being attributed to be a dysfunctional reaction. In sum, the focus of the
interview should take into consideration how the attitudes and treatment by
others contribute to or present as the primary problem for which the applicant is

seeking services. Services targeted at removing social inequities should also be included as part of these applicants' treatment plans.

Finally, we want to re-emphasize that when applicants are not fluent in the primary language spoken in the setting in which the practitioner works, they should ideally work with practitioners who are fluent in their native language (e.g., Spanish, American Sign Language). When this is not feasible (e.g., practitioner who only speaks English is the only one serving a rural community), qualified interpreters and translators should be provided for the applicant. Likewise, these applicants should be referred to other professionals for additional evaluations who are fluent in their native language or qualified interpreters or translators should be provided for any appointments that are scheduled with other service providers for further evaluations. Again, in line with principles of the working alliance, applicants should be actively involved in decisions regarding how to address language barriers that may exist between themselves and practitioners.

APPLICATION

Having multicultural attitudes, knowledge, and skills does not necessarily translate into the application of these competencies into culturally competent interviewing.[23] Wilson, et al.[23] recommended several strategies that go beyond awareness to consistently implementing competencies in practice. They noted that each practitioner carries "self-baggage" related to diversity issues and to begin, they should ask themselves "Am I putting my awareness, knowledge, and skills into action?" This question should be asked before and after each interview to identify areas in which practitioners need additional training. Arredondo, et al.,[1] describe culturally skilled practitioners as those that actively pursue continuing education, consultation, and training experiences to improve their knowledge and skills in working with culturally different populations. These practitioners also know when to refer clients/patients to qualified individuals or resources. Healthy supportive conversations about diversity issues and areas in which practitioners have intentionally or unintentionally undermined the working alliance with individuals whose cultural identities differ from their own should occur in a supportive environment with supervisors and co-workers. These conversations can also point out areas of need for further professional development so that practitioners validate service recipients' perceptions of bias and include in treatment plans social justice and advocacy practices to reduce disparities.[23]

A final consideration regarding multicultural competencies is that even the most culturally competent practitioners can unintentionally violate cultural norms and say things or behave in ways that may be culturally offensive to clients/patients. In the context of a strong working alliance, when the service recipient knows that the practitioner has the service recipient's best interests at heart and values and respects her or him, the service recipient is likely to forgive the practitioner and understand that these statements or acts were not meant to be disrespectful. Also, in strong working alliances, practitioners (a) observe applicants' reactions to their questions, comments, and behaviors and (b) invite applicants to educate practitioners about culturally appropriate interactions.

All practitioners, including the most effective, culturally competent professionals, can confront challenges in conducting intake interviews. Each applicant is unique, and even practitioners who consistently use best practices in interviewing can be confronted by situations that take them off guard. Although it is impossible to describe all the challenges that may occur, we next describe common challenges for interviewers and offer suggestions for how to respond to these challenges. These challenges include (a) responding to applicants who have negative anticipations about services, the practitioner's ability to help them, and the outcomes of services; (b) interviewing individuals who do not perceive their participation in treatment as voluntary; (c) establishing rapport with both applicants for services and their parents/legal guardians who attend intake interviews; (d) interviewing applicants whose basic needs are not met, and (e) appropriately responding to "no shows" for intake interviews.

CHALLENGES IN CONDUCTING THE INTAKE INTERVIEW

The intake interview can be a stressful experience for clients/patients. Oftentimes, they have no idea what to expect, experience anxiety about meeting a stranger who is going to ask them to divulge personal information, and have doubts that the practitioner will be able to help them. Likewise, the intake interview has the potential to be a stressful experience for the practitioner. Practitioners, like applicants, do not know what to expect, can experience anxiety about meeting a stranger, and may also have concerns about their abilities to help applicants for services. In some cases, practitioners may have heard negative comments about applicants from referral sources or other service providers who have worked with the applicant. Negative comments from others can result in negative expectancies about the upcoming interview. In these situations, practitioners must be conscientious about setting negative anticipatory biases aside so that they can make their own independent judgments that are uninfluenced by what others have said. Strategies described in the section on mentally preparing for the interview can be used for this purpose. Additional challenges arise when applicants present with negative anticipations about working with the practitioner, do not perceive their participation in the intake interview as voluntary, bring family members or legal guardians to appointments who do all the talking, have unmet basic needs, or fail to show up for appointments.

APPLICANTS WITH NEGATIVE ANTICIPATIONS

In a survey of the preferences and anticipations of individuals who had applied for vocational rehabilitation (VR) services but had not had an intake interview yet, Koch[10] found that a substantial number had negative anticipations before they even met with a VR counselor. Among the negative anticipations reported were that they were going to have to deal with a lot of unnecessary red tape (bureaucratic delays in the process), would be deemed ineligible for services or have to wait for an unnecessarily long time to receive an eligibility decision, would have their names placed on lengthy waiting lists, initiation of service plans would be stalled, have to wait for extended periods of time to receive services, be denied services that they desired, and would be not have their treatment goals and desired outcomes supported by the case manager. These negative anticipations may arise from a variety of sources including prior negative experiences with counselors, social workers, human service workers, and health care providers; or accounts they have heard from others about their own negative experiences.

When individuals arrive at intake interviews with preset negative anticipations, unique challenges arise for the practitioner. Foremost among these challenges is to prove negative anticipations wrong and to reinforce applicant preferences. Koch, Williams, and Rumrill[13] suggested using an expectations-based approach to interviewing that requires practitioners to ask applicants about both their preferences (e.g., what they *want* to occur in terms of interactions with case managers, services to be provided, treatment goals) and their anticipations (i.e., what they *think* will occur). Gathering this information will help the practitioner and applicant to construct the working alliance in a manner that incorporates applicant preferences into treatment planning and counters the applicant's negative anticipations.

INVOLUNTARY APPLICANTS

Individuals who are not voluntarily seeking services or do not perceive their participation as voluntary can also present unique challenges for the interviewer. These individuals may be court-ordered or referred to a probation/parole officer or addictions treatment program as a condition of their probation or parole. They may be referred to a vocational rehabilitation specialist by the Social Security Administration and fear losing their benefits if they do not participate in the intake interview. Others may be involuntarily admitted to psychiatric facilities because they pose a threat to themselves or others. Transition age youths may be referred for services by their transition team and may believe they had no say in the decision for a referral.

A strategy for addressing the issue of perceived or actual "forced" participation in services is for practitioners to openly acknowledge that they understand the individual is not there out of personal choice and to discuss how to work together to make the experience worthwhile. For example, the interviewer may state, "I understand that you are here as a condition of your parole rather than personal choice, but let's figure out a way to make our time together worthwhile. Do you have any ideas?" An accompanying approach is motivational interviewing.[16]

> *Motivational interviewing is a collaborative, goal-oriented style of communication with particular attention to the language of change. It is designed to strengthen personal motivation for and commitment to a specific goal by eliciting and exploring the person's own reasons for change within an atmosphere of acceptance and compassion.*[16, p.29]

Motivational interviewing is based on the premise that change involves a developmental process and that applicants for medical, health care, and human services are at different stages in terms of their readiness for change. Individuals who are not voluntary referrals may not perceive a need to change. Motivational interviewing is focused on working with these clients from where they are at. Interview questions and intake planning are then targeted at facilitating movement towards readiness for change and personal investment in taking the steps necessary to make changes in their lives. Readers are referred to Miller and Rollnick[16] for additional information on motivational interviewing and techniques used in motivational interviewing.

APPLICANTS ACCOMPANIED BY PARENTS OR LEGAL GUARDIANS

Practitioners are likely to encounter situations in which parents, legal guardians, primary care givers, or other individuals attend intake interviews with the applicant for services and do all the talking for the applicant. The practitioner asks the applicant a question and these individuals respond with an answer, not allowing the applicant to speak for him/herself. In other cases, family members may think that the applicant is in need of services, but the applicant does not believe she or he needs services. Likewise, individuals who have power of attorney for the applicant may indicate the applicant needs services, but the applicant does not perceive this need to be present. These situations can be frustrating; however, the practitioner should be empathic with parents or legal guardians who have often had to fight for services for their children or elderly family members. Practitioners should also be aware that trust must be built with parents, family members, and legal guardians as well as with the applicant so that everyone understands that the case manager has the applicant's best interest at heart. Once this trust is built, practitioners can then educate family members and significant others about the importance of allowing the applicant to speak for him/herself and to gain experience with taking ownership of decisions affecting his or her life. Finally, practitioners do not want to alienate parents/legal guardians who can be instrumental in supporting the service recipient to achieve his or her case management goals. It might take several interview sessions for parents and legal guardians to accept that the applicant's goals are of primary importance. Multicultural competencies of practitioners must be used to develop an understanding of how decisions are made (i.e., independently or collectively with the family) and to use culturally appropriate approaches to assist the applicant with decision-making. Of utmost importance, however, is to prioritize the choices of the applicant for services while educating them about alternative options if better choices exist.

In cases in which adult children and elderly family members have not had opportunities to make their own decisions, decision-making training may be an important service to consider for inclusion in the treatment plan. In discussing whether the applicant wants to participate in services and exploring treatment options, practitioners must be aware of acquiescence, especially when these individuals have had little experience with making their own decisions. Gaining trust with applicants and increasing their comfort level with stating their own choices can begin by showing an interest in what interests them. Then, the practitioner can work with the applicant to build her or his decision-making skills by starting with small choices and slowly graduating to bigger choices.

APPLICANTS WITH UNMET BASIC NEEDS

Another challenge for service providers arises when conducting intake interviews with individuals who report that their basic needs (e.g., food, water, shelter, medical needs, safety) are not being met or applicants who are in such distress that they have difficulty participating in the interview. If individuals who present for intake interviews are homeless, experience food insecurity, are not taking needed medications, cannot access needed medical care to treat and manage their health conditions, and/or have had their utilities suspended due to inability to pay for these services or cut off due to natural disasters, practitioners will need to assist these applicants with obtaining immediate assistance in response to these unmet basic needs from either the practitioner or other community service providers before the individual is capable of committing to active participation in treatment planning and execution. If individuals are put on waiting lists for services to meet their basic needs, case managers should explore all alternatives for temporarily meeting their basic needs (e.g., stay with relatives or friends, use food banks, access temporary emergency assistance from case manager's agency or other agencies). Practitioners should also advocate for more immediate assistance by engaging in efforts such as negotiating with power companies to restore electricity or contacting organizations such as the Red Cross, churches, synagogues, mosques, and other religious organizations for assistance. They should also continue to follow up with these applicants until needed assistance is provided.

When individuals exhibit substantial distress during the intake interview, practitioners need to stop interviewing and shift to active, empathic listening using techniques such as minimal encouragers and reflection of feelings (e.g., "I hear grief in your voice when you talk about your divorce."). Active listening, while providing hope and encouragement that the situation can change and making necessary referrals to address the source of distress, can provide these individuals with substantial relief. In such situations, the practitioner will also want to ensure that eligibility decisions and service provision are provided in an expedient manner. Practitioners may be able to gather enough information to open the case and proceed with next steps or it may be necessary to immediately refer the applicant for community services and schedule a second interview with the practitioner as soon as possible.

BALANCING THE NEED TO INPUT DATA INTO CLIENT TRACKING SYSTEMS WITH CONDUCTING THE INTERVIEW

The requirement to spend most of the intake interview inputting data into computerized client tracking systems may not be conducive to establishing a positive working alliance. This requirement often demands the practitioner to focus his or her attention on the computer rather than the applicant. Several strategies can be implemented to ensure that attention is focused on the applicant rather than the computer. For example, forms with information needed to input into computer programs can be provided to applicants to complete prior to the intake interview. Applicants may be asked to come in early to complete forms in the waiting area before meeting with the practitioner. Another strategy that has been used in health care, human service, mental health, and rehabilitation settings is the group orientation. During the group orientation, an agency representative explains the program, discusses what to expect when individuals meet with a practitioner for the intake interview, answers questions, and assists applicants with completing forms prior to their interview. Collaborative documentation (CD) is an innovative alternative that has been implemented in mental health settings and is recommended by Sheehan and Lewicki[21] as a promising practice that could be implemented in a variety of health and human service settings. CD is a practice that involves both the practitioner and applicant in developing intake summaries, completing progress notes, and completing intake questionnaires. In CD, the practitioner reserves time at the end of the interview to collaboratively develop an intake summary with the applicant and to input information into the computer. CD reinforces active client involvement and ownership of the process, which is a necessary component of the working alliance. Additionally, it enables the practitioner to develop better rapport with the applicant because the applicant has input into all aspects of the intake interview and jointly develops information to be entered into computer programs. Preliminary research on CD indicates that it improves client satisfaction with services. CD also improves practitioners' job satisfaction because they can spend more time with service recipients and less time doing paperwork.[21]

"NO SHOWS" FOR APPOINTMENTS

A major source of frustration for many practitioners is high rates of "no shows" for intake interviews. However, when an applicant does not show up for an interview, the practitioner should not automatically assume that the applicant is unmotivated or uninterested in services. Practitioners should contact those who do not show up for interviews to determine why and if they would like to reschedule the appointment. Many reasons rather than lack of interest may explain why the individual did not show up. Among these are cognitive impairments that may affect memory and result in forgetting the appointment, anxiety about meeting with the case manager, transportation issues, exacerbation/flare up of symptoms on the day of the scheduled appointment, or an inability to contact the case manager if scheduling conflicts occur. By contacting applicants when they have missed appointments, practitioners communicate that they care about these individuals, are invested in working with them, and are determined to take actions to ensure that these individuals can attend appointments (e.g., contacting them with appointment reminders, providing transportation assistance, discussing and alleviating their anxieties about meeting the practitioner, coming up with strategies for rescheduling appointments for those with episodic conditions).

One strategy that is becoming more common is the concept of "open access" wherein an agency has both a trained interviewer as well as backups (i.e., counselors, practitioners, and staff members who have training in the interviewing process).[6,17] In open access, like medical walk in clinics, individuals can come in during a predetermined set of hours to have an interview completed. They complete necessary paperwork and are seen as soon as possible. This approach has been shown to reduce the number of "no shows" for intake interviews.

CASE STUDY
INTAKE INTERVIEW WITH JOY

DEMOGRAPHIC INFORMATION

Joy is a divorced, 37-year-old white female with two children ages 16 and 12. She is the sole provider for her two children and receives no child (i.e., court-ordered payments to support one's minor child or children) or spousal support (i.e., alimony) from her ex-husband with whom she and her daughters have no contact. Joy lives in a three-bedroom house with her children and has a monthly mortgage of $1,200.00. Her primary source of income is from her current job which pays her an annual salary of $76,000.00. Joy has comprehensive medical insurance that covers her two children and herself. Joy does not have any family members living in her community, but her two brothers and her parents live in a city that is a 2.5-hour drive from her home. Her mother visits at least once a month to help Joy out with various household chores, shopping, other errands, and cooking and freezing meals that can later be heated up.

DISABILITY INFORMATION

Joy has been living with chronic pain for the past five years. The pain started in her neck and shoulders. After several weeks of continuous pain, she saw her primary care physician who prescribed muscle relaxants. When these failed to relieve her pain, he referred her for physical therapy, but this also did not help, and Joy began experiencing pain in other parts of her body. After then consulting several different medical and health care specialists who ran various medical tests and put her on a course of various treatments (spinal manipulations, massage therapy, acupuncture, heat and cold compressions) none of these treatments provided anything but temporary relief. Joy was told by these specialists that they could not find anything wrong with her and she was subsequently diagnosed with unexplained medical symptoms. Her primary care physician then suggested the problem could be stress-related and it was recommended that she sees a mental health professional for counseling and stress management. Joy follows through with this recommendation, knowing that her pain was real and "not in her head." However, she could learn some coping strategies from the psychologist to whom she was referred. Finally, after reporting to her primary care physician that none of these referrals resulted in relief of her pain and that the pain was becoming worse and spreading to other parts of her body, she was referred to a rheumatologist (i.e., a physician who specializes in in the diagnosis and treatment of arthritis and other diseases of the joints, muscles and bones). The rheumatologist diagnosed her with fibromyalgia. Fibromyalgia is a chronic condition that is believed to result from abnormal pain processing and causes widespread pain, fatigue, and sleep difficulties.[5] Fibromyalgia can also be accompanied by significant emotional and physical distress. The rheumatologist prescribed Cymbalta and Lyrica to reduce her pain as well as Trazodone to help her sleep. The rheumatologist also recommended she participate in light exercise such as taking daily walks. Joy indicates that the medications have helped to reduce her pain, but she still experiences significant pain, especially at the end of a long work day, when she doesn't get enough sleep, when the weather changes, or when she is under pressure to meet work deadlines. Joy indicates that she does not exercise due to lack of time and energy.

Joy describes many symptoms of her fibromyalgia, in addition to pain, that interfere with her ability to carry out daily activities such as working, spending quality time with her children, preparing meals, and doing household chores. Both of her children are active in athletics, and she is usually unable to attend their sporting events. Joy's symptoms include fatigue, upset stomach, appetite loss, restless legs syndrome, memory problems, difficulties with concentration, irritability, anxiety, and frequent headaches. She indicates that by the end of the workday, she is in too much pain and is too exhausted to cook meals for herself and her children. She often immediately goes to bed when she returns from work, and her oldest daughter brings her dinner in bed. Additionally, she spends most of many weekends in bed and has unpredictable "fibro flares" that incapacitate her. Joy indicates that she feels extremely guilty that she is unable to take better care of her children and that she puts so much responsibility on her oldest daughter.

EMPLOYMENT AND EDUCATIONAL BACKGROUND

Joy is currently employed as an account manager for a large international company that sells personal care, house cleaning, and a variety of other products. She has been working for the company for eight years and indicates that she loves her job but is having difficulty keeping up with the fast pace and demanding schedule of her position. Joy is part of a sales team and manages an account with a large retailer. Her position requires her to assist the retailer with marketing of her company's products, develop business plans, recommend pricing, secure merchandizing, assist the retailer with creating displays of merchandize, and distribute new items developed by her company. Her position requires long working hours, substantial computer work, weekly team meetings, and frequent conference calls and in person meetings with her customers.

Joy has always received very positive annual performance reviews. However, she is having increasing difficulty keeping up with the work pace, has begun making careless mistakes on written reports and projects, forgets meetings, has trouble recalling clients' names, and experiences increasing pain and fatigue as the work day proceeds. She indicates that she has also begun to obsessively worry when thinking about her future and has begun to dread going to work. Joy indicates that, with two children to support (both of whom she hopes will eventually go to college), a mortgage to pay, and the need for health insurance, she has no choice but to continue working full time despite her pain. Subsequently, she experiences significant anxiety about her ability to continue working and has begun dreading going to work each day whereas she always looked forward to each workday prior to the onset of her chronic pain.

Joy received a Bachelor's degree in Marketing. Prior to her position with her current employer, she worked in a variety of clerical and receptionist positions. After her divorce, she began college while continuing to work, and obtained her bachelor's degree because these positions did not provide her with enough money to support her family. She acquired her current position after completing an internship with the company during the final semester of her Marketing degree program.

OBSERVATIONS

Joy arrived on time for her appointment, was dressed in business attire, and was articulate, actively engaged in the interview, and appeared to be highly motivated to work with the VR counselor to achieve her goal of continued employment with her current employer. Joy did indicate some signs of distress such as fidgeting with her hands and her eyes welling up with tears when discussing her fears about her ability to continue working. She also rubbed her neck and shoulder several times during the interview, and when asked if she was in pain and needed a break to stretch or walk around, she indicated that yes, she was always in pain, but that rubbing her neck helped, and she wanted to continue with the interview rather than taking a break.

CLIENT PREFERENCES FOR SERVICES

Joy indicates that she was referred to her state's vocational rehabilitation (VR) agency by a member of a fibromyalgia support group she attends. Joy would like to continue working in her current position but fears that the symptoms of her fibromyalgia will prevent her from keeping up with the fast work pace. She indicates that, overall, she enjoys her job and needs the health benefits it provides for herself and her children. If she is unable to continue in her current positions, she would like to explore other job opportunities with the same company that would enable her to use her talents but are slower paced. Joy indicated that if it is determined that she should change positions; she would need a position with comparable salary.

NEXT STEPS

After the intake interview, the VR counselor and Joy agree to the following next steps: (a) refer Joy for a comprehensive medical examination with her primary physician, and (b) schedule a comprehensive evaluation with a rehabilitation psychologist who specializes in working with individuals with chronic pain. The purpose of the evaluation will be to determine if she could benefit from mental health services and/or referral to a psychiatrist for medications to treat her anxiety. Because Joy would like to continue in her current position or be transferred to another position in her company, the case manager contacted the coordinator of Retaining a Valued Employee (RAVE), a program that provides a rapid response to assisting employees with disabilities who are at risk of job loss. The RAVE coordinator scheduled a meeting for the following week with a RAVE counselor to be attended by both Joy and the VR counselor. Joy *agreed to develop a comprehensive description of all her job duties before the meeting so that (a) she, the case manager, and the RAVE counselor can begin to explore potential accommodations (e.g., flex time, work from home, teleconferences to reduce travel, transfer to another position) that would enable her to continue working for her current employer and (b) explore with Joy if she would like to set up a meeting with her supervisor and RAVE counselor to discuss potential job accommodations.*

DISCUSSION QUESTIONS

1. Discuss how intake interviews in the settings where practitioners in your field work can be structured and conducted in a manner that establishes the foundation for a positive working alliance? What are barriers that may need to be ameliorated in these settings to conduct interviews in this manner?

2. How can you mentally prepare for the intake interview?

3. What are important multicultural considerations that should be incorporated into the intake interview in the settings where practitioners in your field work?

4. In addition to the challenges described in the chapter that can occur in the intake interview, what are additional challenges that professionals in your field may encounter?

5. What are examples of interview questions you could ask to gather the information in Joy's intake interview report?

6. What biases related to gender, gender roles, and Joy's reported disability might interfere with a practitioner's ability to establish a positive working alliance with Joy? What should a practitioner do if he or she has these biases?

7. People with chronic pain conditions such as fibromyalgia often experience misunderstanding, disbelief about their conditions, invalidation of the severity of their symptoms, and attributions of their symptoms as being "all in their heads." If a client/patient with fibromyalgia (or another medical condition that is often invalidated by others) brought up these experiences in the intake interview, how would you respond?

CONCLUSION

Conducting the intake interview in a professional and caring manner is one of the most important tasks that practitioners in health care and human services will undertake. The intake meeting with an applicant and the subsequent interview sets the tone for establishing a positive and productive working alliance. It is important to create rapport and establish trust right from the beginning of the intake interview so that appropriate goals can be set and progress toward achieving treatment goals can occur. Skilled interviewers know how to structure interviews, use effective interviewing skills, and determine the need for additional evaluations. This knowledge and accompanying skills enable the practitioner and applicant to develop a comprehensive understanding of the applicants presenting problem(s), coping abilities, desired services, and preferred treatment outcomes. Skilled interviewers also consistently strive to further develop their cultural competencies so that they can effectively serve a wide range of individuals from different backgrounds. Furthermore, they are aware of potential challenges in the intake interview and strategies to address these challenges and reduce barriers to establishing positive bonds with applicants, carrying out the tasks of the alliance, and realizing individualized treatment goals.

REFERENCES

[1]Arredondo, P., Toporek, M. S., Brown, S., Jones, J., Locke, D. C., Sanchez, J. and Stadler, H. (1996). Operationalization of the Multicultural Counseling Competencies. AMCD: Alexandria, VA

[2]Baruth, L. G., & Manning, M. L. (2016). *Multicultural counseling and psychotherapy: A lifespan approach*. Routledge.

[3]Bordin, E. S. (1979). The generalizability of the psychoanalytic concept of the working alliance. *Psychotherapy: Theory, Research & Practice, 16*(3), 252.

[4]Chan, F., Shaw, L. R., McMahon, B. T., Koch, L., & Strauser, D. (1997). A model for enhancing rehabilitation counselor-consumer working relationships. *Rehabilitation Counseling Bulletin, 41*, 122-137.

[5]Centers for Disease Control and Prevention (2017). *Fibromyalgia*. Retrieved from https://www.cdc.gov/arthritis/basics/fibromyalgia.htm

[6]Ghorob A, & Bodenheimer T. (2012) Sharing the care to improve access to primary care. *The New England Journal of Medicine, 366*(21), 1955–1957. doi: 10.1056/NEJMp120275.

[7]Groth-Marnat, G. (2009). *Handbook of psychological assessment*. NY: John Wiley & Sons.

[8]Integrative Trauma Treatment. (2011). *Containment imagery*. Retrieved from https://trauma101.com/ufiles/a-container.pdf.

[9]Ivey, A. E., Ivey, M. B., & Zalaquett, C. P. (2013). *Intentional interviewing and counseling: Facilitating client development in a multicultural society*. Nelson Education.

[10]Koch, L. C. (2001). The preferences and anticipations of people referred to a vocational rehabilitation agency. *Rehabilitation Counseling Bulletin, 44*(2), 76-86.

[11]Koch, L.C., & Rumrill, P.D., Jr. (2005). Interpersonal communication skills for case managers. In F. Chan, M. Leahy, & J. Saunders (Eds.), *Case management for rehabilitation health professionals* (2nd ed.; vol. I; pp. 122-143). Lake Zurich, IL: Vocational Consultants Press.

[12]Koch, L. C., & Rumrill, P. D. (2016). *Rehabilitation Counseling and Emerging Disabilities: Medical, Psychosocial, and Vocational Aspects*. NY: Springer Publishing Company.

[13]Koch, L. C., Williams, C. L., & Rumrill, P. D. (1998). Increasing client involvement in vocational rehabilitation: An expectations-based approach to assessment and planning. *Work: A Journal of Prevention, Assessment, and Rehabilitation, 10*(3), 211-218.

[14]Leahy, M. J., Chan, F., Sung, C., & Kim, M. (2013). Empirically derived test specifications for the certified rehabilitation counselor examination. *Rehabilitation Counseling Bulletin, 56*(4), 199-214.

[15]Lusk, S. L., Koch, L. C., & Paul, T. M. (2016). Recovery-Oriented Vocational Rehabilitation Services for Individuals with Co-Occurring Psychiatric Disabilities and Substance Use Disorders. *Rehabilitation Research, Policy, and Education, 30*(3), 243-258.

[16]Miller, W. R., & Rollnick, S. (2013). Motivational interviewing: Helping people change (3rd Ed.) New York: The Guilford Press.

[17]Murray M, Berwick DM. Advanced access: reducing waiting and delays in primary care. *The Journal of the American Medical Association, 289*(8):1035–1040. doi: 10.1001/jama.289.8.1035.

[18]Office of Disease Prevention and Health Promotion (2016). Quick guide to health literacy. Retrieved from https://health.gov/communication/literacy/quickguide/factsbasic.htm

[19]Roessler, R., Rubin, S., & Rumrill, P. (in press). *Case management in rehabilitation counseling, 5th edition*. Austin, TX: Pro-Ed.

[20]Savickas, M. L. (2015). *Life-design counseling manual*. Lexington, KY.

[21]Sheehan, L., & Lewicki, T. (2016). Collaborative Documentation in Mental Health: Applications to Rehabilitation Counseling. *Rehabilitation Research, Policy, and Education, 30*(3), 305-320.

[22]Sue, D. W. (2010). *Microaggressions: More than just race*. Retrieved from https://www.psychologytoday.com/blog/microaggressions-in-everyday-life/201011/microaggressions-more-just-race

[23]Wilson, K. B., Pitt, J. S., Raheem, M. A., Acklin, C. L, & Wilson, J. M. (2017). Multicultural counseling competencies: Why is it difficult to apply what we know…? In Leavitt, L., Wisdom, S., & Leavitt, K. (Eds.), *Cultural Awareness and Competency Development in Higher Education* (pp. 237-254). Hershey, PA: IGI Global.

[24]Young, M. E. (2009). *Learning the art of helping: Building blocks and techniques* (4th ed). Upper Saddle River, NJ: Pearson Education, Inc.

CHAPTER 4

MEDICAL, PSYCHOLOGICAL, PSYCHOSOCIAL, PSYCHOEDUCATIONAL EVALUATIONS

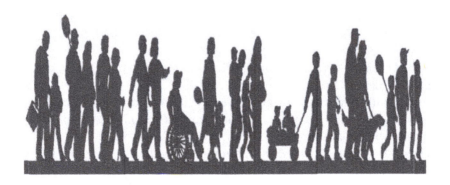

SI-YI CHAO

DEANA LACY MCQUITTY

ABSTRACT

When clients seek human services consisting of medical, psychiatric, psychological, educational, vocational, social, political, and financial services, the goal of human service professionals is to help the client figure out the appropriate treatments and to implement a treatment plan of achieving needs and expectations of the client. To implement an effective treatment plan, it is often the case that human service practitioners use information gathered from medical, psychological, psychosocial, and psychoeducational evaluations. The purpose of this chapter is to provide an overview of commonly used evaluations and to discuss critical issues with interpreting the evaluation results. An accurate and holistic evaluation of the client's relevant information can facilitate success and an appropriate and accessible treatment plan which can bring positive outcomes for the client.

CHAPTER HIGHLIGHTS

➢ Evaluation procedural safeguards;

➢ Comprehensive evaluation process;

➢ Multicultural considerations during the evaluation process.

LEARNING OBJECTIVES

➢ To examine holistic concepts of evaluation.

➢ To explain the details of the evaluation process.

➢ To acknowledge the considerations of evaluation interpretation.

➢ To discuss multicultural considerations affecting evaluation results.

INTRODUCTION

Professionals or case managers of human services provide holistic biopsychosocial evaluations that consist of medical, psychological, social, vocational, educational, economic, and cultural aspects of clients.[12,17] A holistic biopsychosocial evaluation guides human service professionals in making levels of care decisions, treatment plans, individual intervention strategies, and community resource coordination for clients from pediatric through the geriatric populations. Additionally, human service professionals should re-evaluate their clients regularly to follow up on the progression of ailments and treatment outcomes.[2] There are six goals to a comprehensive evaluation:

1. to help human service professionals understand concerns, needs, and expectations of clients;

2. to increase clients' self-awareness of their strengths and weaknesses;

3. to determine other potential opportunities for clients (e.g., vocational rehabilitation, transitional education development, community integration activities);

4. to discuss and make a treatment plan with achievable goals;

5. to access an appropriate and focused service program for clients;

6. to collaborate multidisciplinary resources by referrals to other professionals who can assist the comprehensive assessments, testing, and treatments for clients.[2,16,20]

This chapter focuses mainly on human service professionals conducting a comprehensive evaluation including medical, psychological, psychosocial, psychoeducational domains. The role of the human service professional is to facilitate the evaluation procedures and establish shared goals with clients.

EVALUATION PROCESS

PREPARATION FOR ELIGIBILITY: FOSTERING RELATIONSHIP BUILDING

During the process of medical, psychological, psychosocial, and psychoeducational evaluations, themes of rapport building, empathy with clients and family, and cultural responsiveness are essential to the initial phases of eligibility for services and are deemed appropriate by the human service professional. Such themes suggest that in addition to the clinical and technical skills needed as a human service professional, interpersonal communication skills when interacting with clients and families is equally critical. Paul[13] states "our ability to listen actively and nonjudgmentally, our capacity for empathy and perspective taking, and our skill in absorbing and sharing information will serve as the linkage between research, experience, and client perspective."[13, p.204] The evaluation process is multifaceted with the goal of facilitating services for both the client and the agency.

The human service professional's ability to build rapport with the client as a working alliance, to collect information from the client, and to explain administrative and service processes for the client, begins the initial process for eligibility.[6] The preparation for eligibility will help the human service professional understand the basic background information including diagnosis, current conditions, reasons for referral, and the corresponding client information that the referred agency would like to receive.[2] Obtaining background information and developing trust with the client can facilitate the eligibility process for both the client and the human service professional. While the intake interview was covered in the prior chapter, Chapter 3, we will turn our attention to briefly highlighting the intake interview with an evaluation focus.

EVALUATION BY INTERVIEW

Case managers in the human service field gather necessary information from clients by interviewing either via phone, face-to-face, or video conferencing mediums. The interview can be a structured conversation process with clients who will narrate their concerns, their past and current conditions of diagnosis and treatments, their functional limitations, their psychological and psychosocial status, their environmental conditions, their support system, and their expectations of services. Based on time, the interview process (on average) may last 45-60 minutes per session. Human service professionals may use open-ended or closed-ended questions for evaluations. Gathering information from the client helps the human service professional recognize the client's major concerns. After reviewing the major concerns, the human service professional then determines if the client needs other specific and formal medical, psychological, and vocational assessments or tests. Additional information about the intake interview skills is illustrated in Chapter 3, *"The Intake Interview."*

During the evaluation process, it is important for the human service professional to gather both verbal and non-verbal information from the client. The human service professional can do this by observing the client's facial expressions and nonverbal behaviors, by talking to the client, and by interacting with the client (see Chapter 1). The observational and communicative information helps the human service professional determine:

➤ if good rapport has been built with the client;

➤ the clients' willingness to collaborate and engage in treatment;

➤ the client's level of overall functioning;

➤ the consistency between clients' descriptions and behaviors in their daily living, school, and work envrionment.

Observations can help the human service provider analyze and recommend the appropriate service plans for the client. With the client's permission, the human service professional can also use additional resources to gather information about the client by speaking with family members, personal care providers, friends, caseworkers, social workers, or other professionals to facilitate the interview process. Also, the human service professional can utilize accommodations to complete the evaluation process, like augmentative and alternative communication (AAC), Braille, reader, interpreter, computer screen, pictures, and paper documents. For example, the human service professional can play a tape recording, provide a magnifier, or Braille evaluation tools for individuals with low vision or who are blind. The alternative accommodations provided by human service professionals can facilitate efficient interaction and communication.

FORMAL (NORM-REFERENCED) AND INFORMAL (CRITERION-REFERENCED) ASSESSMENT MEASURES

After interviewing the client, human service professionals can decide whether to use formal (norm-referenced), informal (criterion-referenced) assessment tools, or both. Norm-referenced tests involve comparing a client's performance to a sample of individuals who are similar to the client. Such similarities include gender, age, ethnicity, and intellectual abilities. Unlike norm-reference tests, criterion-referenced tests do not compare an individual's performance to others. Instead, criterion-referenced measures compare the client's skills to certain predetermined expectations. Such predetermined expectations involve assessing the individuals' own strengths and weaknesses. Information related to the client's strengths and weaknesses provides the human service professional with a critical analysis of physical, psychological, intellectual, and vocational domains. For example, if human service professionals would like to understand the cognitive functions of clients, the clients might be referred to a neuropsychologist or school psychologist for the administration of the Wechsler Adult Intelligence Scale (WAIS) to understand the cognitive function levels of the client compared to the population of similar age and gender.[15] Additional information about assessment instruments, tools, and how to utilize and interpret results can be found in Chapter 12, *"Assessment for Case Management."*

REFERRAL PROCESS

After the preparation and evaluation stages, the human service professional should have enough information to determine what level of care (e.g., types of treatments and treatment settings) is the most appropriate for the client. After the appropriate level of care is determined, the human service professional works with the client to make a referral for treatment services. However, if the human service professional feels that there is a need for additional information, the human service professional should take the responsibility to obtain permission from the client and explain the reason(s) for seeking additional information (i.e., medical, psychological, psychosocial aspects).[6] Human service professionals can select a trusted and appropriate professional to conduct further assessments. The additional information from other professionals can help ensure that the client is referred to the appropriate services which can increase the likelihood that the client experiences positive service outcomes. Additional information about the referral process of human services can be found in Chapter 11, *"Referrals in Case Management."*

BUILDING A QUALITY WORKING ALLIANCE

In emphasizing the holistic evaluation approach, human service professionals in each type of human service agency should network for referrals with other professionals to build a collaborative transdisciplinary team.[16] Generally, a good working alliance emphasizes the rapport and service quality between the human service provider and the client. Here, a quality working alliance which is extended the definition would also include other relevant human service professionals who provide the information, specific assessment and treatments to this client. The working alliance between various human service professionals can facilitate appropriate and holistic human services and treatment plans for the client. Team members in the human and allied health professions working alliance can include medical professionals (e.g., physician, physiatrist, psychiatric, physical therapist, occupational therapist, speech-language pathologist, nurse, dietician), mental health professionals (e.g., psychologist, neuropsychologist, vocational counselor, school counselor, substance abuse counselor), and social resources (e.g., social worker, community resources, recreational and leisure agency, self-help group, attorney). Consequences of a lack of a collaborative transdisciplinary team of human service providers can lead to less accessibility of appropriate treatments for clients, or a duplication of services. For example, it is often the case that mental health counseling services are separate services from substance abuse counseling services–even in cases where some individuals need both. It is likely that the client will see two counselors: one for mental health and the other for substance abuse. If the mental health and substance abuse counselors do not collaborate, it may be that the client is addressing the same issues in both treatments that can lead to client frustration and poor service outcomes. It is necessary that human service professionals build a working alliance of collaboration and consultation with other professionals to increase the likelihood that a holistic concept of treatment is being used and increase the likelihood that the client is receiving high quality services.

PROGRESS MONITORING AND FOLLOW-UP

Two critical aspects of the evaluation process are progress monitoring and follow-up. Human behavior is dynamic and complex, therefore, it is highly likely that the client's needs will change throughout the evaluation process. Progress monitoring involves a continuous assessment of how the client is doing in services. Progress monitoring can be done by reviewing case notes, treatment plans, consulting with other service providers, consulting with family members, or updating initial evaluations. Follow-up refers to contacting other professionals or agencies that are involved with the client in order to gather information about any additional evaluations that were performed, the client's level of engagement, and the client's progress. The follow-up information can help the human service professional determine if additional supports, services, or evaluations are needed for the client. The information gathered from following up and progress monitoring will enable the human service professional to determine if the current supports and services are meeting the client's needs, or if additional supports and services are needed.

COMPREHENSIVE EVALUATIONS

Before addressing the different aspects of evaluations, human service professionals need to acknowledge the International Classification of Functioning, Disability, and Health (ICF). The ICF emphasizes a biopsychosocial framework of evaluation and intervention for people who need health care and human services.[18] The World Health Organization announced the ICF model in 2001 that combined the medical model and social model of rehabilitation and human services. The medical model asserts the diagnosis and pathology of disability; the social model advocates participation and inclusion of social activities (e.g., studying at school, employment, attending churches, buying groceries, traveling, recreational activities, etc.). The ICF model innovated the classification system which coded each person's health condition with:

➢ body functions and structures;

➢ activities and participation;

➢ context with personal factors; and

➢ environmental factors.[21]

Human service professionals evaluate their client's health and functional status. Additionally, human service providers consider the effects of personal and environmental factors for the client.[17] Gradually, human service professionals are including more and more aspects related to a holistic view of an individual during the evaluation process in order to deliver more comprehensive programs for the client.[4] Let us highlight the critical aspects of a medical evaluation.

MEDICAL EVALUATION

The main purpose of a medical evaluation is to examine clients' physical, mental, or emotional health. It is important for the human service professional to consider the health, functioning, and limitations of each client in order to ascertain quality of life indicators. Some quality of life indicators that are ascertained from medical evaluations include: independent living, education, employment, recreation, participation in social activities, and wellness. Information is gathered for the medical evaluation including medical history and the current medical diagnosis with any functional limitations, symptoms, prior medical treatments, prescribed medications, contraindications of diseases or chronic disorders, and residual functional capacities of the client. The main idea of the medical evaluation is to ascertain how much information the client knew about his/her own medical condition, the impact that the medical condition has on the client's activities of daily living, education, and vocational pursuits. The results of the evaluation enable the human service professional to plan for the next steps in the evaluation process and to secure other resources the client may need if found eligible for services.

When the medical evaluation is complete, a diagnosis is often made and documented with each diagnosis having a specific code. There are three main coding systems that are commonly used in medical evaluations:

> The International Classification of Diseases (ICD-10-CM);[23]

> World Health Organization Diagnostic Assessment Schedule (WHODAS 2.0),[22] and

> the American Psychiatric Association's Diagnostic and Statistical Manual of Mental Disorders[1] (DSM-V).

ICD-10-CM, the medical diagnosis assessment adopted by the World Health Organization (WHO) provides codes of diseases/disorders, symptoms, abnormal findings, and an etiology and external factor of diseases and injury. WHODAS 2.0[22] is an assessment tool that integrates the levels of individuals' major life functions (e.g., Cognition, Mobility, Self-care, Getting along, Life activities, and Participation domains). DSM-V[1] is a universal diagnostic classification for mental health and psychiatric disorders and provides five dimensions (axes) of codes including definitions of mental and psychiatric disorders, symptoms, medical conditions, environment stressors, assessment of functions for the utilization of diagnosis, and treatment recommendations.

The purpose of the coding systems is so that medical providers can keep data on the types of medical conditions that exist and the medical provider can bill (i.e., receive payment) for services that are provided. The following dimensions of medical diagnoses and symptoms, treatments and other services, and functional capacities outline information gathered by the human service professional.

MEDICAL DIAGNOSIS AND SYMPTOMS

The purpose of gathering information from the medical evaluation is to help human service professionals understand the client's general health conditions. When looking at symptoms and the diagnosis of a health-related condition, there are several factors that the human service professional should be attentive to:

➢ the time of condition onset (i.e., when the medical condition occurred);

➢ symptoms;

➢ etiology (i.e., factors that cause the medical condition);

➢ the severity of condition;

➢ contraindications and complications;

➢ treatment; and

➢ life-long progress.

The following questions can be used to ascertain important information from a medical evaluation:

➢ What are your previous and current major health conditions (e.g., disability, chronic disorders, injuries, mental health disorders, substance abuse disorders, etc.)?

➢ When were you diagnosed?

➢ Who gave you the diagnosis?

➢ What are the symptoms of your health condition?

➢ What caused your health conditions?

➢ How severe is your disability(ies)/chronic disorder(s)?

➢ Who are your healthcare consultants (e.g., physician, psychiatric, dentist, nurse, therapists, dietician, etc.)?

➢ How quickly did your medical condition progress (e.g., acute incidence, chronic, temporary dysfunction, lifelong dysfunction, slow progressive, rapid progressive, controlled by medication and treatment, uncontrolled by medication and treatment, etc.)?

➢ Do you have any co-occurring health conditions (e.g., cardiopulmonary disease, HIV/AIDS, cancer, substance abuse disorders, mental health disorders, etc.)?

➢ Do you have a family history of medical conditions (e.g., hypertension, diabetes, Rheumatic arthritis, genetic disorders, mental health disorders, autism spectrum disorders)?

MEDICAL TREATMENTS AND OTHER HEALTHCARE SERVICES

➢ What medications are you currently taking?

➢ How is your medication prescribed?

➢ Do you take your medications as prescribed?

➢ What medications have you taken in the past?

➢ Are your medications working for you?

➢ Are you experiencing any side effects from your medications?

➢ Does anyone administer your medications?

➢ What are current and past treatments, therapies, and services received (e.g., hospitalization, detox treatment, counseling, psychotherapy, self-help sobriety group, physical therapy, occupational therapy, speech therapy, music therapy, dietary practices, exercise prescription, recreational activities, health care education, etc.)? And, how frequent of receiving the treatments and services?

FUNCTIONAL CAPACITY OF CLIENTS

➢ Are you experiencing any limitations in your functioning?

➢ In what areas of your daily living do you feel you function well?

Based on the above information, the human service professional can gather information about the diagnosis, medical health conditions, treatments, and functional limitations of the client. While most of what is covered in a medical evaluation is physical, we cannot overlook the emotional and psychological components of a holistic evaluation process.

PSYCHOLOGICAL EVALUATIONS

The purpose of the psychological evaluation is to understand the mental and emotional conditions of the client.[20] The human service professional can observe, listen, and talk with the client to determine the client's attention, communication, expression, and comprehension of the human service professional's questions, behaviors, and performances to establish a baseline to understand the client's cognitive, behavior, and affective (emotional) functioning. Psychological evaluation can help the human service professional learn more about the personal conditions and coping skills of the client.[20] The following are dimensions of the psychological evaluation.

COGNITIVE EXECUTIVE FUNCTIONS
The purpose of cognitive evaluation is to understand the client's intellectual level, learning ability, and information processing capabilities. The human

service professional can design several simple questions to identify the client's cognitive functions that are adopted from the mini mental status evaluation (MMSE).[3]

➢ Are the cognitive functions influenced by the disability(ies)/chronic disorder(s)?

JUDGEMENT. What should you do if the traffic light is red at the intersection?

ORIENTATION. Orientation to name, place, time and location

LONG-TERM MEMORY. Do you remember the last time you visited a doctor's office?

SHORT-TERM MEMORY. Did you have breakfast/ lunch today? What did you eat?

CALCULATION. 100-7-7-7-7-7=?, asking the client use 100 to subtract 7 for five times.[3]

COMMUNICATION. Please name a "pen" and a "watch."[3]

➢ What are your strengths and limitations in learning something new?

EMOTIONAL CONCERNS

The purpose of evaluating the emotional and mental health conditions of the client is to understand how the client's emotional wellbeing impacts his or her daily living activities. When the human service professional understands the emotional conditions of the client, the professional can adjust how he or she interacts with the client. For example, a human service professional may use a soft and empathetic tone if the client is expressing hurt or sadness. Analyzing the trend of the client's emotional status can help the client develop appropriate coping strategies to manage and stabilize his/her emotional status. The following questions are important:

➢ How have you been feeling in the past day/week (e.g., anxiety, depression, phobia, obsessive ideas, extreme mood change, hallucination, delusion, sleep disturbance, and other psychiatric symptoms)?

➢ What time of the day do you tend to feel at your best?

➢ Do you have thoughts of harming yourself or others? (*If yes, proceed to the next two questions*).

➢ Do you have an active plan to harm yourself or others? If so, what is your plan?

➢ Do you have the means to carry out harming yourself or others?

> *(Please note that asking about suicidal ideation does not mean that you will trigger the person to carry out the act. In many instances, people want to talk about their thoughts of harming themselves).*

➢ What are some ways that you cope with your stressors? *(Client's may have healthy ways of coping, such as deep breathing, meditating, engaging in self-care, or they may have unhealthy coping mechanisms such as self-harm, drinking, or using substances–to name a few).*

BEHAVIOR

The purpose of evaluating the client's behavioral patterns is to understand the factors that lead to the behavior and the subsequent consequences of his or her behaviors on self or others. Suppose a client informed the human service professional that he or she cuts him or herself. The human service professional would want to gather information about: What triggers the cutting behavior; what does the client think and feel during the cutting behavior; and, how does the client feel after the cutting behavior. By gathering information related to the cutting behavior, the human service professional can help the client develop coping mechanisms for his or her triggers to help reduce the likelihood that he or she will engage in the cutting behaviors. The human service professional can also help the client develop alternate behaviors instead of cutting (e.g., using a marker to draw on the skin instead of cutting). The following questions can be used to evaluate the behavioral patterns of the client:

➢ Do you have any behavior issues resulting from your disability(ies)/ chronic disorder(s) (e.g., impulsive, antisocial or obsessive behaviors, etc.)?

➢ Has there been a time that you harm yourself or other people? If so, when?

➢ Have you ever received behavioral health services? If so, when did you receive the services and what type of service did you receive?

Based on the above information, the human service professional can gather comprehensive information about the client's level of cognitive functioning, mental and emotional concerns, and behavioral conditions. In many aspects, the psychosocial evaluation might consider both medical and psychological elements, to name a few.

PSYCHOSOCIAL EVALUATIONS

The purpose of a psychosocial evaluation is to reveal information about the client's interaction and participation with the environment including family, school, work place, community, and society.

FAMILY

The purpose of a family evaluation is to understand the client's family conditions. The information includes the medical history of the family, the families' care competencies (e.g., knowledge of disability and chronic disorder, knowledge of resources, and care skills), the culture and characteristics of the family, the relationship between the client and the family, and the psychological adaptation of the family. Asking the client the following questions can gain information about the family in the psychosocial evaluation:

> How is the relationship with your family?

> Does your parent/guardian/family have any medical/mental health history? What type of diagnosis/ disability did the parent/guardian/family have?

> Does your family have the knowledge and caring skills for disability(ies)/chronic disorder(s) (e.g., including the diagnosis, symptoms, progress, contraindications, complications, medication, resources, treatments, etc.)?

> How does your family perceive you?

> How is your family's adapting to your disability (e.g., denial, shock, depression, anger, acceptance, and adjustment)?

> What are your family's coping strategies (e.g., attending any self-help group, stress relief program, etc.)?

INTERPERSONAL INTERACTIONS

The purpose of gathering interpersonal interaction information is to understand the relationship and social interaction between the client and other individuals. The context of interpersonal interaction includes the client's social interactions, engagement with his or her family, participation and involvement in the community, school, and workplace. The following questions provide information regarding the client's interpersonal interactions:

> Do you have any personal support system or primary care provider(s) (e.g., from the family, spouse, partner, peers, friends, classmates, teachers, colleagues, neighbors, volunteers, allied health professionals, etc.)?

> Do you have any limitations while interacting with other people?

> Did you attend a self-help group for your disability(ies) or chronic disorders (e.g., Alcoholics Anonymous)?

➢ What kinds of community activities are you involved in (e.g., church, volunteer, service group, recreational activities, leisure)?

➢ Do you attend any community activities? If so, how often do you go to each community activity?

➢ Do you have any difficulties while attending and being involed in community activities?

INDEPENDENT LIVING

Within the independent living domain, the human service professional gathers information about the client's activities of daily living and ascertaining whether the current living arrangement is safe (e.g., does the client have enough food to sustain them on a daily basis and adequate financial resources). Independent living involves *activities of daily living (ADL)*[9,10] that consists of mobility, bathing, dressing, toileting, personal hygiene and grooming, transferring to bed/wheechair, continence control, and eating.

Other independent living skills, called *instrumental activities of daily living (IADL),*[14] consist of cooking, driving, using the telephone or computer, shopping, keeping track of finances, and managing medication. The following are questions that can gather valuable information about the client's ability to live independently:

➢ Do you have enough money to pay for groceries, rent, car payment, insurance, living expenses?

➢ Do you consider your current living condition to be safe for you and/ or your kids?

➢ How do you support yourself financially (e.g., from family, friends, the community, agency, insurance company, and/or social welfare, etc.)?

➢ Do you have any problems with the activities of daily living (e.g., mobility, bathing, dressing, toileting, personal hygiene, transferring, eating, preparing meals, buying groceries, driving, using phone and computer, money management, medication management, etc.)?

➢ Who helps and provides assistance for your independent living (e.g., spouse, child, family, neighbor, friend, peer, volunteer from the community, personal assistant, etc.)?

➢ Do you need any accommodations for your activities of daily living (e.g., environmental accommodation, assistive device, etc.)?

EDUCATIONAL

The purpose of gathering educational information is to understand the
education level and expertise of the client. By gathering educational
information, the human service professional can gain a better understanding of
the client's acquired knowledge and skills. Having a better understanding of the
client's acquired knowledge and skills can help the human service professional
determine what resources the client may benefit from to aid in vocational
development including knowledge and skills mastery and relevant transferable
skills for employment. The following questions might be asked:

> ➤ Did you graduate from high school or college?

> ➤ If so, what school did you graduate from and what year?

> ➤ What was your major in school?

> ➤ Are you interested in pursuing higher education?

For the school-age client (i.e., children and adolescents), the human service
professional needs to consider the learning conditions at school. The following
questions might be asked:

> ➤ What grade are you in?

> ➤ Do you get along well with your teachers?

> ➤ Do you get along well with your peers?

> ➤ Do you have an individualized education plan (IEP)?

> (Note: *An IEP is an education plan that is developed for students
> with disabilities that details what the student's educational needs
> are, the team of professionals that will help the student meet his or
> her needs, what services will be provided to help meet the student's
> needs, and how progress on the needs is being monitored*).

> ➤ If so, what is included in your IEP?

VOCATIONAL

The purpose of evaluating the client's vocational conditions is to recognize
previous work experience, the client's interests, working attitude, and working
abilities. Human service professionals will explore the potential development of
vocational skills or the possibility of returning to work by the results of the
client's vocational information. The exploration also includes transferable skills
(i.e., skills that can be used in several aspects of personal and professional areas
of life, (e.g., teamwork, communication skills, writing skills, etc.) and physical
capacities for work. The following questions can provide valuable information
under the vocational category:

> ➢ What kind of jobs did you have previously?

> ➢ What are your strengths and weakness? (e.g. working attitude, working skills, knowledge, etc.)

> ➢ What kind of occupations are you currently interested in?

> ➢ What kind of experience and skills do you have that relates to the job you are currently interested in? What are your job expectations? (e.g., wages, benefits, work environment, workload, the relationship with colleagues, etc.)

> ➢ Do you have any job seeking skills? (e.g., search job posts, complete resume, job interviewing skills, etc.)

> ➢ Do you know of or need any job training resources?

ENVIRONMENT

Gathering environmental information from the client can help the human service professional understand the client's need for environmental accommodations. Environmental information can also help the human service professional gain a better understanding of clients' knowledge of relevant legislation, agencies, and community resources that can facilitate obtaining reasonable accommodations. The following questions can help the human service professional gather critical information about the client's environment:

> ➢ Do you use any assistive devices (e.g., cane, walker, manual wheelchair, electric wheelchair, augmentative and alternative communication (AAC), service dog)?

> ➢ Do you need environmental accommodations and services at home, school, or at your work (e.g., ramp, elevator, braille sign, rails, large space in bathroom and restroom, automatic door, academic tutor for people with disability, note taking, taping recording of academic classes)?

> ➢ Do you know where you can find information on resources that can help you obtain reasonable accommodations in employment (e.g., Job Accommodation Network (JAN) which is a website that provides the accommodations for various disability types; the local State-Federal Vocational Rehabilitation (VR) Agency which is an agency that provides supports and services for people with disabilities)?

> ➢ Do you need training to help you use your assistive devices (e.g., how to manipulate the electric wheelchair, AAC, etc.)?

LEGAL

Gathering information about the client's legal history enables the human service professional to obtain information regarding the client's criminal record, criminal history, any current legal responsibilities (e.g., having to pay child support, payment of fines), and any current legal obligations (e.g., court-mandated treatment, conditions of probation and parole). There are times when the legal status of the client creates barriers to obtaining supports, services, education, or employment (e.g., a client might not be able to obtain employment that is outside of walking distance due to not have a license resulting from a DUI (driving under the influence). Another example of potential barriers caused by the client's legal history may be that the client wishes to pursue higher education, but due to a drug-related felony (i.e., a serious crime related to drugs), he or she is disqualified from federal student financial aid. The following questions can be useful in obtaining information related to the client's legal history:

- Do you have any criminal records (e.g., DUI by alcoholism, illicit drug usage, probation or parole, history of incarceration, pending charges, any domestic court involvement, any involvement with the department of children and family services, etc.)?

- Are you currently on probation or parole? If so, who is your probation or parole officer?

- How long are you on probation or parole?

- What are the conditions of your probation or parole?

- Were you ever incarcerated? If so, for how long and at what level (i.e., local, state, federal)?

CULTURAL

The client's culture is a broad category that encompasses several dimensions, especially for clients from underrepresented groups (e.g., disability, gender, being a member of the LGBTQ population, people of color). First, the human service professional must take into consideration the society that the client lives in. The social cutlture includes roles, relationships, customs, heritage, languages, communication style, religion, beliefs, interaction patterns, attitudes, education, social norms, expected behaviors, etc.[7]

Second, the human service professional must pay attention to the personal characteristics of the client which includes gender, age, race and ethnicity, sexual orientation, socioeconomic status (SES), geographic living area (city, suburban, rural area), or the presence of a disability. The personal characteristics of the client (i.e., the client's phenotypes) may lead to disparities between the human service professional and the client. The disparities may result from distinct cultural viewpoints, lack of knowledge and awareness of other cultures, or prejudice, bias, and discrimination toward the client. Therefore, it is critical that the human service professional recognizes that there are several demographic variables to take into consideration while working with clients, especially clients of underrepresented groups (e.g., women, people of color, people with disabilities, the member of LGBTQ group).

It is imperative that the human service professional is:

➢ aware of cultural differences that exist;

➢ understand the impact of these cultural differences, and

➢ understand how the human service professional's culture can impact the evaluation process.

We will see later in this chapter that not connecting culture (e.g., gender) to the evaluation process can lead to misinterpretation and misdiagnosing a client. Based on the information mentioned, the human service professional can gather information to further understand how the client establishes a relationship with other people and the community and if the client received the sufficient social resources.

PSYCHOEDUCATIONAL EVALUATIONS

Psychoeducational testing is an evaluation to determine the academic and educational needs of school-aged clientele. To ensure that intellectual and academic needs are being met to assure school success, this evaluation is a critical component. School psychologists are the primary group of health and human service workers who administer psychoeducational evaluations. School psychologists are qualified human service professionals in providing children and adolescent mental and behavioral health services. These specialized instructional support professionals serve as members of school teams that support students' ability to learn and teachers' ability to teach. School psychologists apply expertise in mental health, learning techniques and interventions, and student behavior within a multi-tiered system of support. The multi-tiered system of support includes administrators, teachers, family members, and any other health and human service provider who is working with the client (e.g., therapists, social workers, case managers).

The purpose of the multi-tiered system of support is to help children and youth succeed academically, socially, behaviorally, and emotionally. Many public school systems adopt the multi-tiered system of support to meet the needs of students. The multi-tiered framework promotes school improvement through engaging research-based academic and behavioral practices. School psychologists' professional standards call for collaboration with families, school staff, community stakeholders to meet the everchanging needs of clients and families within the academic setting and community wide.

The *Weshler Intelligence Scale for Children-Fourth Edition* is a common formal assessment used to assess the general intellectual and cognitive abilities of children ages 6 years 0 months to 16 years 11 months. It is important to have knowledge regarding the cognitive ability of students since they are expected to perform like their same aged peers in academic domains such as reading, writing, math, science, and social studies.

The *Woodcock-Johnson Tests of Achievement* are used to measure levels of achievement in reading, mathematics, written language, and knowledge. The measures of achievement in reading, mathematics, written language and knowledge provide a general knowledge and skill set for the student as it relates to their ability to comprehend oral and written language, identify letter and sounds, understand basic math calculations and applied problems in math, and analyze sentence structure through writing samples, dictation, proofing, and writing fluency skills. Based on the information presented, the human service professional can use the intellectual and academic data with the school aged population to develop the student's IEP (discussed earlier in this chapter) to help meet the client's unique cognitive needs in the academic environment.

MULTICULTURAL CONSIDERATIONS DURING EVALUATION

Providing culturally sensitive service delivery for all clients is increasingly critical due to the changing demographics in the United States. Paul[13] stated that "By the year 2050, it is predicted that the percentage of culturally and linguistically diverse individuals will increase as the percentage of individuals of European descent declines. Additionally, the percentage of individuals of Asian descent will double and the percentage of individuals of Hispanic descent will increase by 6%. Likewise, the percentage of African American in the U.S. population will increase by 3%; the percentage of Native Americans will increase to just above 1%; the percentage of European Americans will decrease, forming slightly over half the population."[13, p.290] These statistics suggest that as human service professionals who provide evaluation services, the need to incorporate cultural sensitivity and cultural responsiveness as best practice standards is imperative to ensure that appropriate diagnoses, assessments, interventions, and service coordination are made.

When the human service professional reads the evaluation results or selects the assessment tools for a client, it is vital to take into consideration the diverse backgrounds of all their clients [e.g., gender, race and ethnicity, sexual orientation, socioeconomic status (SES), geographic background, and type of disability]. Within the evaluation process, it is necessary for the human service professional (the evaluator) to be well grounded in the multicultural competencies including awareness, knowledge, and skills.

If handled appropriately, both a firm understanding and application of the multicultural competencies will facilitate positive evaluation outcomes for all populations. For example, if the evaluator does not consider sample representation (e.g., gender) for selected evaluation tools, clients can be misdiagnosed and inappropriately placed, leading to possible hardships for the client and their families. In many human and allied health professions, misdiagnosing a client might be considered unethical. If the human service professional is aware of and understands the importance of clients' backgrounds (e.g., gender, race, sexual orientation, disability status), then competent multicultural skills can be applied to gather information that might facilitate the outcomes that both client and agency can be proud of. By understanding and applying the multicultural counseling competencies, the human service professional can build a trusting, empathetic, and validating atmosphere for the client to disclose his or her needs, current personal health conditions, cognitive and emotional status, environment conditions, and expectations of service during the evaluation.[19] Thus, it is important for the human service professional to be able to ask the right questions and have positive verbal and nonverbal behaviors to encourage the client and increase the likelihood that the evaluation tools will be used and interpreted appropriately.

The following examples demonstrate the need for human service professionals as evaluators, to be multiculturally competent during the evaluation process. Clients with diverse backgrounds (e.g., race, gender, sexual orientation, and disability) are impacted in a negative way during the information exchange and interpretation from many human and allied health professionals. The first outcome we will look at is individuals with mental illness.

DISABILITY. Happell et al.,[5] examined interactions between individuals with mental illness who sought pain management services and the professionals in the medical health care system. When the client with mental health concerns had physical symptoms of acute pain and chronic pain from injuries, the medical health care professionals overshadowed his/her real physical health conditions and interpreted the symptoms as mental illness during the evaluation process.[8] In this study, the allied health professionals believed that the client with mental illness was exaggerating the severity of his or her pain, or that the client was making up the pain. The client who had mental health concerns felt frustrated and helpless toward physicians and allied health care professionals by perceiving less professionlism, prejudice, and discriminatory attitudes from the professionals because of inaccurate assumptions about their mental illness. As illustrated many times in research studies, misdiagnosis can result when a human service provider does not have the skills to integrate culture into the evaluation process. This among other studies support that people with disabilities face discrimination with being misdiagnosed on a regular basis.

RACE/ETHNICITY AND GENDER. This example is about an Asian American female client, Ruby, who sought counseling services to deal with her depression and anxiety. Ruby's case manager's name is Cathy (European American). As background, Ruby's depression and anxiety resulted from the stress of her responsibilities in taking care of her family that included her parents-in-law, husband, and three children. The racial differences between Ruby (Asian American) and the case manager (European American), Cathy, may lead to both the client and the provider having different worldviews of female roles and responsibilities, depending upon where they reside geographically. Additionally, Cathy may suspect that Ruby internalizes all this responsibility and pressure on herself. Furthermore, it is conceivable that Cathy might believe that if Ruby thinks more about herself instead of her family and her children, she will release the stress and eliminate the symptoms of depression and anxiety. Cathy may say to Ruby, "you make yourself depressed and anxious because you think that you are a super mother. You cannot do everything. It is not all your responsibility to care for your family and your children. You should be concerned with yourself first." At the end of the day, Ruby will perceive that Cathy is not sensitive to her culture and the responsibility that comes with putting family above all else.

Women from Asian cultures have traditional concepts about morality and putting the family and children first instead of themselves. In contrast, many providers in North America may assert that Asian (American) women, for example, should be independent and have autonomy to pursue their dreams and achievements while providing little or no attention to their extended families. This racial/ethnic bias will surface if Cathy is not aware that the social culture and morality of many Asian countries should be considered when working with Asian immigrants or Asian American. Again, when human service professionals lack cultural competencies, including awareness, knowledge and skills, clients may not come back because of this mistreatment. When looking at evaluation outcomes, it is conceivable that having a disconnect with other cultures will lead to misinterpreting diagnostic information. Positive outcomes are likely when the human service professional understands the evaluation process and culture. Please refer to Chapter 2, *"Multicultural Considerations in Casement Management"* for additional knowledge to enhance your multicultural competencies during the case management process.

CASE STUDY
RITZ

Ritz is a 28-year-old Latina female who acquired a spinal cord injury two years ago. Ritz has been in the United States for 10 years. She came to the United States when she was 18 years old for her college education. She was an employee of an international company for 6 years after graduating from the college. Two years ago, Ritz was in a car accident. She was binge drinking earlier that evening. Because of the car accident, Ritz became a T8 level incomplete spinal cord injury patient, which meant that she was paralyzed from the waist down. Because of her injury, Ritz now requires the use of a wheelchair. After Ritz was discharged from the hospital, she took the accessible bus to the rehabilitation center for an independent skill training program and attended it regularly for one and half years.

Ritz began to re-learn how to care for herself, how to live independently, and how to get around in the community. However, Ritz made these efforts to train herself and expected that she could recover as normal as before the accident. However, Ritz started to have difficulty mentally adjusting to the permanence of her disability. The realization that she will need to adjust and adapt to her disability for the rest of her life began to make her feel frustrated and depressed. During her outpatient rehabilitation treatment, Ritz usually felt depressed about her physical recovery and unemployment status, so she returned to consuming alcohol at least four times per week for one year.

Recently, Ritz stopped the outpatient rehabilitation treatment for six months and stayed at home because she felt that her outpatient rehabilitation treatment was useless. Recently, Ritz found that the drinking led to several adverse effects instead of helping her mental health condition. Ritz noticed that the strength in her upper limbs was decreasing as well as an increase in the severity of her nerve pain, especially in the morning. Her emotional status sometimes appeared manic and sometimes depressed.

Ritz decided to seek assistance at a behavioral health agency because she would like to stop drinking. Tim is a 50-year-old European American male, who provides evaluations at the behavioral health agency. He interviewed Ritz and conducted a general biopsychological evaluation to ascertain more information in order to make an informed decision about Ritz's eligibility for services at the center.

CASE STUDY
DISCUSSION QUESTIONS

1. What are the purposes of medical, psychological, psychosocial, and psychoeducational evaluations for the client?

2. How should Tim conduct a comprehensive evaluation including medical, psychological, psychosocial, and psychoeducational information for Ritz?

3. What are the steps that a human service professional should follow during the initial evaluation process?

4. Why is it important to build and establish an effective interpersonal relationship as a human service professional?

5. What special considerations should the human service professionals or case managers pay attention to during the evaluation process?

CONCLUSION

The goal of evaluations for human service professionals is to gather information about the client and build a holistic profile to provide an appropriate and achievable service plan for the client. The holistic evaluation includes information about the client's medical, psychological, and psychosocial aspects by asking the client questions. Human service professionals need to construct the individual comprehensive evaluation by observation, listening, inquiring based on the needs, expectations, and goals of the client.

After the evaluation, the human service professional can decide if the client needs to receive detailed information about cognitive function levels, physical functional capacities, or vocational competencies and performances by referral to other professionals. If human service professionals need to know specific information, (i.e., cognitive function, emotional function, behavior analysis, vocational rehabilitation, or physical capacities of the client), the professional should recommend a referral to an external health and human service provider and explain the purposes of the referral to the client.

It is necessary for human service professionals to build a good working alliance with clients, other multidisciplinary professional consultants, and follow-up the dynamic changes in clients' medical, psychological, psychosocial, and psychoeducational conditions.

In summary, the human service professional should follow holistic evaluation results to assist clients in accessing appropriate treatments and to get better daily living, educational, vocational performances, social participation, and quality of life outcomes.

REFERENCES

[1]American Psychiatric Association. (2013). Diagnostic and statistical manual of
    mental disorders: DSM-5 (5th ed.). Arlington VA: American Psychiatric
    Publishing.

[2]Escorpizo, R., Brage, S., Homa, D., & Stucki, G. (2016). *Handbook of
    vocational rehabilitation and disability evaluation*. Switzerland: Springer
    International Publishing.

[3]Folstein, M., Folstein, S.E., McHugh, P.R. (1975). "Mini-Mental State" a
    Practical Method for Grading the Cognitive State of Patients for the
    Clinician. *Journal of Psychiatric Research, 12*(3); 189-198

[4]Fontes, A., Botelho, A., & Fernandes, A. (2014). A biopsychosocial evaluation
    method and the International Classification of Functioning, Disability, and
    Health (ICF). *Educational gerontology, 40*(9), 686-699.

[5]Happell, B., Ewart, S. B., Bocking, J., Platania-Phung, C., & Stanton, R.
    (2016). 'That red flag on your file': Misinterpreting physical symptoms as
    mental illness. *Journal of Clinical Nursing, 25*(19/20), 2933-2942.
    doi:10.1111/jocn.13355.

[6]Hilsenroth, M. J., & Cromer, T. D. (2007). Clinician interventions related to
    alliance during the initial interview and psychological assessment.
    Psychotherapy: Theory, Research, Practice, Training, 44(2), 205-218.
    doi:10.1037/0033-3204.44.2.205.

[7]Hutchins, A. M. (2013). Counseling gay men. In C. C. Lee (Ed.), *Multicultural
    issues in counseling: New approaches to diversity* (4th ed., pp. 171-193).
    Alexandria, VA: American Counseling Association.

[8]Katz, J., Rosenbloom, B. N., & Fashler, S. (2015). Chronic pain,
    psychopathology, and DSM-5 somatic symptom disorder. *The Canadian
    Journal of Psychiatry, 60*(4), 160-167.

[9]Katz, S., Ford, A.B., Moskowitz, R.W., Jackson, B.A., Jaffe, M.W. (1963)
    Studies of illness in the aged. The Index of ADL: a standardized measure of
    biological and psychosocial function. *JAMA, 185*, 914–919.

[10]Keith, R.A., Granger, C.V., Hamilton, B. B., & Sherwin, F. S. (1987). The
    functional independence measure: A new tool for rehabilitation. *Adv Clin
    Rehabil, 1*, 6-18.

[11]Lawton, M.P., & Brody, E.M. (1969). Assessment of older people: Self-
    maintaining and instrumental activities of daily living (IADL).
    Gerontologist, 9, 179-186.

[12]Lazarus, A. L., & Lazarus, C. N. (2005). Clinical purposes of the multimodal
    life history inventory. In G. P. Koocher, J. C. Norcross, S. S. Hill (Eds.),
    Psychologists' desk reference (2nd ed., pp. 232-235). New York, NY:
    Oxford University Press.

[13]Paul, R. (2014). *Introduction to Clinical Methods in Communication
    Disorders, 3rd Ed*. Baltimore, MD: Brookes Publishing Co.-added reference

[14]Peterson, D. B. (2015). Diagnostic assessment in clinical counseling. In M. A. Stebnicki (Ed.), *The professional counselor's desk reference* (2nd ed.). New York, NY: Springer Publishing Company. Retrieved from http://proxy.lib.siu.edu/login?url=http://search.credoreference.com/content/entry/sppcd/diagnostic_assessment_in_clinical_counseling/0?institutionId=3648

[15]Reynolds, C. R., & Suzuki, L. A. (2013). Bias in psychological assessment: An empirical review and recommendations. In J. R. Graham, J. A. Naglieri, I. B. Weiner, J. R. Graham, J. A. Naglieri, & I. B. Weiner (Eds.), *Handbook of psychology: Assessment psychology* (pp. 82-113). Hoboken, NJ: John Wiley & Sons Inc.

[16]Roessler, R., & Rubin, S. E. (2006). *Case management and rehabilitation counseling: procedures and techniques*. Austin, TX: PRO-ED.

[17]Saleeby, P. W. (2007). Applications of a capability approach to disability and the International Classification of Functioning, Disability and Health (ICF) in social work practice. *Journal of Social Work in Disability & Rehabilitation*, 6(1-2), 217-232.

[18]Smedema, S. M., Sharp, S., Thompson, K., & Friefeld, R. (2016). Evaluation of a biopsychosocial model of life satisfaction in individuals with spinal cord injuries. *Journal of Rehabilitation*, 82(4), 38-47.

[19]Sue, D. W., & Sue, D. (2016). *Counseling the culturally diverse: Theory and practice (7th edition)*. Hoboken, NJ: John Wiley & Sons.

[20]Weed, R. O., & Berens, D. E. (Eds.) (2009). *Life Care Planning and Case Management Handbook (3rd edition)*. Boca Raton, FL: CRC Press.

[21]World Health Organization. (2001). International classification of functioning, disability and health (ICF). Switzerland: Author Geneva.

[22]World Health Organization. (2012). Measuring health and disability: Manual for WHO Disability Assessment Schedule (WHODAS 2.0). Switzerland: Author Geneva.

[23]World Health Organization. (2014). International classification of diseases, tenth revision, clinical modification (ICD-10-CM). Switzerland: Author Geneva.

CHAPTER 5

POSSIBLE BARRIERS IN CASE MANAGEMENT

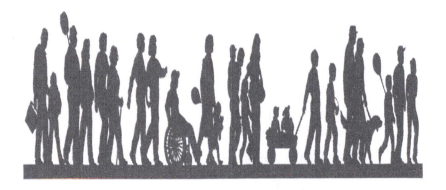

BRYAN O. GERE

AMBER KHAN

ABSTRACT

Human services agencies serve clients with diverse physical, mental, and social needs. An individual that receives services from a health or human service agency is referred to as a client or consumer. Case management practice is used in human service agencies to coordinate services such that clients have a single point of contact responsible for facilitating their multiple needs. However, many client populations in the United States (U.S.) who present themselves for services in human service agencies face significant barriers in accessing comprehensive and quality case management services. This is especially the case for clients from underrepresented populations (e.g., people with disabilities, women, racial & ethnic groups of color, and persons with different sexual orientations). This chapter is unique because the following areas will be discussed: (1) what factors might preclude some populations from equally accessing and benefiting from human services, and (2) what can be implemented to decrease the likelihood of factors that preclude some clients from participation in case management. Cases and discussions are provided in the chapter to increase understanding of the issues and to stimulate critical thoughts on practical measures that can be used by practitioners in addressing these barriers as they emerge in their everyday practice settings.

CHAPTER HIGHLIGHTS

➢ Human Services Case Management: A Response to Diverse Human Needs.

➢ Personal Factors of Service Providers and Clients that impede the Case Management Process.

➢ Environmental factors that impede the Case Management Process.

➢ Addressing Barriers in the Case Management Process.

LEARNING OBJECTIVES

➢ Understand the complexities of socio-political, cultural, and economic forces in access to human services within the United States.

➢ Understand the role that personal and environmental factors in precluding some populations from equally accessing and benefiting from human services in the United States.

➢ Identify measures that can be implemented to address barriers and facilitate better outcomes through the case management process.

98

HUMAN SERVICES CASE MANAGEMENT: A RESPONSE TO DIVERSE HUMAN NEEDS

Perhaps you are currently working in human services or are preparing for a career in the human services field. For those that are already working in human service organizations, you may already be familiar with some or most of the different client populations. Human service client populations include the elderly, homeless, immigrants, people from low socioeconomic background, people with addictions, people with criminal records, individuals with psychiatric and mental illness, and veterans with physical or mental disabilities as well as those returning to civilian life. Based on the client population, specific focal needs could be gainful employment, self-care, independent living, accommodation, treatments for medical and psychological problems, rehabilitation, reintegration into society, and so on.[13] Clients' needs are diverse and complex and require individualized, comprehensive, and focused interventions to achieve quality service outcomes. Case management enables practitioners in human service agencies to provide coordinated services that address clients' many health and social needs. In your role as a case manager in a human service agency, you will work collaboratively with the client and their family or support system (group of people that provide physical and emotional support), to identify their specific needs and develop a plan for intervention services.

The specific steps that are involved in facilitating the case management process depend on the client population and the circumstances of the client. However, even with the best efforts, some clients may not achieve the expected outcomes due to personal and environmental barriers in the case management process. The impact of personal and environmental barriers may be more visible among some client populations than others. Nevertheless, there is an expectation that service providers achieve quality outcomes with their clients. When service providers are aware of the barriers that clients face in attempting to achieve established goals and objectives, then it is likely that they will address these barriers to provide better case management outcomes. Using case management in human service agencies to successfully respond to the diverse needs of clients must begin with an understanding of the possible barriers that clients experience in the case management process.

Central to the barriers in case management is the issue of access to services in the U.S. for people with human and social service needs, particularly among the underrepresented populations.[9] Clients' needs or presenting problems are often a reflection of the client population, how they are located within the society, and their relationship with socioeconomic and political institutions. For instance, homelessness reflects the interaction between personal circumstances, problems with the structure of the society and the failure of the institutions within the society. Individuals that are homeless are typically poor, or have low incomes. In some cases, structural racism impacts the ability of some client populations to access good jobs that allow them to meet their basic needs such as housing. For instance, structural racism has seriously disadvantaged many formerly incarcerated individuals from becoming gainfully employed even after obtaining the necessary vocational training post-incarceration. Previously incarcerated persons are more likely to experience discrimination from employers or other ongoing challenges with law enforcement. Historical factors have also shaped and continue to shape the needs of most client populations that receive services in the U.S.[18] As an example, many low-income families in the U.S. have been pushed into homelessness due to gentrification or the practice whereby homes or neighborhoods are renovated or upgraded to middle class tastes leading to increase in rents and property values that are beyond the means of low income families.

Although, the specific barriers that clients face in human services settings may differ depending on the client population, there are some commonalities in these barriers. Specifically, barriers are evident in two main domains: personal and environmental. For example, personal factors that serve as a barrier in case management in human service agencies include race or ethnicity, gender, socioeconomic status, disability impact, level of education, prior work experience, and the absence of family and other support systems.[7,8,9] Included in environmental factors are agency factors, human service system, cultural factors, systemic barriers, racism, and legal issues.[15,17] In many client populations, a combination of personal and environmental barriers are often present. For clients from underrepresented populations, addressing these obstacles is critical in ensuring client's maximum participation and improving service outcomes.

PERSONAL FACTORS OF SERVICE PROVIDERS AND CLIENTS THAT IMPEDE THE CASE MANAGEMENT PROCESS

While there are countless factors that might impede the case management process, this chapter will cover only a few. The personal attributes of the client and the service provider can impact communication and interactions that take place in the case management process. The ability of clients to connect with the service provider and to articulate their needs is as important as the ability of the service provider to interact with and gain understanding of the client's needs. Personal attributes can contribute to or detract from the ability of clients and service providers to work collaboratively towards the achievement of case management goals.

RACE AND ETHNICITY

The case management process can be impeded due to differences in the race and ethnicity of service provider and the client. Cross-cultural issues in the case management relationship could create problems in the working relationship between the service provider and the client as well as their family or support system. Differences in life experiences, values, and worldviews could create problems with their interactions and expectations from the case management process. From the clients' perspective, there could be a lack of understanding of the role of the service provider or distrust in the abilities and competence of the service provider. Similarly, service provider's implicit or explicit bias towards clients from different racial or ethnic backgrounds could affect their interactions and communication with the client or their family members.[18] Rosenthal[15] investigated the extent to which European American vocational counselors' demonstrated bias in their general evaluation, perceptions of psychopathology, and estimates of educational and vocational potential of African American clients. The author found that African American clients were judged more negatively than European American clients. Whereas implicit bias occurs at the unconscious level, explicit bias occurs on a conscious level. For instance, counselor's unconscious fears related to national security can cause them to perceive their Muslim clients of Middle Eastern origin as a national security threat. It is therefore important for case managers to seek out information about clients especially under conditions of uncertainty so that they can avoid the dangers of operating with assumptions that can activate bias.

More importantly, there are also cultural differences between client and agency culture (e.g., the case management milieu). For instance, in many human service organizations, there is emphasis on formal communication and interaction patterns. Clients are expected to meet with the service providers at specific times and services are delivered according to laid down procedures. When case managers get too accustomed to this culture, they can work with the assumptions that clients are used to it as well. Sadly, clients from diverse racial and ethnic groups can feel more disconnected from the case management interventions or the process itself, when they are not properly educated about the case management process and the goals/outcomes.

GENDER

Gender is another personal factor that impacts the interactions and communications between clients and service providers. Gender influences how both the service provider and the client form impressions and stereotypes about each other. Strong and confident women may be misperceived as stubborn or uncooperative, whereas soft-spoken men may be considered weak and lacking ambition. Some human service workers may convey narrow ideas about gender roles, and consider clients who do not conform to traditional roles as being pathological. For instance, men may be stay at home fathers, and women could be the primary providers for their families. Relative to gender roles, our focus as service providers is also to understand how traditional gender roles within our clients' families' impact the ability of clients to show up for services based on an agreed schedule. Compared to men, women tend to have more family responsibilities that can impact their schedules and the extent of their active participation in case management services.[10]

Inability to understand gender-related behaviors such as the desire to voluntarily seek services or clearly articulate needs could lead providers to draw faulty conclusions about the client. For instance, men often have a responsibility to provide most of the financial support for their families. If they are unable to do so due to life circumstances such as chronic illnesses, disability, a history of incarceration, unemployment, or homelessness, they may feel a sense of shame to seek help. When men present for human services, they are often reluctant to self-disclose their true conditions or express their needs to the service provider. Compared to women, men are more likely to have the need to appear invulnerable or self-sufficient.[10] Among the homeless, men are often reluctant to disclose their true conditions and to ask for help due to a sense of shame.[2] It is therefore important to develop a good rapport and to assist men to move beyond difficulties with openly disclosing their needs.

Gender-based discrimination is also common in service delivery leading to poorer outcomes for some client populations. In their study, Gere and Flowers[8] found that compared to males, female clients in the VR program, with psychiatric disabilities, had a lower weekly earning at the time of closure, this difference is a result of the quality of placements between males and females. Compared to their male counterparts, female clients may need more environmental and transitional support to achieve quality employment outcomes. It is therefore important for case managers to understand the unique challenges that female clients face and to provide ongoing support to improve the service outcomes.

SOCIOECONOMIC STATUS

Socioeconomic status (SES) refers to the economic and social position of a person compared to others within their society. Many of the clients serviced in human service organizations are from low SES backgrounds. Fujiura[6] observed, "If you have a disability and you are from a minority group, odds are that you and your family live in poverty, and that you will be poorer than others of your own race and class." [p.71] Minority groups are likely to live in poverty due to lack of access to opportunities, and discrimination. As a result, persons with disabilities make up a significant portion of persons that participate in public safety net programs such as Supplementary Nutritional Assistance Program (SNAP), Temporary Assistance for Needy Families (TANF), and Supplementary Security Income (SSI). SES factors do not only account for the significant gap in health and social conditions, but could also be responsible for the disparities in case management outcomes. Clients that are from low SES backgrounds lack basic resources in their immediate environment to facilitate the case management process. Within their environments, persons from low SES backgrounds may not have access to basic infrastructures such as telephones, computers, internet connections, and transportation systems that can assist them to be in regular contact with the service provider or other agencies connected with providing needed assistance. Individuals from low SES are thus disadvantaged in their ability to engage in and complete required processes and tasks that facilitate the case management process.

Appio, Chambers, and Mao[2] found that therapists held negative biases against low income clients and tend to perceive low income clients more negatively than they do upper-SES clients. Within the service environment, the difference in the SES between the service provider and the client could also create problems with interactions and communication. The way the service provider asks or responds to client's questions, amount of time spent on client's questions and concerns, the degree of assertiveness or expressiveness in the dialogues, information giving, and the amount of support provided during the case management meetings reflect the differences in SES backgrounds between service providers and the clients. Some clients, from lower SES backgrounds, may feel uncomfortable when we ask them personal questions, such as questions that tend to make them feel inferior. For instance, asking a client who is a U.S. citizen, their ancestry or where they were born. It is therefore not surprising that occasionally some clients may be guarded when it comes to disclosing personal information or discussing issues that are of an intimate nature.

DISABILITY IMPACT

The presence of disability can impact the interactions and communications between the service provider and the client receiving case management services. Disability impact refers to how the disability affects the daily functioning of the disabled person. The ability of clients to clearly articulate their needs towards the development of a case plan, become fully involved, and cooperate with the case manager to facilitate the case management depend on the impact of the disability. Achieving successful service outcomes has remained elusive for many clients who receive services in human services agencies due to the presence of a disability. In many cases, the impact of the disability necessitates greater flexibility in working collaboratively with the client to develop the case plan and to operationalize the plan. Depending on the extent of the disability, some clients may require significant and ongoing support in the areas of transportation, symptom management, and disability related care.[4,7,12] Others may find difficulty in meeting or managing the interpersonal and communication aspects required to complete most of the processes activities that are involved in case management.

LEVEL OF EDUCATION

Client's low level of education can serve as a barrier in the case management process. For instance, persons with disabilities (especially those with learning or multiple disabilities), and individuals from low SES backgrounds are more likely to be educated in restrictive environments in their early years of schooling.[7] Persons educated in restrictive environments may receive inadequate services compared to their counterparts. Having a low level of education may expose individuals to low-quality curriculum and instruction, complete fewer assignments, have poor social experiences, are likely to have significant deficits in language development, reading performance, and social interactions.[7,9] When people have a low level of education they may, for example lack simple literacy (reading and writing) skills needed to process information about the activities, services/processes that are involved in facilitating their needs through the case management process. The case management paperwork in most human services agencies are written using clinical or professional terminology. Although case managers often do their best to explain information in lay terms for the client, many clients still struggle with having a firm grasp of the depth of the information due to their limited education. In addition, clients may also lack the vocabulary to clearly articulate their concerns to other professionals to whom they are referred to as part of the case management process. When there is a lack of understanding of the processes or interventions, clients may become dissatisfied with the interventions provided by the service providers and exit the agency unceremoniously.

PRIOR WORK EXPERIENCE

Employment is a critical need of many clients in human services and some case management environments are targeted at providing some type of employment outcome. Several client populations, such as homeless, immigrants, people with addictions, criminal records, psychiatric and mental illness, unemployed persons, veterans, and others, often require some type of employment related services. The Bureau of labor statistics[3] reported that among unemployed persons 87.7 percent had no prior work experience. For young people with disabilities, prior work experience helps them to build useful skills and exposes them to contacts other than their immediate family, friends, and teachers or instructors. In a study examining post-secondary employment outcomes for young adults with severe disabilities, Carter, Austin, and Trainor[4] found that both paid school-sponsored work and paid community employment were associated with post high school employment. Employers often look favorably on individuals with prior work experience because they are likely to have soft skills in addition to job specific knowledge, skills, and aptitudes.[12] For instance, the ability to interact successfully with other employees or supervisors in the workplace as well as with customers served by an organization is valued by many employers. Individuals with prior work experience are more likely to have better interpersonal and communication skills and can work with others as a team or in a group setting. Within teams, such employees can maximize their areas of strengths while compensating for their weaknesses. In a recent study, Wehman, et al.[19] found that young people with Autism Spectrum Disorder who participated in internships, were not only able to gain and retain competitive employment but also successfully communicate with co-workers and demonstrating appropriate social and work skills.

FAMILY AND SUPPORT SYSTEM

Case management service outcomes can be greatly enhanced by the presence of an adequate social support for the client. Social support refers to psychological, moral, and physical support provided for an individual by members of their immediate family or friends. Individuals that emerge from smaller households, have a small support system, which can become a barrier in achieving case management goals. The attitude of the immediate family toward the client, their needs, and their willingness to support the client with the necessary material and moral support may also be a significant factor in the case management process. For instance, family attitudes towards participation in treatment programs for substance abuse can constitute a barrier towards the facilitation of case management services. In their study, Kail and Elbereth,[10] reported that Latino family members considered having a daughter in a drug rehabilitation program as an embarrassment to the family. This is because there is an expectation that Latinas with substance abuse problems rely on a supportive network of female family members and friends rather than on strangers. Further, when family members reinforce dependency attitudes in some clients, such clients may not follow through with the completion of tasks directed by the case manager towards addressing their needs. More importantly, the absence of a viable family or support system significantly hinders case management as clients lack the wherewithal or encouragement to work on assigned tasks to achieve established case management goals.

ENVIRONMENTAL FACTORS THAT IMPEDE THE CASE MANAGEMENT PROCESS

MICRO-CONTEXTUAL FACTORS

Micro-context or organizational level factors include norms and expectations within the organization that shape social interactions at the organization level. For instance, agency practices, and policies and procedures affect decisions that are made in the case management system. For example, policies that specify that only the most vulnerable or severe individuals should be provided services automatically preclude others whose conditions do not fit into such descriptions from receiving services or only receiving partial service.

Further, agency policies that prescribe specific behaviors as conditions for receiving case management service may sometimes inadvertently impede the case management process. For instance, agencies that cater to the needs of persons with substance abuse often have policies that place emphasis on client behaviors such as regularly showing up for an appointment, discontinued substance use, and a willingness to commit to change as conditions for continuing to receive case management services. These policies may serve as barriers to some clients who are unfamiliar with the process and are genuinely struggling to adhere to policies due to personal factors that are outside their control, such as problems with transportation and the lack of a support system. Relative to service provision, an important barrier in the case management process is lack of multicultural competence or the ability to serve individuals from diverse backgrounds. Even as the diversity within the client populations that are served in human service agencies continue to change rapidly, the approach to case management has remained largely the same. Service providers may not have gained cultural competence or training to work with diverse populations. This can impede their interaction and treatment of clients that are different from them regarding their gender, race, ethnicity, and sexual orientation. Even with prescribed ethical conducts, service provider's attitudes, behaviors, and conducts continue to reflect discrimination and thus create barriers for underrepresented groups.

MACRO-CONTEXTUAL FACTORS

Macro-contextual factors refer to factors within the larger environment that affect the case management process such as sociopolitical, legal, and cultural factors. Although these factors exist outside the organization, they have a strong influence on the organization and its activities. In recent years, there have been significant budget cuts and reductions for many government agencies and programs. Recently, President Donald Trump proposed a budget reduction of nearly 18 percent for the Department of Health and Human Services.[11] This reduction will significantly impact the funding for many human service programs. More importantly, the reduction will lead to the decrease or elimination of some essential programs that constitute a major part of client service needs. For instance, the proposed budget cuts will defund or eliminate programs that target poverty such as the Low-Income Home Energy Assistance Program and the Community Services Block Grant.[11] Another sociopolitical factor is opportunity structure within the environment. Opportunity structures emphasize how available opportunities within a given society, are determined by institutions within the society. Thus, opportunity structures can enhance or limit access to resources for many client populations served in human services agencies. Many underrepresented populations contend with a restricted opportunity structure due to legal obstacles. For example, reentering ex-offenders face significant barriers in obtaining social support, public assistance, as well as in finding stable employment.[16] Employers typically require criminal background checks on those they are hiring which restrict the ability of ex-offenders to get employed.

Cultural factors such as discriminatory attitudes within the wider society towards many client populations served in human service agencies constitute a barrier to having positive case management outcomes. Negative perceptions of many client populations impact their access to vital services that are part of their treatment or service plan. For instance, systematic stereotypes and perceptions often impact selection decisions leading to unemployment of persons with disabilities. When using systematic stereotypes with persons with disabilities, employers may assume that the absence of certain physical characteristics may impact their ability to successfully perform their jobs. The same is also the case, when some employers make assumptions about clients' past behavior. For instance, employers often assume that ex-offenders are likely to reoffend if they are employed in their organizations, and that this may affect the reputation of their organization. Shapiro[17] noted that employers' prejudices such as beliefs about the inability of a disabled person to do the work might result in unemployment. However, biases and prejudices may not be solely connected to the abilities of persons with disabilities, employers may also have other concerns such as costs of accommodation, and fear of legal liability due to accidents or incidents involving such employees with disabilities.

ADDRESSING BARRIERS IN THE CASE MANAGEMENT PROCESS

Addressing the barriers in the case management process requires an understanding of the personal and environmental factors that impede the process. Relative to personal factors, it is important for service provides to develop a good working relationship. This can help to facilitate the collection of information that assists in gaining intimate knowledge of the client's background and their needs. Some clients may have limited or low education levels. Other clients may come from households with members with low educational achievements. For clients with the aforementioned backgrounds, it may be necessary to provide supplementary education that can improve their capacity to benefit from vocational rehabilitation services. Supplementary education includes opportunities for learning and development that takes place outside of the regular school environment, time, or schedule. Supplementary education can be provided in areas of intellectual and personal development for many client populations. For instance, exposure to work environments and work behaviors, orientation to the use of libraries and other community resources can address significant gaps in knowledge about how to address their needs. As well, supplementary education provides grounds for the development of social networks to receive additional education in a particular subject matter or skill.

Understanding the lived experiences of consumers can help set the stage for the development of a strong working alliance. Additionally, consumers' worldview and assumptions regarding case management outcomes should be explored in-depth as these are inextricably linked to the level of motivation and commitment to achieve desired goals and objectives. As previously mentioned, there is a need for service providers as part of the case management process to be knowledgeable about the SES of not only the client but also the immediate and extended family (other relatives e.g. grandparents, uncles and aunts). Such knowledge assists the human service worker particularly the case manager to work with other professionals, and community or government agencies to obtain support services or vital resources in the areas of transportation, supplementary income, symptom management, disability related care, and other areas of need through advocacy. However, the greatest support system for consumers in the case management process is their immediate family and friends.[9] It is also important for service providers to facilitate independence in the clients by providing opportunities to learn the necessary day-to-day skills.[13, 14] This can empower the clients, post-completion of the program, to access these resources on their own and live independently in the community. Given the increasing diversity of the clients that are serviced, there is also a need for case management to be delivered in a culturally competent manner.

The environmental barriers in the case management process can also be addressed at the onset or throughout the case management process to achieve better outcomes for the clients. It is also imperative that clients are oriented to available resources and supports in the community. Case managers should also advocate on behalf of the client with employers, community resources, and various government departments. To ensure availability and accessible service providers should form partnerships with community organizations, as well as integrate their services into their programs. Working with employers and community stakeholders, service providers can address social and health disparities that impact incentive for employment. Barriers from Micro-contextual factors can be addressed via the intentional use of multicultural techniques and practices such as showing acceptance and respect for differences, adapting services to client needs, and so on.

CASE STUDY
ROBERT

Robert is a 37-year-old African American male who was recently diagnosed with Depression. Until very recently, Robert was employed in the retail industry, maintaining a mortgage and salary. All of this changed when he unexpectedly lost his wife to breast cancer six months ago, which resulted in intense grief, severe anxiety, restlessness, and depression. Feeling overwhelmed with negative emotions, Robert turned to heavy drinking, and ended up losing his job, and his car. At the brink of losing his home, due to unemployment, Robert arrives at a community agency, which specifically helps those recovering from substance abuse to obtain employment. Jenna is the case manager who is assigned to work on Robert's case. Jenna is a 24-year-old White female and a recent graduate of a counseling program. Although she has worked with substance abuse clients before, Jenna is not too familiar with grief counseling and especially for clients, like Robert, who are lacking transportation to get to counseling and to a place of employment.

CASE STUDY
DISCUSSION QUESTIONS

1. What are some of the barriers in the case of Robert?

2. What are some of the key areas that the case manager will have to map out for Robert to get the resources and help that he needs?

3. What are some ways that Jenna can remove, if at all, or alleviate some of the barriers that are present in this case?

4. What is a good approach to understanding the factors that impact Robert?

CONCLUSION

The client populations that are served in human service agencies have diverse needs. Case management services assist human service agencies in facilitating clients' needs in a focused and coordinated manner. However, many clients face significant barriers as they navigate the service system. Personal and environmental factors can impede the case management process and negatively influence outcomes. The impact of these factors is amplified when considered along *race* and social *groupings*. For underrepresented groups, systemic racism, and structural inequality compound the counter productive outcomes these and other groups face. Systemic racism is racism that is deeply rooted in the structures and social relations within a society as well as institutions within a society and manifested through discriminatory policies and practices that result in inequalities. Similarly, structural inequality deals with a condition where one group of people within a society is conferred a higher/preferential status over others such that they have more rights and opportunities compared to others. Within the U.S. society, the influence of systemic and structural racism may affect individuals from some social or racial groups more than others. Therefore, it is critical for case managers to work collaboratively with consumers to identify specific barriers for each consumer, and can assist the case manager to advocate/network for resources to address these barriers. As more human service agencies face problems with resource constraints because of budget cuts and increased service demands, it is imperative that case managers develop creative ways to maximize existing resources and to ensure that all client groups have access to resources or services that they need. More importantly, there is need for heightened interprofessional collaboration–different professionals working together as a team to achieve set objectives, –as well as cooperation between the multiple agencies that provide services to address human and social service needs.

REFERENCES

[1]Amato, F., & MacDonald, J. (2011). Examining risk factors for homeless men: Gender role conflict, help-seeking behaviors, substance abuse and violence. *The Journal of Men's Studies, 19*(3), 227-235.

[2]Appio, L., Chambers, D. A., & Mao, S. (2013). Listening to the voices of the poor and disrupting the silence about class issues in psychotherapy. Journal of clinical psychology, *69*(2), 152-161.

[3]Bureau of Labor Statistics. (2015). Persons with a disability: Labor force characteristics -2014. summary. Retrieved from https://www.bls.gov/news.release/

[4]Carter, E. W., Austin, D., & Trainor, A. A. (2012). Predictors of postschool employment outcomes for young adults with severe disabilities. *Journal of Disability Policy Studies, 23*(1), 50-63.

[5]Escorpizo, R., Brage, S., Homa, D., & Stucki, G. (Eds.) (2015). Challenges and Opportunities. *Handbook of Vocational Rehabilitation and Disability Evaluation* (pp. 545-557). Springer International Publishing.

[6]Fujiura, G. T. (2000). The implications of emerging demographics: A commentary on the meaning of race and income inequity to disability policy. *Journal of Disability Policy Studies, 11*(2), 66-75.

[7]Fouad, N. A., & Byars-Winston, A. M. (2005). Cultural context of career choice: meta-analysis of race/ethnicity differences. *The Career Development Quarterly, 53*(3), 223-233.

[8]Gere, B. O., & Flowers, C. R. (2016). Vocational services and outcomes of psychiatric clients in state-federal VR Program. *The IAFOR Journal of Psychology and the Behavioral Sciences 2*(2), 30-46. doi.org/10.22492/ijpbs.2.2.03

[9]Hasnain, R., Sotnik, P., & Ghiloni, C. (2003). Person-centered planning: A gateway to improving vocational rehabilitation services for culturally diverse individuals with disabilities. *Journal of Rehabilitation, 69*(3), 10-17.

[10]Kail B. L., & Elbereth, M. (2002). Moving the Latina substance abuser towards treatment: The role of gender and culture. *Journal of Ethnicity in Substance Abuse,1*(3),3-16.

[11]Los Angeles Times. (2017). Trump budget envisions big cuts for health and human services. Retrieved September 29, 2017 from http://www.latimes.com/politics/washington/la-na-essential-washington-updates-trump-budget-envisions-big-cuts-for-1489664310-htmlstory.html

[12]Madaus, J. W., Gerber, P. J., & Price, L. A. (2008). Adults with learning disabilities in the workforce: Lessons for secondary transition programs. *Learning Disabilities Research & Practice, 23*(3), 148-153.

[13]Martin Jr., E. D. (2007). *Principles and practices of case management in rehabilitation counseling.* New York, NY: Thomas.

[14]Roessler, R. T., & Rubin, S. E. (2006). *Case management and rehabilitation counseling: Procedures and techniques.* Austin, TX: PRO.

[15]Rosenthal, D. A. (2004). Effects of client race on clinical judgment of practicing European American vocational rehabilitation counselors. Rehabilitation Counseling Bulletin, 47(3), 131-141.

[16]Schmitt, J. & Warner, K (2011). Ex-offenders and the labor market. *Journal of Labor and Society. 14*(1),87-109.

[17]Shapiro, J. P. (1994). No pity: People with disabilities forging a new civil rights movement. Three Rivers Press.

[18]Sue, D. W., & Sue, D. (2016). *Counseling the culturally diverse. Theory and Practice. (7th ed.).* Hoboken, NJ: Wiley & Sons Inc.

[19]Wehman, P. H., Schall, C. M., McDonough, J., Kregel, J., Brooke, V., Molinelli, A., Ham, W., Graham, C. W., Riehle, J. E., Collins, H. T., & Thiss, W. (2014). Competitive employment for youth with autism spectrum disorders: Early results from a randomized clinical trial. *Journal of autism and developmental disorders, 44*(3), 487-500.

CHAPTER 6

FAMILY CONSIDERATIONS IN CASE MANAGEMENT

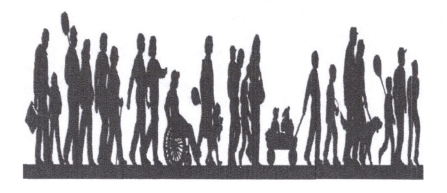

KEITH B. WILSON

CARRIE L. ACKLIN

ABSTRACT

FAMILY. Depending on how we define family, we all have one! Yes, we all have a family; no qualifiers! The importance of family influence on how we act, behave, and what we value, or not, is all documented throughout the ages. As we will highlight in this chapter, the structure and function of families have changed depending on the circumstances and political nature of religion, history, and time. Thus, families can be complicated because of the different layers, values, customs, and traditions throughout the different time periods in a given historical context. While many family values and structures, that are represented in the United States (U.S.), might be as unique as a fingerprint, it is essential to acknowledge that all families in the U.S. are not alike. Likewise, families outside of the U.S. borders represent other family structures (e.g., values, customs) that many human service providers are sure to encounter given the contemporary changes in the U.S. demographics over the last decade or so. The demographic transformation is scheduled to continue as providers of human and allied health services will continue to be faced with populations of clients that have minimal resemblance to the dynamic "norms" of what family structure is in the U.S.

CHAPTER HIGHLIGHTS

➢ Overview of family and the complexity of family structures;

➢ Defining family based on geography;

➢ Understanding how to work with families when contextualizing the broad sense of the word "diversity."

LEARNING OBJECTIVES

➢ To understand and define what a family is.

➢ To recognize that the diversity within the family can present an opportunity to resolve possible conflicts within the family.

➢ To apply a variety of techniques and approaches to facilitate services for all families.

INTRODUCTION

Like a sweet, firm piece of fruit with several layers, there are several layers of peeling that will reveal the fruits of our labor (pun not intended). Even before we take a bite of the fruit, the smell heightens our senses. As we bring the piece of fruit closer to our mouths, the saliva production begins to increase as we anticipate the first bite of the fruit. So, it is with families and the case management process. Many encounters with families at an initial intake bring excitement and a new beginning to facilitate services for our new client(s) and their families. Although this fruit and family analogy might be awkward for some to grasp, there are similarities that bare presenting:

Both a piece of fruit and families are layered. As with a piece of fruit, once you bite or peel back the layers, you really do not know what you are going to get until the big reveal (i.e., bite into or peel back the fruit to see or taste if the fruit is what you expected it to be). As with families, we understand that families present one way on the outside and can be something entirely different once you start to peel back the superficial layers of pleasantries during the first encounter. For example, there might be physical abuse happening in a family, yet the family conceals the abuse when they arrive for services. What a family presents initially might be considered one layer. The first layer is peeling back the fruit.

It is not until the case manager starts to ask questions like: Why is Jim talking for Susan when the questions are directed at Susan? It is common knowledge that one trait of a dysfunctional family might be to silence other family members. Muting or talking for other family members to take away their voice and exert power and control is a potential layer of that family. Peeling away the layers of the family will lead the case manager to understand behaviors of a family that might be counterproductive to some of its members. As would be expected, some families might need more peeling than others. Oh yes, family members can be very protective of the family unit by symbolizing to the case manager, "I want you to stop peeling" by avoiding questions, changing the subject, becoming defensive, or changing the body language from open to defensive (e.g., crossing arms and legs, turning away, giving "intimidating looks" to other family members), to name a few.

What you expect might not be what you receive. We assume, most of us have had this experience with fruit or other tangible related produce. As with this piece of fruit analogy, before one starts to peel away the layers of the fruit, there is usually an expectation of what the fruit might taste like based on how the fruit looks or smells on the outside. Once the peeling is over, a bite into the fruit might reveal an unexpected foul taste. "OK, that was unexpected given how nice the fruit smelled or looked on the outside. A family may give the impression that everything is not only great for the family, but there are no conflicts or family disagreements, EVER. Yes, the EVER is your first clue that by its nature of living together with different personalities, having conflict within the family is not unavoidable and unrealistic to expect. Thus, after questioning one family member about the continued visits to the emergency room, he/she revealed that the physical and emotional abuse has been consistent for the past 15 years. What you see or what you are presented with may not be what is truly occurring within a family. Case managers must use all their senses to detect ways they can peel back the layers of the client and the families of their clients. In our opinion, this is the art of working with families in a case management context.

Because of the brief analogy between a family unit and fruit, it is crucial to note not only how diverse families are in the U.S., but across the globe. In this chapter, we highlight a brief history of the family structure in the U.S., the diversity of family structures both in the U.S. and other places in the world, and the reason why understanding the expectations of families and family values can facilitate the work of both the client, family of the client, and the agency delivering case management services. While families in the U.S. and other parts of the world can be as complex and diverse as a fingerprint, there are key areas of focus that can facilitate positive outcomes for all families seeking case management services in the human and allied health services.

UNITED STATES DEMOGRAPHICS

As many readers of this chapter are aware, the demographics of the U.S. are shifting to include more populations that have family structures that might be preconceived as different from what is considered "typical" in the U.S. We are using the word "typical" VERY loosely in the context of the U.S. population which now calls home for many from the Asia, Africa, and South America continents.

When looking at the United States Census Bureau[1] information, we know that about half of the U.S. population is female. Additionally, the population in the U.S. is expected to grow to approximately 450 million by 2050 due to the migration patterns of people coming to the U.S. As the U.S. demography shifts; there will be more women represented in the workforce. Not only is it essential to look at how gender is changing the landscape of the U.S. population, but people who are part of other underrepresented groups are increasing as well. For example, in 2010, 16% of the population identified as either Latino or Hispanic in the U.S. By 2060, it is projected that one-fifth of the individuals in the U.S. will be 65 years or older. Additionally, one third of the population that is expected to increase will be Asian, Hispanic or Latino; African Americans will increase by 15%; individuals who are classified as Alaskan Native or Native Americans are likely to increase, along with Pacific Islanders and Native

Hawaiians. If these projections are correct, more than half of the population in the U.S. will be members from underrepresented groups.[1] While there are many skills case managers need to provide quality services for all clients, the changing demographics will increase the necessity for acquiring skills that will facilitate services for all clients seeking services for themselves and their families.

FAMILIES IN THE CONTEXT OF CASE MANAGEMENT

Family. Depending on how we define family, we all have one! There is no qualifier for having a family or not. We all do have a family. We all have a unit that we were born to or raised by that is considered our family unit. In the context of this chapter, a family can have a biological link or not. One thing is for sure, who we are or what we call family can influence the way we think, act, and behave. As Michael Teachings [2] reported, "One of the strongest influences in the lives of many is our family." Our birth order, the traits of our guardians (e.g., parents, family members who raised us), the way we interacted with our siblings (or other family members of a similar age such as cousins or friends), the education that was available to us, or the community that we lived in. All of these factors shape what we value and how we view our world and people in our world.

Our parents and guardians taught us specific values, beliefs, and behaviors that are considered acceptable or unacceptable. The process of learning how to survive in one's own group (in this case, one's own family) is called encultration. Enculturation is a set of values, beliefs, and behaviors that are taught to us and teaches a person the "right" and "wrong" way of behaving. For example, it is often the case that parents of children of color have a conversation with their children about how to act and how to not react when stopped by a person of authority (e.g., Police). Why? The reason is that reacting to a situation in a "wrong" way could be a matter of life or "accidental" death. Many parents who are not part of underrepresented groups do not have these conversations with their childern. Why? Because their childern do not face these particualr curricustances when dealing with law enforcement. It would be easy for case managers to pathologize childern of color as paranoid if they do not understand the context in which families of color exist in the U.S. Therefore, it is of paramount importance that the case manager understands the dynamic of the family and how the family dynamics shape not only the family's worldview, but the worldview of the client.[2]

Indeed, it is difficult not only to change things that happened to us as kids, but it is also impossible to unring that bell. The bell representing counterproductive behaviors our clients might perceive happened to them as children. However, we can assist our clients to reframe many of the adverse activities that happened to them as a child. In many of our clients, these adverse experiences in childhood shaped thoughts and behaviors long after childhood.

Accordingly, our job as case managers might be, depending upon the context that case management is being carried out, to decrease the effects of the perceived adverse actions projected on them as a child so that our clients can live a more fulfilled and productive existence. In the end, certain interventions at the hands of the case manager can facilitate positive outcomes for our clients, despite what happened our clients in their childhood.

For example, I remember a story of a young girl (Sofia) asking her Mother (Isabella) why she did not like to eat squirrel. Isabella replied: "I just do not like the taste of squirrel." As Sofia got older, she discovered that her Mom, Isabella, never had eaten squirrel. So, how could her Mom not like the taste of squirrel if she had never tasted squirrel before? Well, after a Sunday afternoon dinner with her grandmother (Isabella's Mom) years later, it was disclosed by her grandmother that she did not like squirrel either. Neither Sofia's Mom nor grandmother ever tasted squirrel, but still did not like it. It appears that many women in her family did not like squirrel because their mothers did not like squirrel. Our family can have a profound impact on not only what we like to eat, but our values about others living in our community.

While this illustration might be simple and harmless, there are many family traditions that are counterproductive (e.g., physically abused children tend to grow up committing the same abuse) to our client's mental and physical health. It is within this context that case management and families are linked forever. We all have families, many who raised us the way they were raised. Sometimes, it is not a healthy act to continue traditions that cause us, and others, psychological or physical pain and discomfort. Many human and allied health providers will validate that various concerns our clients display during the case management process are part of the lingering effects of childhood trauma (e.g., sexual abuse) which continue to guide our client's behaviors and thoughts as adults.

Understanding the link between family and the transmission of unhealthy family traditions can be the first step in supplying needed resources to facilitate positive outcomes for all clients, despite the trauma that may present during the case management process. Services that are sensitive to the trauma that a client and his or her family experienced is referred to as trauma informed care.

According to the Substance Abuse and Mental Health Services Administration,[3] trauma informed care is a type of evidenced based service provided to clients and families that focuses on four main aspects:

> "Realize the widespread impact of trauma and understands potential paths for recovery;

> Recognizes the signs and symptoms of trauma in clients, families, staff, and others involved with the system;

➤ Responds by fully integrating knowledge about trauma into policies, procedures, and practices; and

➤ Seeks to actively resist re-traumatization."[p.1]

By providing trauma informed care, the case manager can help clients and families work together to facilitate positive outcomes (e.g., increased communication, reduction in re-traumatization, improved relationships) between the client and the family.

HISTORY OF THE AMERICAN FAMILY

Justice Sandra Day O'Connor reported that the changes in demographics during the last century make it very challenging to identify what an average American Family is.[4] Indeed, the American family structure has evolved over time. In the early years, the United States' family consisted of a wife, husband, and the biological children of the two. During this time, Blacks were forbidden to marry. Additionally, those who could marry did in many cases and stayed married until the death of their mate. It is important to note that once married, many people not only stayed married, but divorce was rare.[5] This was the beginning of what many would call the Nuclear family expectations when marrying. However, the nuclear family can include children who are biological or non-biological. When we look back into the history of the American family, marriage was common among those who could get married, and divorce was uncommon.

Marriage was critical in the way roles were carried out in the early family in the U.S. Husbands and wives of the times had very rigid roles they performed based on their gender. While many did get married, marriage was limited to individuals considered heterosexual. Because of the unyielding gender norms of the time, it was forbidden for women to own property or enter into contracts with others. Wives were considered subordinate to husbands and were relegated to taking care of the children and other household responsibilities.[5] In contrast, husbands were the providers and had authority over their wives and others residing in the household. They were managers of the finances and had the right to engage in sex with or without the permission of the wife. As we can see, not only were Blacks limited by the customs of that time by not being able to marry, but women were also marginalized in a way that many might view today as sexist. During certain times in our history, families and the roles of men and women had different meanings and expectations.

FAMILY STRUCTURE

It is essential for case managers to understand not only family structure, but how a certain family structure might function because of its structure and expectations. Because of the increasing diversity of cultures in the U.S., case managers will be presented with different family structures that might not align with the family structures they are familiar with. Thus, it is all too easy to make counterproductive judgments about a person because of the family structure they inherited or choose to create because of traditions and customs. There are countless types of family structures all over the world and our clients can come from many different types of family structures. The following is not an exhaustive list, but represent some common family structures that many providers will encounter as case managers in the human services.

NUCLEAR FAMILY

The nuclear family is thought of as two parents with children.[6] There can be one or several children in this family structure. Like the nuclear family, the extended family might have key family members either living within or outside of the house that may share some kinship.

EXTENDED FAMILY

The extended family refers to many kinships (e.g., aunts, uncles, grandparents) either living in the same residence and have influence over persons residing in or outside the residence.[6] In many instances, grandparents raise the children with very little supervision from parents. In this example, the child will grow up with the values and beliefs of the grandparents.

SINGLE PARENT FAMILIES

Because of various circumstances (e.g., the spouse being killed in the military, unwanted union, divorce), many clients come from a single parent household. Depending upon the reason, many single parents may face many struggles.[6] For instance, many single parent households experience financial hardships, especially if the head of the household is female. Considering the context, it can be difficult for many women for various reasons. One reason could be the sexism that exist in our society. For example, on average, women make approximately 80 cents to every dollar that males make.[7] Many single families may become step families because of the blending together of two or more units. Stepfamilies.

STEPFAMILIES

In past generations, stepfamilies were less frequent.[6] A step family can be defined as a family that might have two single parents with children, coming together to form a single-family unit. What about families with people who may have disabilities?

119

FAMILIES WITH DISABILITIES

Disability can be defined as "a physical or mental impairment that substantially limits one or more major life activities."[8 para.2] A family with one or more people with disabilities can create unique challenges for the family. For example, having a child with a disability often means that the parents or caretakers need to take extra time to attend doctor's appointments or school appointments to discuss how the child's needs are being met. It is also important for the case manager to understand how the family views the disability. Family responses to disability can be positive or negative. An example of a positive response to disability in the family would be providing a stable and supportive home environment (e.g., not shaming the person with the disability). A negative response might be that the family views the disability as a burden (e.g., thinking that a person with dyslexia is not as smart as a person without the dyslexia). The overall functioning of the family with a disability depends on how the disability is contextualized. In many respects, how a disability is contextualized will depend on the culture in which the person was raised.

SAME GENDER FAMILIES

Same gender families are families that might have parents of the same gender (e.g., male, female). Same gender families, as with other family structures, might be integrated with other family structures depending upon the context (e.g., race, ethnicity, geographical). A study by Patterson[9] suggested that children of same-sex couples **do not** have differences in adjustment or development. This is an important outcome because case managers are not precluded from projecting their biases on clients based on what they think is the optimal family structure for development.

While there is a difference between family structure (e.g., Stepfamilies) and family values (e.g., the amount of influence a family might have on its members, being interdependent or dependent on the family to make decisions about one's life), it is important for case managers to realize that not all families have identical values. For example, in the Asian culture, generally, families tend to be influenced by both the nuclear and extended family. As a result, many Asian cultures will look at the needs of the family unit before their own personal needs. This family value system from individuals who are from the Asian continent might be applied in the following example. Let's say a case manager strongly suggests that a person who is Asian make the decision to be more independent (e.g., move out of the home, spend more money on themselves for materialistic gains, stop contributing financially to the care of elderly parents (NOTE: married Asian females might be the ones expected to care of aging parents-in-law). Specifically, the hierarchy of siblings and their marital status would decide what male or female would be expected to care for aging parents. More than likely, the suggestions by the case manager might be met with resistance because of the value system of the Asian culture. Simply put, "we" comes before the "I" (collectivism). This philosophy (i.e., values, norms) is different from the values of families in the U.S., in that the U.S. tends to be more individualistic (e.g., European Americans) instead of collectivistic (e.g., Asian Continent or people who are Native American). Understanding the structure, values, and expectations of the family can help the case manager facilitate positive outcomes. However, by not understanding the family structure can lead to poor service quality and harm the family and the client.

Suppose there is a client that has an extended-family structure where aunts and uncles are viewed as having the same amount of influence as the parents. If the case manager undermines the influence that the aunts and uncles have by not giving weight and validation to their influence, the family members may be offended, felt misunderstood, or frustrated with the delivery of the case management process. If the family feels offended, misunderstood, or frustrated, it is unlikely that they will return for services.

While several client variables may cause many case managers to pause when working with clients who might come from diverse family structures (e.g., signal parent, same gender), it is important to not only understand but to apply cultural competence to diverse family structures. In many cases, cultural competence in the family structure context might be not forcing others to yield to family expectations that are most familiar to a certain culture or group. Clients can feel, and many times see, the disconnect between their family values and the family values of the provider. For example, a nonverbal movement of disapproval displayed by the case manager. Another example might be the provider being explicit about the "right way" that the family should act or not act in a given context or situation.

At the end of the day, when the case manager is not validating the client, (i.e., not giving truth to what the client is communicating to the case manager) the relationship tends to be superficial with small talk and pleasantries controlling much of the mood and expectations of the outcomes. Thus, validating family expectations from the client's worldview is not only critical for developing rapport and trust between the case manager and client dyad, but being on the same page tends to yield better outcomes for the provider and client. While there may be numerous client variables that may provide reasons for concerns with case managers, understanding how to give truth to what the client is communicating is a great way to start. Now, let's look at a case study that connects many of the outlined concepts in this chapter.

CASE STUDY
AKI LEE

A case manager (Rashaad Jones, African American male) is meeting his new client (Aki Lee, Asian American female) for the first time to determine if she is eligible for services at a community mental health center. Aki arrived on time for the session and was happy to feel

121

welcomed by Rashaad. During the session, Aki voiced concerns that she is feeling frustrated because of all the demands being put on her by her family. Aki, continues, "Our parents are aging, and I do not feel that my older brother is feeling all of the expectations to care for our parents." Because Rashaad is somewhat familiar with the Asian culture, he is surprised that Aki voiced this concern during their first meeting. This promoted Rashaad to ask the following question. "What do you expect from your brother?" Aki responded, "Well, I am not really sure at this point. I am just getting tired of all the extra things I must do for our parents." The session continues with Rashaad suggesting the following to Aki. "Why don't you put your parents in a nursing home and let the nursing home take care of them? This way, both you and your brother will not have this obligation, decreasing much of the stress that you are feeling." Aki looked confused once Rashaad completed his thoughts on the matter. At the conclusion of the session, Aki appeared less talkative and withdrawn. However, this did not go unnoticed by Rashaad. After ending the session, Rashaad thought to himself, "Aki must have something on her mind that she did not feel like expressing to me. Most of the people that I know would not put up with what she is putting up with her brother. She should confront her brother about not contributing to the care of their parents."

CASE STUDY DISCUSSION QUESTIONS

1. Do you think the case manager (Rashaad Jones) and client (Aki Lee) have different family values and expectations?

2. What do you think about what the case manager said to the client as the session was ending with the client? [*Why don't you put your parents in a nursing home and let the nursing home take care of them? This way, both you and your brother will not have this obligation, decreasing much of the stress that you are feeling.*]

3. Why do you think the client was "*less talkative and withdrawn*" after the case manager's comments? [*Why don't you put your parents in a nursing home and let the nursing home take care of them? This way, both you and your brother will not have this obligation, decreasing much of the stress that you are feeling.*]

CONCLUSION

We all come from and have a "family." While some of us would rather not claim our families for one reason or another, we all have a family unit that we have inherited via biological connections or formed based on the union of adults with prior children, for example. Early in the history of the United States, families were considered a vital union that formed how husband and wives separated responsibilities. Based on the norms in the early history of the United States, black slaves could not get married. Additionally, women were subordinate to their husbands in the right to own property and being able to take another person to court. Today, families are more diverse because of the increase in migration of other ethnicities and cultures coming to the United States. Yielding both a diversity of family values and structures and an expansion of how family values are viewed. To be an effective case manager, it is important to understand and apply a broader net on how family's functions. Why? Because of the influence of the family unit on the lives of most clients, understanding the power, influence, and expectations of families can facilitate better outcomes for all the clients we serve. This is an ideal that we must strive to achieve in the human and allied health services environments.

REFERENCES

[1] U. S. Census Bureau. (2012a). *U.S. Census Bureau projections show a slower growing, older, more diverse nation a half century from now*. Retrieved from https://www.census.gov/newsroom/releases/archives/population/cb12-243.html

[2] Michael Teachings. (n.d.). *Family Influence*. Retrieved from http://www.michaelteachings.com/family_influence.html

[3] Substance Abuse and Mental Health Services Administration. (2015). *Trauma-informed approaches and trauma-specific interventions*. National Center for Trauma-Informed Care and Alternative to Seclusion and Restraint. Retrieved from https://www.samhsa.gov/nctic/trauma-interventions

[4] Grossman, J. (2015). Family Law's Loose Canon. Texas Law Review, 93(3), 681.

[5] Joslin, C. G., The Evolution of the American Family (December 21, 2009). 36 SUMMER-Human Rights 2 (Summer 2009); UC Davis Legal Studies Research Paper No. 200. Available at SSRN: https://ssrn.com/abstract=1526839

[6] Meyerhoff, M. (2017). Understanding family structure and dynamics. Retrieved from https://health.howstuffworks.com/pregnancy-and-parenting/understanding-family-structures-and-dynamics-ga.htm

[7] Institute for Women's Policy Research. (2017). *Pay equity and discrimination*. Retrieved from https://iwpr.org/issue/employment-education-economic-change/pay-equity-discrimination/

[8] U. S. Department of Justice. (2009). *A guide to disability rights law*. Retrieved from https://www.ada.gov/cguide.htm

[9] Patterson, C. J. (2006). Children of lesbian and gay parent. *Association for Psychological Science, 15 (5)*, 241-244.

CHAPTER 7

ETHICS AND FACILITATING SERVICES FOR CLIENTS

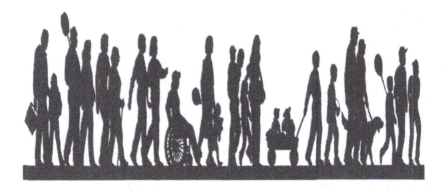

SARA P. JOHNSTON

MICHAEL T. HARTLEY

ABSTRACT

Human service professionals are required to make decisions that affect the quality of life and well-being of their clients. The process of decision-making can be difficult, and agency guidelines often do not provide sufficient guidance. In addition, many decisions require human services professionals to balance the moral, ethical, and legal aspects of the various stakeholders to make the best decision in each case. To enhance decision-making and manage the conflicts inherent in ethical dilemmas, human service professionals can benefit from understanding how to consult professional resources as well as trusted colleagues to obtain facts as well as different perspectives. This chapter will describe how to: (1) recognize the ethical, moral, and legal aspects of an ethical dilemma; (2) how to effectively use consultation to improve decision-making in ethical dilemmas, and (3) how to advocate to promote client welfare during the case management process.

CHAPTER HIGHLIGHTS

➤ Moral, ethical, and legal considerations;

➤ Ethical principles;

➤ Ethical decision-making model;

➤ Consultation.

LEARNING OBJECTIVES

➤ Identify an ethical dilemma and define ethical principles;

➤ Understand moral, ethical, and legal considerations as they relate to an ethical dilemma;

➤ Describe the steps in an ethical decision-making model;

➤ Define consultation;

➤ Describe the benefits of consultation and explain the process of consultation;

➤ Describe how consultation can enhance human service professionals' ability to manage conflicts inherent in ethical dilemmas and improve advocacy skills.

INTRODUCTION

What is ethics? What is ethical decision making? This chapter seeks to answer those questions as well as provide the reader with practical applications of ethics, ethical decision-making, and consultation as it applies to human service professionals.

Many people confuse ethics with religion. While it is true that traditional religious values such as "Thou shall not kill," and "Love your neighbor" inform ethics, ethics is broader in that it covers both religious and non-religious individuals. Others confuse ethics with the law. Again, while it is true that ethics informs laws and legal systems, ethics is broader than any one set of laws. Ethics may also deviate from the law. The Civil War in the United States was the result of a conflict between those who believed that slavery should continue to be allowed under the law and those who believed slavery was wrong and should be abolished. Finally, people often assume that societal norms are ethical. However, history shows us that societal norms may reinforce stereotypes about and discrimination against certain groups of people. For example, in the mid-20th century, white supremist movements in the South and in Germany encouraged the rise of the Ku Klux Klan and the Nazi regime, respectively. The Nazis and the Ku Klux Klan used negative societal beliefs about groups of individuals, including Jews, people with disabilities, and racial/ethnic minorities, to promote a political and economic agenda that encouraged discrimination, hatred, and violence against targeted groups of people. More recently, the U.S. has witnessed a conflict between individual and societal norms regarding the shootings of African American men by police officers, which resulted in the "Black Lives Matter" movement, and the right of children of illegal immigrants to live and work in the U.S. under the Deferred Action for Childhood Arrivals (DACA) program, which the current presidential administration seeks to end.

DEFINITION OF ETHICS

For purposes of this chapter, ethics is defined as long-held standards of right and wrong that govern human behavior. Ethical standards provide guidance to individuals on what to do ("Do good") and what not to do ("Do not harm"). Ethical standards are based on broader ethical principles– autonomy, justice, fidelity, beneficence, non-maleficence–which will be discussed in more detail later in the chapter. Ethics also refers to the development of individual ethical standards. Individual ethical standards may differ from societal ethical standards, which means that, in some situations, individuals must choose between following societal standards at the expense of their own standards and vice versa. Ethical standards are dynamic, not static. This means that individuals must regularly assess their ethical standards. The regular assessment of ethical standards assists individuals in making consistent, well-reasoned decisions. Ethical decision-making is the process of evaluating and choosing the most ethical course of action in each situation.[10]

Often, the process of ethical decision-making becomes difficult and agency guidelines may not provide sufficient guidance. In such cases, it is important that human service professionals make use of intuitive and critical-evaluative levels of ethical decision making, thus incorporating both conscious and non-conscious thoughts and emotions.[6] However, this is easier said than done and it is, therefore, important that human service professionals consult with professional resources as well as trusted colleagues to obtain both facts as well as different perspectives regarding how to manage the conflict inherent in an ethical dilemma.[3]

Human service professionals often struggle with ethics and ethical decision-making when faced with a difficult decision in a case. Difficult decisions include emotional or sociocultural aspects that tug at the heartstrings or produce feelings of anger or outrage. Individuals who pursue careers in the human service field are natural advocates who strive to be fair and just in their interactions with others. However, without an understanding of how to advocate effectively for their clients, human service professionals may inadvertently violate agency policies, professional codes of ethics, and in some cases, break the law.

The next section of the chapter will introduce you to the moral, ethical, and legal considerations that undergird the decisions we make at the client, agency, and public policy levels of practice.

MORAL, ETHICAL, AND LEGAL CONSIDERATIONS IN ETHICAL DECISION-MAKING

Throughout the day, each of us makes countless decisions—some minor, such as where to eat lunch, and some major, such as whether to apply for a new job or resign from a current job. Thus, the process of decision-making should not be unfamiliar to human service professionals. What may be unfamiliar, and perhaps uncomfortable, is decision-making that involves a controversial or traumatic situation involving clients, the agency, or the larger community. When making difficult decisions, it is important to understand how and why we make a decision; in other words, where the decision originates from. It's also important to understand what the consequences of the decision may be.

MORAL, ETHICAL, AND LEGAL STANCE

Difficult decisions originate from one of three stances: moral, ethical, and legal. These three stances, or groups, are what we use to justify the decisions that we make. Each of the three stances derives from a specific body of knowledge or code.

MORAL STANCE. The moral stance derives from individual, societal, and religious values (e.g., "Thou shall not kill"). Morals inform ethics, but, again, ethics is broader than one set of morals or one religion. For example, Buddhist, Christian, Islamic, and Native American religions all prohibit the intentional taking or harming of a life. However, there may be differences among religions with respect to whether or not there are any exceptions to the prohibition against the intentional harming or taking of a life.

ETHICAL STANCE. The ethical stance derives from ethics and ethical standards. There are five ethical principles that are commonly found across professions: Do no harm (non-maleficence); Do good (beneficence); Be fair (justice); Allow individual choice (autonomy); and, Be loyal (fidelity). Professions, such as medicine, nursing, counseling, and human services, incorporate ethics and ethical standards into a formalized code of ethics, which governs their behavior in their practice as professionals. For example, the codes of ethics for medicine, nursing, counseling, and human services all contain an ethical standard that requires the professional to practice in a way that will not harm the patient or client–non-maleficence (Do no harm).[10] Some professional codes of ethics may contain more than five ethical principles. For example, the counseling profession has added a sixth ethical principle, veracity (truthfulness). [1, 4]

LEGAL STANCE. The legal stance derives from the law and legal standards. For example, intentional homicide violates both state and federal laws. Keep in mind that both morals ("Thou shall not kill" and ethics and ethical standards ("Do no harm," non-maleficence) inform laws that prohibit the intentional harm or killing of an individual.

It is important to consider that morals, ethics, and laws may vary by groups of individuals; geographic location (within the same country and between countries); and by culture. For example, Western cultures may have very different morals, ethics, and legal standards concerning individual rights and independence than do cultures that place more importance on collective or interdependent relationships.

ETHICAL DECISION-MAKING

Ethical decision-making requires that decision-makers are clear about the stance they are taking–moral, ethical, or legal. The stance a person takes in a situation dictates the consequences as well as the protection from consequences of taking that stance. Consequences may be intrinsic or extrinsic. Let's work through a case example to understand how stance may affect the decision in the case as well as the consequences of the decision.

CASE STUDY
CARA

Cara is an 18-year-old client who receives counseling for anxiety and depression at a community agency. Cara would like to begin dating a young man in her freshman Biology course; she thinks that getting out more on campus will help her feel less isolated. Joe, the human services professional who is working with Carla states that he will not encourage Cara to date because "dating may lead to sex, and sex among unmarried adults is illegal." Joe goes on to state that if he supports Cara's decision to date, it would be unethical because he would be violating the ethical principle of "Do no harm" (non-maleficence). He claims that he is taking both an ethical and legal stance regarding his decision about Cara, and asks his supervisor to support his decision. Joe's supervisor counters that she believes he is confusing an ethical and legal stance with a moral stance. She explains that there are no laws in the state prohibiting pre-marital sex among consenting adults, and that the client is of legal age. In addition, she reminds Joe that the agency's code of ethics states that client choice is respected and encouraged (autonomy). In this case, the supervisor is correct, Joe is confusing a moral stance about pre-marital sex with an ethical and legal stance, because there are no ethical standards or laws prohibiting an adult client from engaging in premarital sex. To continue working effectively with Cara, Joe will need to assess the consequences of basing his decision about Cara's dating on a moral stance.

Intrinsic and Extrinsic Consequences in Decision-making

In the case above, Joe's decision to take a moral stance in this situation may have several consequences for himself, the client, and the agency. For example, the consequence to Joe is that in supporting the client's choice to date, he is violating his morals, which may be emotionally difficult and stressful for him. An individual may feel guilt or shame when violating his or her own morals. This is an example of an intrinsic consequence, which is simply a consequence that originates from within an individual. On the other hand, if Joe chooses not to support the client's choices because of his moral stance on pre-marital sex, he risks violating the agency's code of ethics and the client's legal rights. Joe's decision to take a moral stance in the case may cause the agency to discipline or fire Joe; and/or the client may file a grievance or a lawsuit against Joe and the agency charging that the agency did not respect her choice or autonomy. These are examples of extrinsic consequences, which are consequences that originate from outside an individual.

Resolving Moral, Ethical, and Legal Conflicts

Ethical decision-making skills are improved when human services professionals must have a clear understanding of the moral, ethical, and legal stances in a case, as well as the potential consequences for taking a stance in a case.

Many times, human services professionals may know which decision is the best decision in a case, yet conflicts among morals, ethics, and laws often make it difficult for human services professionals to "do the right thing." Human services professionals who are unable to negotiate conflicts among morals, ethics, and values, may become frustrated, cynical, and dissatisfied with their work when they find themselves making decisions that go against what they feel is the right decision in a case. Learning how to resolve moral, ethical, and legal conflicts in a human service setting may improve service delivery and reduce the risk of professional burnout.

The first step in resolving moral, ethical, and legal conflicts is reflection. As the case of Joe and Cara demonstrates, human service professionals may confuse a moral stance with a legal or ethical stance, which may lead to decisions that are at best based on faulty assumptions or incorrect information, and at worst not in the best interests of the client. Human services professionals must take the time to reflect on the stance that underlies each decision they make to ensure that they are not confusing stances or missing information that could affect their stance. Upon reflection, Joe realizes that his objection to Cara's dating derives primarily from a moral stance, specifically, his religious beliefs that premarital sex is immoral.[6]

The second step in resolving moral, ethical, and legal conflicts is to determine if the conflicts can be resolved by additional education and training, counseling and guidance, additional supervision, consultation with supervisors and other colleagues, or, as a last resort, client referral. To continue working effectively with Cara, Joe must be able to resolve any potential conflicts between his own morals and the ethical and legal requirements he is bound to by the agency and the laws of the state. Joe must determine if he is comfortable in setting aside his own religious beliefs about dating and premarital sex to support Cara's choice to date. Joe may be unable to set aside his religious beliefs. In that case, Joe must decide whether he is able to continue working with Cara, and, more broadly, working for the agency, or remaining in the human services field.[10]

Joe may decide that he is able to resolve the conflict between his morals and the ethical and legal requirements that he is bound to uphold in his work. He may seek support and guidance in working through the conflict through counseling or through consultation with his supervisor or colleagues. We will discuss consultation in more detail later in the chapter.

Conversely, Joe may decide that he is unable to resolve the conflict between his morals and the ethical and legal requirements he is bound to uphold in his work. Joe may request that Cara be referred to another human services professional. There may be consequences to this decision, however, because Joe may be bound by professional, agency, and legal codes or requirements that prohibit human services professionals from using the referral process to discriminate against a client or group of clients who are members of a legally protected class of individuals (e.g., gender, race/ethnicity, age, sexual orientation, or religion). If Joe states that he is unable to work with Cara due to his religious beliefs, Cara may perceive Joe's refusal to work with her as discriminatory. Cara may have grounds for filing a complaint against Joe and the agency charging that she was not treated fairly because of her gender.[1]

The situation may be further complicated if Cara informed Joe that she was interested in dating a woman in her biology class, and Joe is a member of a religion that believes same-sex relationships are a sin. In this case, Joe and his supervisor may need to determine if there are policies or codes at the agency level and laws at the state or national level which protect Cara's rights as a member of the LGBT community. The supervisor may decide that Joe's religious beliefs prevent him from providing appropriate services to clients in accordance with agency policy and state laws, and Joe may be fired. Joe, however, may believe that he is being discriminated against based on his religious beliefs and contest his firing.[7]

Ultimately, Joe makes the decision to work through his conflict through additional supervision and consultation. As he has worked through the conflict between his morals and his ethical and legal responsibilities to the client and the agency, he has discovered that he still has concerns that if he supports Cara's decision to begin dating, there is the potential that she may be exposed to situations that she is not emotionally ready for, which may exacerbate her symptoms of depression and anxiety. He is struggling with how to balance respecting his client's choices (autonomy) with his duty to protect her from harm (non-maleficence). Joe must resolve this conflict between autonomy and non-maleficence before advising Cara on her decision to begin dating.

ETHICAL DILEMMAS

When a conflict occurs within the confines of a profession, such as law, medicine, nursing, psychology, and human services, such a conflict is termed an ethical dilemma. An ethical dilemma is a case or situation that involves a conflict between two or more ethical principles.[1, 4, 10] Ethical principles are derived from morals that society, as a collective body, deems important and necessary for the well-being of its members or citizens. Morals inform ethical principles that individuals and societies use to guide behavior. Ethical principles are often codified into ethical codes, such as the *American Counseling Association (ACA) Code of Professional Ethics*[1] and the *National Organization for Human Services Ethical Standards for Human Services Professionals*.[8] Members of these health and human service organizations must adhere to the code in their professional practice. Ethical principles are also the foundation of many procedures, policies, and laws that form our institutions and government. For example, the ethical principle, "Do no harm" (non-maleficence) forms the basis for laws that prohibit individuals from intentionally or unintentionally harming other human beings. As a review, there are five ethical principles that are commonly found across professions: Do no harm (non-maleficence); Do good (beneficence); Be fair (justice); Allow individual choice (autonomy); and, Be loyal (fidelity).[10]

MULTICULTURAL AND STAKEHOLDER CONSIDERATIONS

Ethical dilemmas often involve controversial or traumatic situations, such as abortion, euthanasia (assisted suicide), and the rights of individuals from the LGBT community to marry or have the right to serve in the military. Ethical dilemmas involve morals and values–both individual morals and values and societal or collective morals and values. For example, individuals living in individualistic societies (e.g., the United States) are more likely to value independence, which may lead to a collective societal view, supported by legislation, that individuals should not rely on government to fund their retirements; rather, individuals should be responsible for setting up their own retirement plans and save for them. In contrast, individuals living in a collectivist society (e.g., Norway) may have access to "cradle to grave" government programs that reflect the societal view that government has the responsibility to care for its citizens throughout the lifespan. Societal views on the proper role of government in providing for its citizens may be influenced by individual and societal morals.[5, 7, 10]

Human services professionals must not assume that the client shares the same individual and societal morals as the human services professional. Human services professionals must assess and respect the client's worldview and refrain from imposing their worldview on the client. Every ethical dilemma has the potential to incorporate several worldviews, including the worldviews of the human service professional, the client, the client's family, the agency, the community, and the government and legal systems. Differing worldviews are often referred to as "stakeholder perspectives." Stakeholders are defined as any person, persons, agency, institution, or government who has an interest in the outcome of an ethical dilemma. In the case example above, the stakeholders would include Joe, Cara, the clients' family (if the client is underage), the supervisor, the agency, the community, and the legal system.[5, 7, 10]

An ethical decision-making model can be useful in working through the conflicts among morals, ethics; conflicts between ethical principles; and for understanding stakeholder perspectives.[10]

ETHICAL DECISION-MAKING MODEL

An ethical decision-making model consists of a series of steps that facilitate decision-making. An ethical decision-making model contains the following four steps:

> Determine whether an ethical dilemma exists.
  a. Is there a conflict between two or more ethical principles?
  b. If yes, what are the principles in conflict, and why are they in conflict?

> Examine contextual issues
  a. What are the potential sources of bias, sociocultural considerations, or multicultural considerations?
  b. Who are the stakeholders, and what are their perspectives?

> Formulate a course of action.
  a. Gather all data, consult with supervisors and colleagues.
  b. Make a decision.

> Implement and evaluate the course of action.[5, 10]

It is important to note that ethical decision-making often involves choosing from several courses of action, none of which offers a perfect solution to the dilemma. Ethical decision-making requires decision-makers to be comfortable with ambiguity. In other words, the most ethical course of action may not be black or white, but grey.[10]

Joe uses the ethical decision-making model to assist him in working through the ethical dilemma in Cara's case. First, Joe determines that there is a conflict between autonomy and non-maleficence. He wants to support Cara's decision to begin dating (autonomy), but not at the expense of potential harm to Cara's mental health and progress in school if she becomes involved in a relationship that ends badly, and that she is not emotionally prepared to handle (non-maleficence).

Second, Joe considers the contextual issues related to the case. Contextual issues include factual information related to policies, codes, and laws that may be important to the case; potential sources of bias, including negative attitudes towards or stereotypes about specific groups of people; and multicultural considerations, such as differing worldviews. Understanding the contextual issues will assist Joe in determining who the stakeholders are in the case. For example, if Cara is underage, Joe would need to determine if there are laws in his state which require Cara's parents or guardians to be informed about matters affecting Cara. Joe will also need to assess Cara's attitudes and beliefs about dating and relationships. Joe should consider if it is important for him to disclose his religious views about dating and premarital sex, which may be a source of potential bias. Depending on Cara's situation, Cara's teachers, guidance counselor, and medical providers may be stakeholders in the case. Joe may need to gather information from them about any educational or medical considerations. Finally, Joe must be aware of any multicultural considerations that may impact Cara's views on dating, relationships, and sex. The more information Joe can gather about the contextual issues in the case, the better informed he will be about client and stakeholder worldviews.[5, 7, 10]

The third step is that Joe will use the information he gathered in Steps 1 and 2 to formulate a plan of action. Joe will meet with his supervisor to go over the details of the case, the dilemma, and the information he gathered. He presents his supervisor with his plan to resolve the dilemma, which is to support Cara's decision to date in a supportive manner that includes providing her with education about dating safety, interpersonal communication skills, recognizing the signs of a potentially abusive or controlling relationship. Joe has decided not to disclose his religious beliefs to Cara at the current time; however, he will have a broader discussion with Cara about her beliefs and values about dating, relationships, and sex. Joe realizes that because he is man, there may be some issues related to sex that Cara may be more comfortable discussing with a woman. Joe will offer Cara the opportunity to discuss any sensitive topics with his supervisor, who is female. Joe will also encourage Cara to discuss birth control with her medical providers if she becomes involved in a sexual relationship. Joe realizes he will need to be mindful of Cara's beliefs and values regarding birth control. Joe believes that his plan of action will allow Cara to make her own choice about dating, relationships, and sex, which respects her autonomy. His plan of action puts protections in place so that Cara is making an informed and educated choice, which addresses Joe's concern about the potential for dating to cause Cara emotional harm which may exacerbate her depression and anxiety.[10]

Before implementing his plan of action, Joe asks his supervisor for her input and feedback. This is known as consultation. Joe is wise to ask his supervisor to consult with him on the ethical dilemma before implementing the plan. His supervisor may be able to point out factual errors, suggest additional resources, and address potential biases.

Human services professionals can gain assistance on how best to complete each of the steps in the ethical decision-making model by seeking additional information from professional resources and from colleagues and supervisors. The process of consultation is important to professional practice; indeed, many professions' codes of ethics recommend consultation to resolve ethical dilemmas and improve service delivery.

CONSULTATION

The process of decision-making may be difficult and agency guidelines often do not provide sufficient guidance. In such cases, it is important that human service professionals make use of intuitive and critical-evaluative levels of ethical decision making, thus incorporating both conscious and non-conscious thoughts and emotions.[6] However, this is easier said than done, and it is therefore important that human service professionals consult professional resources as well as trusted colleagues to obtain both facts as well as different perspectives regarding how to manage the conflict inherent in an ethical dilemma.[3]

With this in mind, consultation is a key component of virtually all ethical decision-making models as well as ethical codes of conduct regulating the behavior of helping professionals.[5] As an example, the preamble of the *Code of Professional Ethics for Rehabilitation Counseling*[4] mandates that "when rehabilitation counselors are faced with ethical dilemmas that are difficult to resolve, they are expected to engage in a carefully considered ethical decision-making process, consulting available resources as needed."[p.3] Representing human service professionals more generally, the National Organization for Human Services (NOHS) *Ethical Standards for Human Services Professionals*[8] includes the requirement of consultation if there are ethical dilemmas involving clients, colleagues, employers, or the profession. As an example, Standard 28 states that "Human service professionals seek appropriate consultation and supervision to assist in decision-making when there are legal, ethical or other dilemmas" (Section: Responsibility to the Profession). While consultation is a critical aspect of ethical decision making, professionals also must take care not to divulge confidential information that could lead to the identification of clients or other persons unless there is a written disclosure. We therefore conclude this chapter with tips regarding how to engage in appropriate and ethical consultation when faced with an ethical dilemma.

DEFINITION OF CONSULTATION

Consultation refers to the deliberate exchange of information and advice to enhance professional practice, treatment of complex cases, management of risk and liability, and professional growth and development.[2] Consultation is an excellent way to monitor effectiveness, generate new approaches to service provision, and to improve clinical competencies. Further, when faced with an ethical dilemma, consultation is used to assess the accuracy of initial intuition as well as to provide a useful resource to increase critical-evaluative thinking, including the use of "professional judgment and to engage in a process of information gathering, analyzing, reasoning, and planning to determine the most ethical course of action in a challenging situation."[9, p.170]

Consultation is particularly important when there may be serious and foreseeable harm to clients and colleagues. In such instances, there are complex ethical obligations related to the five primary ethical principles of autonomy, beneficence, non-maleficence, justice, and fidelity. While the definition of these principles is straightforward, the application to clinical practice is complex, often requiring a social systems approach to account for both socially and relationally influenced factors.[5] A social system approach posits that ethical obligations are social and relational. Hence, there is a need to consider the unique perspectives of diverse individuals who may be impacted by an ethical decision, beginning with the client, moving outward to the treatment team and agency as well as the family and community of the client, and then finally to the role and function of the profession within society. Consultation is thus an approach to broaden the consideration of the contextual forces, rather than a singular focus on an individual practitioner and his or her relationship with an individual client.

SOURCES OF CONSULTATION

The sources of consultation are abundant, and the first step is often confiding in a trusted colleague within the employment agency. Reaching out to a particularly valued colleague who may have a similar personality or viewpoint regarding professional and ethical issues can be a great way to gain information as well as emotional support. At the same time, soliciting advice from professionals with different backgrounds may offer divergent viewpoints and insights. Consulting with multiple colleagues within the employment agency also offers a means to gauge how different professionals within the agency may view both the ethical dilemma as well as the potential course of action.

Supervisors and administrators within the employment are another consultation source. Agency policies tend to be broadly written. Rather than assuming one understands a policy, it is important to clarify with supervisors and administrators regarding how to interpret and implement a policy. Professionals employed by an agency are expected to adhere to the agency policies, and the best way to clarify these expectations is to consult with a supervisor and administer regarding how to interpret a policy.

Consultations within the agency of employment are an excellent starting place because it is the social context in which the problem resides, yet professionals will also want to consult with resources outside of the agency. Lacking the contextual knowledge of the agency, consultations with related professionals outside the agency may be more objective, although based solely on the self-report of the professional describing the situation. Sources of advice from outside the agency could be related professionals in the field as well as professional organizations and credentialing bodies.

Consultations with related professionals working for other human service agencies are also useful, such as previous co-workers or former fellow students from the same professional development program. It is particularly important in such consultations to not divulge confidential information that could lead to the identification of a client unless client consent has been obtained. Such information would be breach of confidentiality unless the client has signed a release for the consultation. Soliciting general opinions on a professional listserv is not recommended, and it is much better to have a one-on-one conversation with a trusted professional that is careful to only provide information for the purpose of the consultation that would not break confidentiality.

Consultation with professional organizations and credentialing bodies is another option. Some professional organizations offer members access to resources to help with ethical decision making, including helplines and advisory opinions. Such resources are an avenue to clarify professional obligations, especially in situations when the professional standards of the field conflict with the policies of the employment agency. In such cases, a professional may need to consider termination of employment if it is not possible to create change within the employment agency.

DISCUSSION QUESTIONS

1. Name the five ethical principles.

2. What is an ethical dilemma?

3. Describe the four steps in ethical decision-making models.

4. How might using an ethical decision-making model assist human services professionals in working through ethical dilemmas?

5. What are some reliable sources for consultation?

6. How might engaging in consultation assist human services professionals in working through ethical dilemmas?

CASE STUDY

The following case example is based on a true scenario that a student faced in a clinical course:

You are a student in the human services field. You are completing your required clinical hours at the local high school. You have been assigned to work with new students who have been categorized as at-risk students. You have been working with a student who has been having difficulty in school. She has recently moved to the city, and this is her first semester at your school. She has high rates of absenteeism, and she has been earning failing grades in more than one of her classes. In one of her counseling sessions with you, she discloses that she would like to quit school to focus on getting a job. She also tells you that she has been working against her will as a sex worker. You suspect your client may be a victim of sex trafficking.

1. What are the potential moral, ethical, and legal stances in the case?

2. What are the consequences of each stance?

3. What happens if there are no laws or ethical standards governing suspected sexual abuse of an underage client, but there is an agency ethical standard that requires you to protect client confidentiality?

4. Who might you consult with to obtain additional guidance about the issues in this case?

5. Are there any local ordinances or state laws in your state that may require you to report your suspicions about sex trafficking to the authorities?

CONCLUSION

Human service professionals are required to make decisions that affect the quality of life and well-being of their clients. The process of decision-making can be difficult, and agency guidelines often do not provide sufficient guidance. In addition, many decisions require human services professionals to balance the moral, ethical, and legal aspects of the various stakeholders to make the best decision in each case. To enhance decision-making and manage the conflicts inherent in ethical dilemmas, human services professionals may benefit from understanding how moral, ethical, and legal considerations, as well as intrinsic and extrinsic consequences, may affect decision-making in each case. Human resources professionals may also benefit by using a decision-making model when faced with an ethical dilemma. Ethical decision-making models provide a framework for understanding the conflict between ethical principles in a case; contextual, stakeholder, and sociocultural factors related to the case; possible courses of action, and a plan for implementing the course of action. Another benefit to using an ethical decision-making model to resolve ethical dilemmas is to minimize potential practitioner bias towards clients who are members of minority groups (e.g., race/ethnicity, gender, age, disability). Ethical decision-making models encourage human service professionals to consult with trusted colleagues, supervisors, and professional resources to obtain facts as well as different perspectives. Some professional organizations offer members access to resources to help with ethical decision making, including helplines and advisory opinions. Such resources are an avenue to clarify professional obligations, especially in situations when the professional standards of the field conflict with the policies of the agency.

REFERENCES

[1]American Counseling Association (ACA). (2014). *Code of Ethics*. Alexandria, VA: Author.

[2]Bowers, M., & Pipes, R. B. (2000). Influence of consultation on ethical decision making: An analogue study. *Ethics & Behavior, 10,* 55–79.

[3]Cartwright, B. Y., Hartley, M. T. (2016). Ethics consultation in rehabilitation counseling: A content analysis of CRCC advisory opinions, 1996-2013. *Rehabilitation Counseling Bulletin, 59,* 84–93.

[4]Commission on Rehabilitation Counselor Certification. (2002). *Code of Professional Ethics for Rehabilitation Counselors*. Schaumburg, IL: Author.

[5]Cottone, R. R. (2001). A social constructivism model of ethical decision making in counseling. *Journal of Counseling & Development, 79,* 39-45.

[6]Kitchener, K. S. (1984). Intuition, critical evaluation, and ethical principles: The foundation for ethical decisions in counseling psychology. *The Counseling Psychologist, 12*(3), 43-55.

[7]Liu, W. M., Toporek, R. L. (2017). Advocacy. In V. M. Tarvydas and M. T. Hartley (Eds.) *The Professional Practice of Rehabilitation Counseling.* New York, NY: Springer.

[8]National Organization for Human Services (NOHS). (2015). *Ethical standards for human services professionals.* Retrieved from http://www.nationalhumanservices.org/ethical-standards.

[9]Shaw, L. R., & Lane, F. (2008). Ethical consultation: Content analysis of the advisory opinion archive of the Commission on Rehabilitation Counselor Certification. *Rehabilitation Counseling Bulletin, 51,* 170-176.

[10]Tarvydas, V. T., & Johnston, S. P. (2017). Ethics and ethics decision making. In V. M. Tarvydas and M. T. Hartley (Eds.), *The Professional Practice of Rehabilitation Counseling.* New York, NY: Springer.

CHAPTER 8

DOCUMENTATION EVOLUTION: ELECTRONIC HEALTH RECORDS

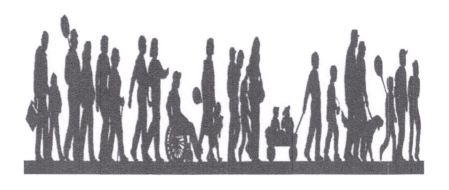

SI-YI CHAO

ALAYNA THOMAS

ABSTRACT

There is an increasing trend of using computer-based infrastructure and software to construct electronic record-keeping systems in the public sector, private practice, and non-profit human service facilities and agencies. Thus, the advance in technology has made electronic record keeping systems an inevitable replacement of traditional paper records. This chapter will introduce the components and items which are included in the record system, functions that can help human service professionals and administrative staff achieve effective and efficient case management by way of a compatible record keeping system. This chapter will also discuss the ethical, confidentiality, and legal considerations while using an electronic record keeping system.

HIGHLIGHTS

➤   The evolution of electronic health records (EHRs).

➤   Selecting an appropriate electronic health records system.

➤   The pros and cons of electronic health records system vendors.

➤   The considerations in electronic health records.

OBJECTIVES

➤   To recognize the need for keeping records for client, stakeholders and human service providers.

➤   To build up the essential items in electronic health records (EHRs) system.

➤   To decide the appropriate record keeping software and services of companies.

➤   To understand the ethical and legal considerations involved when using electronic health records system.

INTRODUCTION

Record keeping is a key component of the case management process.[3] Furthermore, the rise in technology has shown the benefits of technology as it relates to recording client information using electronic health records (EHRs). The use of electronic health records (EHRs) has proven to be so profound that laws such as the American Recovery and Reinvestment Act were enacted.

The American Recovery and Reinvestment Act requires all public and private healthcare providers and other eligible professionals (EP) to adopt and demonstrate "meaningful use" of electronic health records (EHR) to maintain their existing Medicaid and Medicare reimbursement levels. As a result of the American Recovery and Reinvestment Act mandate, research data have shown that seventy-two percent of office-based physicians in 2012 use electronic health records (EHRs) system as compared to approximately thirty-five percent of physicians in 2007.[6] When human service professionals deliver services to clients, the entire process is recorded by paper or electronic system including appointment time, intake interview, evaluation results, assessment tools results, treatment plan, treatment diary (treatment implementation), and so on.

An efficient record keeping system can promote a tight working alliance among staff, professionals, clients, and related stakeholders (e.g., clinic supervisors, administrative supervisors, insurance companies, other funding resources, etc.) and improve the service quality and service outcomes.[2] The human service case manager has access to the progress of the client through his/her records and is able to keep consistent track of the health and treatment conditions of the client. Now more and more human services organizations, facilities, or agencies in the public sector, private practice, and the non-profit sector utilize an electronic record keeping system as a treatment tool to document the information and data regarding the client to assist with the clinical decision-making processes of treatments and services.[8] Therefore, human service professionals need to enhance their knowledge and skills in using EHRs to document, maintain, manage, plan, and evaluate human service performances and outcomes for the clients.

THE EVOLUTION OF ELECTRONIC HEALTH RECORDS

The Healthcare Information and Management Systems Society stated that "Electronic health record is a longitudinal electronic record of patient health information generated by one or more encounters in any care delivery setting." [4, 5, p.2] EHRs system is an integration which consists of a holistic view of clients. EHRs record the personal information of clients, the evaluations from the professionals, the laboratory tests or psychological assessments, the treatment plan and medication, the progress of treatments, and the outcomes of treatment.

Previously, when clients sought human services, they needed to bring their paper documents to the human service provider. When the client had a more extensive medical and behavioral health care history, the paper recording documents became longer which made it hard to transmit between agencies. Utilizing paper documentation made it easy to miss information regarding test results, medication prescription, problem lists, and treatment plans of other involved professionals (e.g., physician, nurse, therapist, psychologist, social worker, etc.).[4] Missing data and illegible handwriting also resulted from the busy and intense service load. In the clinical setting, human service professionals often managed a large caseload, and the professionals could not spend much time to flip through, search, and review the previous records. After the treatment, the professionals often did not have sufficient time to immediately write down the treatment process because of the need to attend to the next client. Human service professionals also became accustomed to storing a tremendous volume of paper records that occupied spaces in these organizations, facilities, and agencies. Frequently, paper documents could not be protected well because of humidity, insects and animal damage, and missing pages. Furthermore, clients' privacy was a risk unless each storage unit for paper records had a lock. The storage of paper records in cabinets proved to be problematic as a result of the need to request permission for keys and limited accessibility to client's overall health records from other providers.[4] When a professional wanted to review the paper records of the client, the professional turned in an application to the storage place for permission. The professional needed to wait to receive the paper record documents from the storage room. Gradually, paper recording was found to be burdensome, time and space consuming, less accessible, and flawed.

The electronic record keeping system is evolving to replace paper documents. A case in point is the 2005 Health Insurance Portability and Accountability Act (HIPAA) which adopted the security rules for health care providers. Human service providers must follow the standards of security protection to manage electronically protected health information (ePHI) of clients in the EHR system. The rules protected accessibility rights of health information and addressed the exchange of private information with other stakeholders (e.g., other professionals, insurers, government, patients and their families, researchers, etc.).[9] In 2009, President Obama announced the Health Information Technology for Economic and Clinical Health Act (HITECH) which stimulated the utilization of EHR systems to improve health care for patients.[16] In 2011, medical service providers who demonstrated the meaningful use of EHRs systems were eligible to receive incentive payments up to 44,000 dollars.[7] The criteria of meaningful use in EHR includes the improvement of care coordination for public health, the improvement of quality and efficiency management of using EHRs, the elimination of health care disparities, the facilitation of clients and families engagement in the care process, and the management of privacy and security of clients' health information. King, Patel, Jamoom, and Furukawa[7] mentioned that seventy-eight percent of physicians improved their patient care by using EHRs. The physician using EHRs system stated that the benefits of EHRs brought positive outcomes of clinical quality, patient safety, and efficiency during the medical healthcare process.[7] The research showed that eighty-one percent of the participants (the physicians) perceived that they can access the health records of the patients in the workplace and home as a clinical benefit. Approximately sixty-five percent of the participants gained benefits from EHRs because the system can alert them to a potential error in medication and lab values.[7] In addition, the current trend of electronic technology affected the acceptance and use of EHRs system and practice management software by human service professionals. Each state in the United States also encouraged behavioral health professionals such as counselors and psychologists to use the EHRs system under HITECH rules. It is hoped that the generalization of EHRs systems not only promotes more human service providers to adopt the EHRs system for case management, but also to construct a comprehensive EHRs system like Health Information Exchanges to transact, manage, and exchange the health information of clients with other stakeholders (e.g., supervisors, insurance companies, other professionals, clients, and related agencies, etc.). The further utilization of EHRs systems brings integration and efficiency of case management and avoids time and cost consumption. It is important to know the resource, HealthIT.gov, funded by the U.S. government provides abundant information to educate the human service providers about the policies, utilization, and management of EHRs. In summation, when compared to paper recording, the electronic record system provides lightweight, time-saving, portable, easily accessible, and highly secure tools for human service case management.

The following goals reflect an efficient and systematic record system:[8]

1. The facilitation of communication between human service providers, stakeholders (insurance companies, funding resources), and service clients. Records help human service providers obtain information about the client and recognize service progress. Human service providers can present records for the client such as past and current biopsychosocial conditions and discuss the possibility of protocol progress.

2. Assist in the development and decision-making of treatment plans, treatment implementing conditions, and the termination of the case.

3. Evaluate the service quality and treatment outcomes.

4. Provide continuing care, treatment, or human services by tracking conditions of the clients.

5. Communicate with the clinical practice supervisor and administrative supervisor to ensure ethical practices of the human service professional.

6. Decrease the waiting time for document agreements and transaction time of paper records to other relevant stakeholders (e.g., other professionals, administrative staff, supervisors, insurance company, and other funding resources).

7. Develop records easy to complete by clicking items, scanning paper documents, and examining results by internet rather than handwriten documents.

8. Decrease the error rates and uncertainty with clear and necessary record items and notes.

9. Provide a database for research purposes such as demographic data, treatment performance appraisal, treatment outcomes, and intervention strategies.[2] Systematic data can assist the human service agency to present evidence-based practice of services and to develop improved services for clients.

10. Most importantly, cost-saving from the elimination of unnecessary paper, storage expenses, and transferring fees.

SELECTING AN APPROPRIATE ELECTRONIC HEALTH RECORDS SYSTEM

Before contracting with the EHR vendor, the human service professional can conduct a needs assessment to figure out how to construct the items in the electronic record system. Needs assessment includes several parts such as the service population, service type, organization employee size, requirements of electronic record systems, the involvement of other stakeholders, and the services provided by the electronic health company.[1] Richards said that "Selecting an ideal electronic record system is like selecting a spouse."[15, p.15] Choosing an appropriate electronic record system takes time based on the needs of the organization and the services provided by the software vendor. If the organization does not conduct a needs assessment and select the appropriate vendor, the collaboration between organization and system vendor will be unproductive. The following items can help human service providers assess the needs of EHRs management and the characteristics that vendors can provide.

Recognize the mission, vision, and value of the organization. It is the foundation of human service professionals to choose the population for whom the human service agency provides services, the stakeholders who are involved in the service process, service activities the agency provides, and the features that improve service quality, service outcomes, and efficiency. The information above helps the human service professionals to construct the customized electronic record system platform.

Think about the organizational structure. A human service agency or facility would like to utilize an electronic record system to manage the service process and outcomes for customers (patients, clients). The agency or facility needs to consider the size, type, and culture of the agency or facility. The organizational structure will aid in evaluating and deciding the appropriate electronic recording system, the accessibility for staff logging into the system, and how to conduct educational courses for the employees and staff to learn about and administer the electronic record system.

The features of an electronic record system. A practice's record management system consists of bill payment, functions of record keeping, software upgrade, and long term technological support services. The following information provides partial features that can be customized based on the needs of the human service providers, the human service agencies, and the population being served.[11]

> ➤ *Diagnostic Codes*: Include the medical and mental health diagnosis and knowledge data base reference information, e.g., the International Classification of Diseases, 10th revision, Clinical Modification (ICD-10- CM); the Diagnostic and Statistical Manual of Mental Disorders (5th ed.; DSM-5); and the related disability measure, the World Health Organization Diagnostic Assessment Schedule 2.0 (WHODAS 2.0); an electronic library, or other customized references.

> ➤ *Service code and procedure code*: The organized and customized categories help the user find the item and fill out the information based on the needs of clients. The codes consist of the eligibility determination, service categories, treatment types, treatment activities, treatment time, service status, payment status of the client, and so on.

> ➤ *Medication lists*: Contains all types of medication names, functions, and side effects.

> ➤ *Social network:* A human service agency collaborates and connects with referral human service agencies and other social resources by an electronic record system. The contact information of the referral agencies and social resources needs to be maintained and updated to provide the correct information for clients.

> ➤ *Intake evaluations, assessment, and plan:* Customize the items of biopsychosocial evaluation, assessment tools, and treatment plan.

➤ *Facilitate engagement of clients/patients*: To utilize an Application (App), software for mobile and tablet devices assists the clients/patients and their families to access personal health management online. Each client has his/her own account number and password to log in the EHRs system for registration, bill-checking, scheduling, and bill payment. Besides, the text function, voice message, email, and phone calls to remind the client about the appointment time can facilitate customer recruitment and enagement.

➤ *Manage appointment schedule:* The calendar schedule of appointments is the reminder (phone call, SMS, or email) for clients and human service case managers of appointment times, online appointment reservation portal, and easy appointment finder.

➤ *Accounting:* Bill payment management, expense tracking, profit and expense, payment balance tracking, payment due time reminder for human service professionals and agencies.

➤ *Customized Insurance Claim Forms:* Transfer claims easily to address requirements of different insurance companies and other thrid party insurers.

➤ *Easy to Use:* Data imput is easy to recognize, organized, and mostly use click function instead of typing notes.

➤ *Easily Correct Mistakes:* The system can help the user to automatically correct mistakes without a complicated adjustment process.

➤ *Export Data:* Any type of document can be exported as PDF, Word, Excel, RTF, etc. which matches the Window Microsoft and Apple IOS system.

➤ *Backup and Restore:* The safe storage of records, the space volume of storage, minimal risk of privacy and missing records.

➤ *Customer support service:* Fast and efficient support service when users of electronic record systems need technical support. Support can also include any user manuals or instructions for reference.

➤ *Update:* Regular updating the software to improve the comprehensive functions and uploading speed to save time. In addition, you need to inquire if the vendor has extra fees for updating EHRs system and software.

➤ *Network Compatible:* Multiple users can access the record system and can upload the record of clients simultaneously.

➤ *Password protection:* The security and safety to store the record data of clients which is Health Insurance Portability and Accountability Act (HIPAA) compliant.

➤ *Additional device accessibility:* Mobile APP (software application) and the cloud provide users easy access into the electronic record system and the ability to check health conditions and current treatment records at any time and any place. Users can use their own mobile devices to detect and follow-up with clients away from the office.

Choosing a vender can be a difficult decision. A good vender of EHRs can satisfy the users' needs and the expectations; whereas a vendor that is not as proficient may cost the user more than money (e.g., losing time and efficacy in serving clients). There is no universal system to fufill all the requirements of each human service provider and agency. Before purchasing the EHRs system software, it is vital to recognize the essential structure of the record system and take advantage of the free test trial provided by the vendor to decide the most appropriate vendor for the electronic record system.[4] Also, the human service provider should discuss and negotiate with the vendor the content included within the contract, how much the system can be customized, support services, updating fee(s), and additional services. The goal of selecting an appropriate vendor is to obtain a beneficial EHRs system with cost-effectiveness and efficiency for the case management process.

THE PROS AND CONS OF EHRs SYSTEM VENDORS

PROS

With the cost of the US national health expenditure currently at 17 percent of the gross domestic product, the stakeholders of the government are now, more than ever, looking for ways to reduce costs while simultaneously increasing quality of care.[12] The utilization of electronic health records has proven to be cost efficient while concurrently increasing the quality of care for clients. Research suggests the efficiency of EHRs is relative to the size of the healthcare facility. Electronic health records are beneficial to healthcare providers as they allow for immediate access to client's medical history. Healthcare providers could have a better understanding of their client and are able to provide higher quality services as healthcare providers recognize and treat medical problems more efficiently. Research also indicates electronic record systems are beneficial to healthcare providers as well as clients due to the elimination of human error. Physicians are infamously known for poor penmanship, thus, the utilization of EHRs will ensure that client's medical records are legible.

CONS

There is a myriad of benefits for human service providers utilizing electronic records systems, however, there still are notable disadvantages. Although healthcare providers have implemented standard procedures to protect the client's identity, due to advances in technology, healthcare providers are perpetually at risk of their databases being compromised. Electronic health records are a new phenomenon. Although, EHRs have been adopted by most healthcare providers, EHRs and their use have not been standardized across the various electronic record software. For example, there are no universal abbreviations for services and/or diagnoses. Therefore, human service providers should consider in depth the advantages and disadvantages of each electronic record system prior to purchasing.

Some useful online sources provide the references to assist decision-making in selecting EHRs vendors. First, GetApp,is a a website that provides the choices, exploration, and comparison of the business software. You can search for electronic records software for human services. Abundant information on vendors, features, ranking, and prices are presented and compared. Another source is a blog entitled *Tame your practice*.[14] The blog provides reviews of EHRs vendors with ranking, advantages, and weaknesses. Based on the rankings shared by the reviewers in GetApp and the blog, five vendors, *Counsol, ClinicSource, SimplePractice, TherapyNotes*, and *TheraNest*, were chosen to present information in tables (*See* Table 1 and Table 2). Table 1 presents the information of Counsol, ClinicSource, and SimplePractice; Table 2 presents the information of TherapyNotes and TheraNest. The information in both tables (Table 1, 2) illustrates the names of vendors, weblinks of the vendors, populations using the software, and accessible devices. It also divides the information into seven domains, Client documents management, Calendar and Scheduling, Account and bill management, Security and law compliance, System management, Expenses, and Pros and cons. Each domain has several sub items that present the functions and platforms provided by the vendors. The main purpose of the tables is to identify EHRs services that vendors can provide, for use in understanding and comparison of systems. If the clinical practitioner would like to build his/her private practice, the practitioner can search for the vendor consultant who can assist the user to choose appropriate EHRs software by understanding the needs and preferences of the user. As you can see, there is a lot of variability from price to what kind of payment the case management software can accept.

TABLE 1

THE COMPARISON OF ELECTRONIC HEALTH RECORDS
SOFTWARE VENDORS

	Counsol	ClinicSource	SimplePractice
Webpage link	https://www.counsol.com	https://www.clinicsource.com/	https://www.simplepracti com/features
People that use the software	Psychologists, Psychiatrists, Counselors, Social workers, and Therapists	Physical therapists; Occupational therapists; Speech-language pathologists; Behavioral health care professionals	Psychologists, Psychiatrists, Counselors, Social workers, and Therapists
Device accessibility	Web-based (web Browser with no software installment); cloud-based, which means the user access with a smartphone, tablet, or computer with internet	Web and cloud-based (web based (web Browser with no software installment)	Web-based (web Browser with no software installment); Mobile App via iPhone/iPad app and android devices
CLIENT DOCUMENT MANAGEMENT			
Customized forms	Customized forms	Customized forms	Lack of integration of progressive notes and treatment plans
Diagnosis code	ICD-10	ICD-10	An ICD-10 list combining with DSM 5; can create mental status test
Document management	Effective document management	Effective document management	Effective document management
Import the data	No information	Easy to import and transfer previous notes and data	No information
Export Data	Easy to select and export the notes and files with any format	Export schedules and notes to a PDF file	Easy to export the notes and files with any format
Backup	Hourly backed up with	Regular Nightly Backups	Routine Backups and Disaster Recovery
CALENDAR & SCHEDULING			
Appointment schedule management	Easy-use and clear interface	Easy-operated Schedule Calendar	Easy-operated Schedule Calendar. Easy-use and clear interface
Incorporation of schedule calendar	iCal	Google calendar, Outlook and iCal	Google calendar, Outlook and iCal
Appointment reminder	Automatically send notification texts, emails and phone calls	Automatically send notification texts, emails and phone calls	Unlimited email, voice, and text reminders for the user and clients

	Counsol	ClinicSource	SimplePractice

CALENDAR & SCHEDULING (Cont.)

	Counsol	ClinicSource	SimplePractice
Client engagement	Client portal, which client can access his/her own account to schedule the appointment, share intake documents, secure messaging, and pay with credit card	None	Client Portal

ACCOUNT and BILL MANAGEMENT

	Counsol	ClinicSource	SimplePractice
Billing statement and reports	Can track daily payment history including agency accounts receivable and payable	Can track daily payment history including accounts receivable and payable	Can track daily payment history including accounts receivable and payable
Tracking and processing client payment	Easy to tract the client's payment conditions and process bill filing.	• Easy to tract the payment conditions, credits and balance of the clients • Easy to process bills.	• Easy to tract the payment conditions, credits and balance of the clients. • Easy to process bills.
Electronic claims	No charges of electronic claims	Electronic billing for 49.95/month	25¢ for each electronic claim (up to 6 sessions per claim); 5¢ for coverage report
Payment options	Integrated credit card services, paypal	Credit card and e-check processing	Credit card

SECURITY and LAWS COMPLIANCE

	Counsol	ClinicSource	SimplePractice
Security	Ensure the protection personal health information of the clients	Ensure the protection personal health information of the clients	Ensure the protection personal health information of the clients
HIAAP compliance	Follow the requirements of HIAAP	Follow the requirements of HIAAP	Follow the requirements of HIAAP

SYSTEM MANAGEMENT

	Counsol	ClinicSource	SimplePractice
Network Compatible	Single location	Single location	Single location
Analysis of data base	None	None	Client demographics; information reports; revenue reports; and referral sources tracking
Customer support service	Good customer support	Good customer support	Good customer support
Updated fee	No information	No information	Need to pay updated fee
Free trail	First 30 days trail. The fee can be refunded with less satisfaction	30 days	30 days
Schedule a demo	https://DrJohnDoe.SecurePatientArea.com	https://www.clinicsource.com/	None

	Counsol	ClinicSource	SimplePractice
EXPENSES			
Price	Starting from standard package $49.95/month with no setup fee. Plus package $64.95/month with no setup fee https://counsol.com/site/package/pricing/	$59.95/month for: • 1 user, • 1 billing location, • 2 hours initial training,1 gigabyte attachment storage, • No setup fees https://www.clinicsource.com/therapy-emr-pricing/	$49 / month Unlimited Non-Clinical Staff users (e.g., receptionists, schedulers, bookkeepers, billers) https://www.simplepractice.com/pricing
Accessible user (employees, staff, billers)	Solo clinical user	$29.95/month for each additional full-time users with unlimited visits	$29/month for each additional clinician
Additional charge		• 1 Billing Location for $29.95/month, • 1 gigabyte attachment storage for $9.95/month • 7¢ for each text and 15¢ for each phone call appointment reminder • 30 minutes Telephone Support for $39.95	
PROS and CONS			
Pros and Cons	Pros: • Customized forms. • Client portal. Cons: • Applying on solo clinical practitioner	Pros: • Good integration of treatment plan and notes. Cons: • But the integrated forms are targeted for therapists instead of mental health professionals, • High cost and many additional charges.	Pros: • Easy-use and clear interface. • Client portal. • Has mobile App. Cons: • The lack of integration between treatment plans and progressive notes

TABLE 2

THE COMPARISON OF ELECTRONIC HEALTH RECORDS SOFTWARE VENDORS

	TherapyNotes	TheraNest
Webpage link	https://www.therapynotes.com/?utm_campaign=Capterra&utm_so	https://www.theranest.com/
People that use the software	Psychologists, Psychiatrists, Counselors, Social workers, and Therapists	Psychologists, mental health care professionals, social worker, behavioral care professionals, group mental health treatment, Marriage & Family Therapists
Device accessibility	Web-based (web Browser with no software installment). Windows, Macs, iPads, iPhone, android devices and other tablets can access	Web and clouded-based (web Browser with no software installment). Mobile App via iPhone/ iPad app and android devices
CLIENT DOCUMENT MANAGEMENT		
Customized forms	Customized forms with full integration	Less integration of progressive notes and treatment plans
Diagnosis code	ICD-10; mental health terms	DSM 5 and ICD 10
Document management	Effective document management	Easy to check and review the incomplete documents
Import the data	No information	Import, transfer and upload the data with any format
Export Data	Easily download or print notes into a PDF	Easily download or print notes into a PDF
Backup	Routine Backups and Disaster Recovery	Data backup in multiple locations
CALENDAR & SCHEDULING		
Appointment schedule management	• Easy-operated Schedule Calendar, Easy-use and clear interface. • To-Do lists for client appointment and agency meeting	• Easy-operated Schedule Calendar. • Easy-use and clear interface
Incorporation of schedule calendar	Google calendar, Outlook, iCal or another compatible calendar software	Google calendar, and iCal
Appointment reminder	Automatic text, phone, and email	Text, phone, and email
Client engagement	Client portal, which client can access his/her own account to schedule the appointment, share intake documents, secure	Client portal

messaging, and pay with credit
card

	TherapyNotes	TheraNest
ACCOUNT and BILL MANAGEMENT		
Billing statement and reports	Can track daily payment history including agency accounts receivable and payable	Can track daily payment history including agency accounts receivable and payable
Tracking and processing client payment	• Easy to tract the payment conditions, credits and balance of the clients • Easy to process bills. • An alert system to remind the bill filing.	• Easy to tract the payment conditions, credits and balance of the clients • Easy to process bills.
Electronic claims	14¢ for each electronic claim	No charges of electronic claims
Payment options	Credit card, debit	Credit card; Online transection
SECURITY and LAWS COMPLIANCE		
Security	Ensure the protection personal health information of the clients	Send messages and share files securely with your clients through the client portal (admission).
HIAAP compliance	Follow the requirements of HIAAP	Follow the requirements of HIAAP
SYSTEM MANAGEMENT		
Network Compatible	Multiple location support, multiple users can access at the same time; home care support	Multiple location support
Analysis of data base	None	Client demographics; information reports; revenue reports; and referral sources tracking
Customer support service	Good customer support	Good customer support
Updated fee	Automatic update	No information
Free trail	30 days	21 days
Schedule a demo	https://www.therapynotes.com/contact/	https://calendly.com/theranest/demo1/09-26-2017?utm_source=theranest&utm_medium=button&utm_campaign=schedule-a-demo
EXPENSES		
Price	$59.00/month for one user https://www.therapynotes.com/about/pricing/	Starting from $29/month (30 active clients) The prices vary by the numbers of active clients

https://www.theranest.com/pricing/

	TherapyNotes	TheraNest
EXPENSES (Cont.)		
Accessible user (employees, staff, billers)	$30/month for additional users	Unlimited users without additional charges
Additional charge	14¢ for each phone and text appointment reminder	None
PROS and CONS		
Pros and Cons	Pros: • Friendly interface. • Integrated forms. • Have reminding system for the user and clients about the appointment and bill filing. Cons: • Have charges on electronic claim.	Pros: • Good price of small business (30 clients). • Easy-use interface. • Client portal. • Mobile App. Cons: • Less integration of treatment plan and progressive notes from different formats.

COMPONENTS OF
ELECTRONIC HEALTH RECORDS

A good electronic health system also needs to consider ethical and legal concerns that may lead to potential adverse consequences For example, the healthcare agency rejects the services for high-risk clients or the insurer raises the premium of the client with multiple disabilities or complicated medical conditions because of the ability of healthcare providers to access client's medical history via the EHRs system.[2] Because of the advantages of easy access and exchange of information in the EHRs system, human service providers should consider the risks and threats of security and privacy issues of electronic personal health information. There is no 100 % guaranteed way to do enough to keep the confidentiality and security of electronic information. It is a vital task of the EHRs system to maintain the privacy and security of clients, and the privacy and disclosure of information to related insurance companies, other involved professionals, and larger health corporations and systems.[13] Also, the EHRs system should adhere to ethical principles of the federal and state government. The laws include methods for obliterating the client's electronic information when the client terminates services. Therefore, human service providers must find a way to balance and stay in compliance with their own professional codes of ethics, legislation, and the agency policies, to minimize harming clients.

The evolving technology, the increasing use of EHRs systems, and the impact of the HIPAA and HITECH lead the Health and Human Services Department (HHS) to revise separate HIPAA rules for electronic record keeping systems.[8] The purpose of the HIPAA Security Rule is to establish standards for technological security, confidentiality, and acquiring private health records during electronic storage, maintenance, and transmission. The HIPPA rules can protect the privacy and security of the client's health information. It is recommended that human service providers discuss with the selected EHRs system vendor the importance of privacy and security while exchanging and disclosing health information with insurers and other professionals. The vendor may design some specific security steps to ensure the confidentiality, integrity, and availability of the client's health information.[4]

Mental health information regarding clients is a different situation. To protect the privacy of clients, when the client has co-occurring medical and mental health issues, the human services provider must acquire permission from the client to disclose either type of information. The human service provider adheres to the nonmaleficence principle, doing no harm toward a client while using the EHRs system.

DISCUSSION

1. The chapter suggests the use of electronic health record (EHR) helps to establish a working alliance and improves service quality. Who is benefitted by this working alliance and improvement in service quality? Why?

2. The chapter suggests electronic health record (EHR) provide a holistic view of the client. According to the chapter, what information is included in a client's EHR?

3. How does the use of electronic health record (EHR) benefit research?

4. What should a human service provider consider when selecting an electronic record system?

5. According to the chapter, what are some disadvantages of electronic record systems?

CASE STUDY
DR. HART

Dr. Hart is an interventional cardiologist in Potomac, MD. Dr. Hart has been in practice for 15 years and he provides specialized care for the heart and cardiovascular system. In speaking with his clients over the years, Dr. Hart noticed that a considerable portion of his clients reported having stress because of the demands of their families and work. Since Dr. Hart had only utilized paper-based documentation, he did not have access to the client's records from their family physician. Therefore, Dr. Hart was not able to confirm his belief that client's environment affected their health. To improve his quality of care, Dr. Hart decided that electronic record software would be a good option. Upon researching electronic record software, Dr. Hart determined the software that would be most suited for his practice would include appointment time, intake interview, evaluation results, assessment tools results, treatment plan, and treatment diary (treatment implementation). To protect his clients, Dr. Hart discussed with the vendor of the electronic health record system the importance of privacy and security in exchanging and disclosing health information with insurers and other professionals. Eventually, Dr. Hart selected an adequate electronic record system. Dr. Hart was now able to have access to client's records from other human service providers and thus have a holistic view of the client.

CONCLUSION

The evolution of EHRs systems brings conveniences for human service case management. Human service professionals can easily access and obtain the health information of the client which allows the client's other human service providers to communicate and enhance the consistency and continuum of services for clients. However, the conveniences also bring threats to confidentiality, privacy, and security of record keeping of the clients' electronic personal health information.[10] Therefore, the human service provider selects an appropriate EHRs system vendor to assist case management by discussion and implementation of its practice software. It is necessary that the vendors understand the needs of users to design a customized platform and mechanism for electronically protected health information of clients. Additionally, the users and vendors need to follow the ethical and legal principles to store, maintain, protect, and exchange the information through EHRs systems. A cost-effective and efficient EHRs system does no harm to clients using human services.

REFERENCE

[1]Adams, A. J. & Culp M. L. (2005). Needs Assessment. In E. J., Bieber, F. M., Richards, & J. M., Walker (Eds.). *Implementing an Electronic Health Record System* (pp. 9-14). London, UK: Springer.

[2]Adler, N. E., & Stead, W. W. (2015). Patients in context—EHR capture of social and behavioral determinants of health. *Obstetrical & gynecological survey, 70*(6), 388-390.

[3]Bieber, E. J., Richards, F. M., & Walker, J. M. (2005). *Implementing an electronic health record system.* London, UK: Springer.

[4]Campbell, R. J. (2015). The electronic health record and the mental health professional. In M. A. Stebnicki, The professional counselor's desk reference (2nd ed.). New York, NY: Springer Publishing Company. Retrieved from http://proxy.lib.siu.edu/login?url=http://search.credoreference.com/content/entry/sppcd/the_electronic_health_record_and_the_mental_health_professional/0?institutionId=3648

[5]Healthcare Information and Management Systems Society (2014). The electronic health record. Retrieved from www.himss.org/library/ehr.

[6]Hsiao, C. J., Hing, E., & Ashman, J. (2014). *Trends in Electronic Health Record System Use Among Office-based Physicians, United States, 2007-2012.* US Department of Health and Human Services, Centers for Disease Control and Prevention, National Center for Health Statistics.

[7]King, J., Patel, V., Jamoom, E. W., & Furukawa, M. F. (2014). Clinical benefits of electronic health record use: national findings. *Health services research, 49*(1pt2), 392-404.

Luepker, E. T. (2012). *Record keeping in psychotherapy and counseling: Protecting confidentiality and the professional relationship*. New York, NY: Routledge.

Lawley, J. S. (2012). HIPAA, HITECH and the practicing counselor: Electronic records and practice guidelines. *The Professional Counselor*, *2*(3), 192-200.

Nielsen, B. A. (2015). Confidentiality and electronic health records: Keeping up with advances in technology and expectations for access. *Clinical Practice in Pediatric Psychology*, *3*(2), 175-178. doi:10.1037/cpp0000096

Marlene, M. M., Pulier, M. L., Wilhelm, F. H., McMenamin, J. P., & Brown-Connolly, N. E. (2004). *The mental health professional and the new technologies*. Mahwah, NJ: Lawrence Erlbaum Associates, Inc.

Otto, P., & Nevo, D. (2013). Electronic health records. *Journal of Enterprise Information Management, 26*(1/2), 165-182. doi:10.1108/17410391311289613

Pope, K. (2015). Record-Keeping Controversies: Ethical, Legal, and Clinical Challenges. *Canadian Psychology-Psychologie Canadienne*, *56*(3), 348-356.

Reinhardt, R. (2017, Jun. 14). *Cloud Practice Management System EHR/EMR – Reviews*. Retrieved from https://tameyourpractice.com/blog/cloud-practice-management-system-reviews

Richards, F. (2005). Vendor Selection and Contract Negotiation. In E. J., Bieber, F. M., Richards, & J. M., Walker (Eds.). *Implementing an Electronic Health Record System* (pp. 15-20). London, UK: Springer.

Simon, L. (2015). Electronic Health Records Technology: Policies and Realities. In, N. A., Dewan, J. S., Luo, & N. M., Lorenzi (Eds.). *Mental Health Practice in a Digital World: A Clinicians Guide*. (pp. 13-36). Switzerland: Springer International Publishing.

CHAPTER 9

FUNDING SOURCES

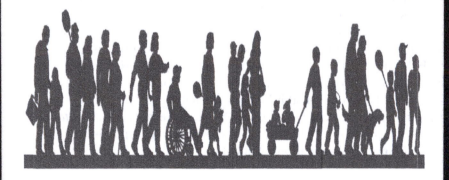

CARRIE L. ACKLIN

ABSTRACT

For people to receive health and human services, there must be some type of funding that covers the healthcare services that the person is seeking. In this chapter, we will look at the various types of funding sources that are available in the health and human services. Specific attention will be paid to the types of public, private, and grant-funded sources. Also included in this chapter is an overview of common terminology that is used when talking about funding sources. Special attention will be paid to how members of underrepresented groups (e.g., women, people with disabilities, people of color) are impacted by the various types of funding sources as well as barriers that members of underrepresented groups face when accessing health and human services.

CHAPTER HIGHLIGHTS

➢ Common terms and definitions that are used when referring to funding sources;

➢ Discussion regarding public, private, and grant-funded sources;

➢ Implications of the various funding sources on members of underrepresented groups.

LEARNING OBJECTIVES

➢ Identify and discuss features and components of public, private, and grant-funded sources;

➢ Identify, define, and explain common funding sources terminology;

➢ Identify and explain issues that are experienced by members of underrepresented groups.

OVERVIEW OF FUNDING SOURCES

Several health and human services that clients' access have been discussed in other chapters. In this chapter, we will examine how various health and human services are paid for. There are several ways that health and human sources are paid for. The entities that pay for services are referred to as funding sources. We will examine three main categories of funding sources: public health insurance, private health insurance, and grant-funded. Further, we will examine:

> ➤ eligibility criteria for each funding source;

> ➤ what services the funding source covers; and

> ➤ costs associated with the funding source.

There are several reasons why having a well-rounded understanding of funding sources is important for the practitioner. First, the types of services that a person is eligible for is largely dictated by the type of funding he or she does or does not have. Second, in many cases, the practitioner (or someone within the practitioner's agency) will have to review the types of services with the funding source. Third, there are times when the amount of services is limited by the funding source (for example, a funding source might only pay for a certain number of sessions in a given timeframe). Fourth, having a well-rounded understanding of funding sources is important because agencies need funding to provide services. First, let's look at what health insurance is.

WHAT IS HEALTH INSURANCE?

Health insurance is a way of covering the cost of healthcare services. As we will see in Part Two of this book, healthcare services can be defined as a broad set of services provided to individuals. Healthcare services can be medical, behavioral, vocational, occupational, or assistive. To receive services, the person must have a way to pay for the healthcare services. There are several ways a person can pay for the healthcare services, one way being through health insurance. It is important to note that health insurance is often referred to as "coverage." Thus, the terms health insurance and coverage can be used synonymously. Health insurance provides coverage for healthcare services; however, the nature and extent of coverage varies depending on the type of insurance. Health insurance can be broken down into two main categories: Public and private (which we will discuss later). Before we move into a discussion about public and private health insurance, here is some common terminology that will be used throughout this chapter that relates specifically to health insurance.

PLAN. A plan refers to what the health insurance will and will not cover. Many health insurance plans include the following: premium, deductible, co-payment, out of pocket expense, benefits, annual maximum limit, and co-insurance. Some insurances also have what is referred to as a lifetime maximum limit (defined below).

PREMIUM. A premium refers to the amount of money that a person must pay to have health insurance. There are two terms that are commonly used: Annual premium and monthly premium. An annual premium refers to the amount of money per year a person must pay to have insurance. A monthly premium refers to the amount of money a person pays per month to have insurance. As we will see later in this chapter, premiums vary based on the type of coverage that the person has. In addition to premiums, most insurance companies have what is called a deductible.

DEDUCTIBLE. A deductible is a set amount of money a person must pay before services will be covered by health insurance. For example, if a person has a $500 deductible, that means that the person must pay for the first $500 dollars of services before the health insurance will pay for the rest. Deductibles vary based on the type of coverage that the person has. Co-payments, much like deductibles, can vary based on the type of coverage the person has.

CO-PAYMENT. A co-payment (often referred to as co-pay) is a set amount of money that the person pays before receiving a service. For example, if a person has a co-pay of $30.00 for a primary care physician appointment, that means that the person must pay the $30.00 before he or she is seen by the physician. Co-pays are determined in a variety of ways. Some insurances pre-determine the amount of the co-pay while other insurances use the person's income to determine the amount of the co-pay. Co-pays also vary based on the type of services that are received. It might be the case, for instance, that a person has a $30.00 co-pay for primary care physician appointments, but there might be a $20.00 co-pay for an individual counseling session. In addition to co-payments, the person might have out-of-pocket expenses.

OUT OF POCKET EXPENSE. An out of pocket expense refers to the amount of money a person pays in deductibles and co-payments each year. Once the person has met their out of pocket expense, he or she does not have to make any other payments toward healthcare services. Thus, the person would no longer have to make a co-payment at his or her appointments.

BENEFIT. A benefit refers to the types of healthcare services that the insurance will cover. There are several types of benefits: medical, behavioral health, dental, and vision (to name a few). Examples of coverage for medical benefits are primary care physician appointments, specialist appointments (e.g., going to the chiropractor, going to a physical therapist, going to an OBGYN), emergency room visits, and hospitalizations. Examples of behavioral health benefits are substance abuse counseling, mental health counseling, case management, crisis intervention, and community support services. Dental benefits cover services that are related to dentistry. This can include routine dental exams, x-rays, fillings for cavities, crowns, braces, or dentures (to name a few). Vision benefits can cover services such as annual eye exams, frames, lenses, and contacts. As shown, there are several types of benefits that health insurance can cover. However, there are times when an insurance company will put a limit on how much of a service a person can access. An example of this is the annual maximum limit.

ANNUAL MAXIMUM LIMIT. An annual maximum limit refers to the amount of services an insurance plan will cover each year. For example, an insurance plan may only cover 30 counseling appointments per year. After the person has used up the 30 counseling appointments, he or she has reached the annual maximum limit and would then pay for the services they received. When a person pays for services, it is often referred to as "self-pay" (which can become quite expensive–discussed in the next section). Some insurance companies have what is called a co-insurance.

CO-INSURANCE. Co-insurance refers to the percentage of health services that the insurance covers. For example, the insurance company may pay for 80% of the cost of services, leaving the additional 20% for the person to pay. Co-insurance is a common method that insurances use to help keep the cost of healthcare down.

LIFETIME MAXIMUM LIMIT. A lifetime maximum limit is like the annual maximum limit in that the lifetime maximum limit refers to the amount of services an insurance plan will cover over the duration of a person's lifetime.

As stated previously, there are several unique terms when it comes to health insurance. It is often the case that many of the insurance terminologies are not readily explained to consumers. Therefore, an essential part of case management is being able to explain insurance terminology to consumers who may not understand what the terms mean. It is imperative for the health and human service provider to understand why having health insurance is so important, as discussed in the next section.

WHY HEALTH INSURANCE IS IMPORTANT: THE RISING COST OF HEALTHCARE

You might be asking yourself why it is important to have health insurance. The answer to this question is complex. In some countries (e.g., Canada), the healthcare system is referred to as Universal Healthcare. Universal Healthcare (a single payer system) is a healthcare system where all healthcare is funded via taxpayer dollars. Therefore, each citizen of the country has healthcare that they do not directly have to pay for (e.g., paying a monthly or annual premium). However, this is not the case in the United States. In the United States, people either:

> meet eligibility criteria for public health insurance which is funded via taxpayer dollars,

> purchase private insurance via the free market (to be explained later),

> receive health insurance via their employer, or

> are uninsured (i.e., do not have any form of healthcare coverage).

Being uninsured can lead to several negative consequences. Suppose there is a person who needs emergency room services, but this person does not have health insurance. An emergency room department cannot deny healthcare services to a person who is uninsured. Therefore, the uninsured person would receive emergency room services, but would also be responsible for paying for the services.

An average emergency room visit can cost thousands of dollars and even more if the person is hospitalized. There are many instances where an uninsured person is not able to cover the cost of healthcare services. Thus, the services go unpaid. When this happens, the cost of healthcare increases. However, this is not the only factor that leads to the rising cost of healthcare in the United States.

Another factor is medical technology. Medical technology is increasing at a very quick pace. As new medical technology is introduced to the health and human services, the cost to use the new technology increases and, the cost of providing healthcare services increases.

It is essential that the health and human service provider has a working knowledge of healthcare coverage, the importance of having coverage, and factors that act as barriers to obtaining healthcare coverage. The reason is that, oftentimes, people seeking health and human services are not aware of their options when it comes to healthcare coverage. The health and human service provider can act as the critical link to the person obtaining healthcare coverage.

Next, we will look at the different types of insurances. The two main categories of health insurance are (1) public health insurance, and (2) private health insurance.

PUBLIC HEALTH INSURANCE

Public health insurance refers to insurance that is paid for via taxpayer dollars. To receive public health insurance, a person must meet certain eligibility criteria. Eligibility criteria is a set of standards and characteristics that a person must possess to receive public health insurance. Public health insurance falls under two main categories: Medicaid and Medicare. Each main category of public health insurance has its own components.

MEDICAID
Medicaid is a type of public health insurance that is provided to individuals and families who fall within a certain income limit. This income limit is often referred to as the "federal poverty limit." The federal poverty limit is an income level that is established by the federal government and represents what is poverty in the United States. The federal poverty limit for a family of four (e.g., two adults and two children) is an annual income of $32,319. To qualify for Medicaid, an individual or family's income must fall

within 138% of the federal poverty limit (i.e., the income of a family of four must be at or below $44,600). Medicaid is a public insurance and is funded through taxpayer dollars. However, we have yet to look at what funding through taxpayer dollars means.

There are two types of income when a person works. The first is referred to as gross income. Gross income refers to the amount of money a person earns during a given pay period (pay periods refer to the length of time a person works before he or she is paid). A pay period is usually bi-weekly or monthly which means that the person receives a paycheck every two weeks or monthly. Suppose that a person earns $600 per pay period. The person will not take home the entire $600 because taxes that are deducted from the paycheck (i.e., federal taxes, state taxes, and (sometimes) local taxes). In addition to these taxes, there are taxes that are taken out of a paycheck that go toward funding Medicaid. The money that is left after all taxes are referred to as net income. Some people feel that it is unfair for working individuals to pay for public insurance, especially if working individuals make too much money to qualify for Medicaid. This assumption can lead to dangerous consequences for members of underrepresented groups.

MEDICARE

Medicare is a second type of public health insurance. However, instead of the eligibility criteria being a certain income limit (as is the case with Medicaid), Medicare is provided to people who are:

➢ 65 years of age and older,

➢ people with disabilities, or

➢ people with end-stage renal disease (kidney failure).

It may be the case that a person meets both the Medicare eligibility criteria and is low-income (the eligibility criteria for Medicaid). People who meet the eligibility criteria for both Medicare and Medicaid are often referred to as "dually-eligible." Medicare is a bit more complex than Medicaid. The reason is because Medicare is broken down into several sections referred to as "parts." Medicare consists of parts A through D.

PART A. Medicare Part A is often referred to as hospital insurance. Part A covers a variety of hospital-based services such as skilled nursing facilities (e.g., nursing homes), inpatient acute care (e.g., hospitalization for a medical condition that has a rapid onset such as a heart attack), inpatient rehabilitation services (e.g., hospital services that help people regain their physical functioning such as walking, eating, dressing), home healthcare (e.g., medical and behavioral healthcare services that are provided to a person within their own home), inpatient behavioral healthcare (e.g., residential psychiatric or substance abuse services), and hospice care (e.g., medical treatment provided to people who are close to the end of their life). Medicare Part A is available to any Medicare recipient regardless of their income level. Other parts to Medicare require that the individual pay a premium based on their income to be covered.

PART B. Medicare Part B is often referred to as supplemental medical insurance. Supplemental medical insurance covers both preventive services and medically necessary services. Preventive care is medical services that are geared toward preventing illness and injury. Examples of preventive care include routine medical screening (e.g., physical exams, bloodwork), vaccinations (such as the flu shot), and cancer screenings.

Medically necessary services refer to healthcare services that are needed to diagnose a condition, or treat a condition. Examples of medically necessary services include medical equipment (e.g., a walker, oxygen tank, breathing machines), some prescription medications, or second opinions before major surgery. Unlike Medicare part A (where the individual does not have to pay a premium to be covered), part B has both a deductible and a premium. The annual deductible is typically about $166 per year followed by a 20% coinsurance. The premium is based off how much a person earns per year. For example, the typical monthly premium for a person or family whose income is less than $85,000 per year is $121. The premium then increases after $85,000.

PART C. Medicare Part C is also called Medicare Advantage. Medicare Advantage is an insurance plan that is available for people to purchase if they are enrolled in both Medicare part A and Medicare part B. Medicare Advantage covers vision, dental, and hearing services in addition to prescription medications. The premiums for Medicare Advantage vary based on where the person lives and may be lower than the premiums for Medicare part B. Typically, the out of pocket expenses for Medicare Advantage are lower than the out of pocket expenses for Medicare parts A and B.

PART D. Medicare part D provides coverage for prescription medications. Prescription medications can either be (1) name brand, or (2) generic. Typically, name brand prescription medications are more expensive than generic brands. Therefore, many insurance plans (in this case, Medicare) categorize prescription medications into what is called tiers. The higher the tier, the more expensive the prescription medication. Conversely, the lower the tier, the less expensive the prescription medication. There are different plans under Medicare part D with each plan having its own premium. The premiums for Medicare part D plans vary and are typically based off the person's income. There is also a deductible for part D coverage. After the deductible is met, the Medicare part D typically covers 75% of the cost of the prescription medication.

Medicaid and Medicare are both public health insurance plans. The distinguishing feature between Medicaid and Medicare is the eligibility criteria. Medicaid provides insurance coverage to individuals and families whose income falls within 138% of the federal poverty limit. Medicare provides insurance coverage to individuals who are 65 or older, people with disabilities, or people with end stage renal (kidney) disease. Approximately 21% of the United States population receives public assistance. However, people who receive Medicaid and Medicare (especially members of underrepresented groups) face certain barriers to healthcare that people with private insurance (to be discussed in the next section) do not. The primary barrier is stigma.

IMPACT OF PUBLIC ASSISTANCE ON UNDERREPRESENTED GROUPS

Take a moment to think about what thoughts, feelings, and emotions come to mind when you read the word "welfare." Were any of your thoughts negative? If so, you are not alone. Many people use the term welfare to refer to people who are receiving public assistance and associate the word "welfare" with negative connotations that are made up of stigma and stereotypes. Here are a few stigmas and stereotypes that are associated with the word "welfare:"

➢ Many people believe that people on welfare are lazy, unmotivated, and unwilling to work.

➢ Many people believe that people on welfare are "addicts" and are abusing the system.

➢ Many people believe that women continue to have children so that they can continue to be on welfare.

These examples are certainly not all-inclusive. However, there are two components regarding stigma associated with receiving public assistance:

➢ Statistics that debunk the stigma, and

➢ how the public-assistance stigma impacts members of underrepresented groups.

DEBUNKING PUBLIC-ASSISTANCE STIGMA. *Many people believe that people on welfare are lazy, unmotivated, and unwilling to work.* According to the United States Department of Agriculture, in 2014 approximately 76% of individuals and families who were receiving public assistance had some form of earned and unearned income. Earned income is income via employment and unearned income is income that is obtained outside of an employment setting. Examples of unearned income are income obtained by annuities, dividends, unemployment compensation, or income from investments. Approximately 1/3 of public assistant recipients have no income. When "somebody knows someone who is lazy and refuses to work" that person generalizes the other person's "laziness" to the entire population of public assistance recipients.

Taking this a step further, people with disabilities have very high employment rates. According to the Bureau of Labor Statistics, approximately 80% of people with disabilities are unemployed. However, what is typically not known is that most people with disabilities want to work, but face systematic barriers to employment. What are those barriers?

First, is how Social Security Disability Insurance (SSDI) is arranged. A person with a disability can only earn so much money before their SSDI benefits are reduced. If a person with a disability makes more money than SSDI allows, then that person is at risk of losing their insurance. Many people with disabilities rely on SSDI for life-sustaining medications and coverage for assistive technology (e.g., prosthetics, walkers, wheelchairs) that they could, otherwise, not afford. You might be asking yourself "but won't the employer provide health insurance for the person?" The answer is yes and no. It is highly likely that the person with a disability may end up in a job where health insurance is not offered. Moreover, many employers are afraid to hire people with disabilities for fear of being sued for not providing accommodations. Many employers also believe that providing accommodations would be far too expensive. However, many accommodations cost little to nothing. For example, an employee with a disability has difficulties standing for long periods of time. A way that an employer can accommodate the employee is by providing a chair or stool for the employee to take periodic breaks from being on his or her feet. In reality, what happens is that there is a lack of awareness of ways to reduce barriers for people with disabilities. They tend to automatically assume that the person with a disability is lazy, unmotivated, and unwilling to work. This assumption is especially true for people with invisible disabilities. Invisible disabilities are disabilities that cannot be seen. Examples of invisible disabilities are anxiety, depression, fibromyalgia, and lupus. People tend to assume that if a person cannot see the disability, then the disability does not exist. To bring this full circle, here is what we've learned about debunking the myth:

What people believe: *Many people believe that people on welfare are lazy, unmotivated, and unwilling to work.*

What we now know:

➢ Approximately 76% of people receiving public assistance have an income and are working.

➢ Many people with disabilities want to work, but face systematic barriers that prevent them from working.

➤ Nearly all the time, accommodations can be provided that cost little to nothing.

➤ Invisible disabilities tend to be more stigmatized than visible disabilities.

What effect does the stigmatizing myth have on people with disabilities? Many people with disabilities are not afforded the same equal opportunity as people without disabilities. The unequal opportunities exist in accessing healthcare and becoming employed.

Here is the next stigmatizing myth: *Many people believe that people on welfare are "addicts" and are abusing the system.*

There is a common phrase that some people tend to use when referring to people on public assistance. Many people hold the belief that "if I must be drug tested at work, they (people on public assistance) should be drug tested to keep their benefits." While many people believe that drug testing public assistance recipients is a logical solution to removing people who abuse the system and save taxpayer dollars, the implementation of drug testing public assistance recipients is counterintuitive—why would it be counterintuitive?

Before answering that question, there are two types of drug tests that can be used. The first is an "instant" test. Think of an "instant" test like a pregnancy test. There is a panel that is placed into a cup with a person's urine in it and the urine is absorbed into the test. The test will show if the individual is positive for substances, and which substances the individual is positive for. However, no test is 100% accurate. There might be times when there is a "false positive." A "false positive" is when the test shows that a person is positive for a substance when that person was not using that substance. How is this possible? False positives occur when certain medications mimic a substance of abuse. How does this happen? Whenever an "instant" test is used, it tests for liver enzymes (enzymes are substances in the liver that helps to break down things like food and medications to help the body's metabolism). There are times when the liver uses the same enzymes to break down medications as it does to break down substances. Therefore, there might be instances when a test shows a positive result when, in fact, it was a false positive. So, what happens when there is a false positive? In many cases, the urine is sent to a lab to be analyzed.

Lab testing is the second type of drug testing and is much more detailed, and means that it is much more expensive. Lab tests can cost anywhere from $50.00-$100.00 per test. Lab tests are often used to confirm or deny the instant test results. The lab testing process can take from two days to two weeks for the results to come back.

Here is why drug testing all public assistance recipients is counterintuitive. As of 2012, there were 52.2 million people (approximately

21% of the United States population) receiving public assistance.[6] Suppose that we drug test ALL 52.2 million recipients. Let's also suppose that we initially use an "instant" test on all recipients. That means 52.2 million people times $20.00 per person, that is over one billion taxpayer dollars. Well, if it leads to removing the people who are abusing the system, isn't it a wise investment? The answer is simply: No. Why? Let's look at some existing research. According to Covert and Israel,[1] in 2014, seven states piloted studies where people receiving public assistance were randomly drug-screened. What was found in all seven states was that the rate of illicit drug abuse among public assistance recipients (which ranged from 0.02% to 8.9%) was lower than the national average rates of illicit drug abuse (9.2%) among the U.S. population[1].

What people believe: *Many people believe that people on welfare are "addicts" and are abusing the system.*

What we know:

➢ The number of people who abuse public assistance is lower than what is generally believed. For example, in a 2014 Massachusetts study of the number of public assistance abusers, it was found that there were approximately $9 million dollars lost due to "welfare fraud."[5] Although $9 million dollars may seem like a lot of money, it is quite small compared to the money that is used to fund public assistance. For example, in 2014, Massachusetts' spending on public assistance was $13 billion dollars[5]. Therefore, less than 1% of all funds that were used to provide public assistance was lost due to "welfare fraud."

➢ The number of people receiving public assistance who use substances is lower than the national average.

➢ Drug testing each recipient is not a cost-effective way to reduce public assistance abuse.

The last stigmatizing myth of public assistance: *Many people believe that women continue to have children so that they can continue to be on welfare.*

According to Gellman,[4] women experience what is termed "dependence" that leaves many women living in poverty. Women may find themselves dependent because of a divorce, having a child, or a death.[4] Gellman explained that women tend to find themselves in a cycle of dependency on the welfare system and noted that women and men receiving public assistance are treated unequally. Gellman asserted that there is a general belief that women are expected to be supported by males. This assumption limits the supports and resources that women may receive while receiving public assistance, such as work-training programs. Further, even if the woman becomes employed, it may be in an occupation where she is paid minimum wage and still needs public assistance to support herself and, if applicable, her children.

It is essential that health and human service providers recognize these factors and how the factors create unique barriers for women who are receiving public assistance. The health and human service provider should be aware how the cycle of dependency creates the stigmatizing myth–that many people believe that women continue to have children so that they can continue to be on welfare. Whereas, women might have more equal opportunities if the cycle of dependency and other systemic barriers were reduced or eliminated.

PRIVATE HEALTH INSURANCE

Currently, private health insurance is available to people who do not meet the eligibility criteria for Medicaid or Medicare. It used to be the case that a person could only obtain private health insurance through their employer. However, currently, people can individually purchase private health insurance (e.g., they do need an employer sponsored insurance plan).

There are two major types of private insurance: individual and family. Individual private insurance only covers the person who is purchasing the insurance. Family insurance covers the person and the person's family members, (i.e., the person's children, domestic partners, spouses, or dependent adults).

The cost of private health insurance depends on:

➢ the number of people in the person's family that are covered,

➢ the benefits that are selected, and

➢ the type of insurance plan that is purchased.

The two major types of health insurance are group insurance and individual private insurance. Group insurance is purchased by an employer and offered to the employer's employees. If an employee elects to enroll in group insurance, the employer will pay much of the monthly premium and the rest of the monthly premium is deducted from the employee's paycheck. There are times when an employee may elect not to enroll in group insurance. This is often referred to as "opting out." Some examples of when an employee might "opt-out" of group insurance:

➢ The employee already has insurance that was purchased on the free market (this is called individual private health).

> ➤ The employee is covered on someone else's insurance plan (for example, a domestic partner or spouse's insurance).

> ➤ The employee meets eligibility criteria for Medicaid or Medicare.

Individual private health insurance refers to insurance plans that are purchased "on the market." Think of "on the market" like going grocery shopping. Much like you would go to the grocery store to get what you need; individuals and families can purchase insurance "on the market." As previously mentioned, it used to be the case that individuals and families could only obtain private health insurance via their employer. However, because of the Affordable Care Act (ACA), private insurance plans can be purchased by any individual or family. The idea behind the ACA is that by making private insurances available to individuals and families, the cost of health insurance would decrease. However, many individuals and families are finding it difficult to cover the monthly premiums of self-insurance. A "safeguard" was written into the ACA that helps individuals and families experiencing financial hardship to afford the monthly premiums by Government subsidies (i.e., Government money that is used to help pay for the premiums) that are available to individuals and families experiencing financial hardship. There is some controversy over the Government subsidies. In some instances, the number of subsidies an individual or family receives might have to be paid back when the individual or family files taxes. Second, many people feel that the Government subsidies cost too much money. The future of the ACA is evolving, and it is uncertain how long individuals and families will continue to be able to purchase insurance on the free market and whether those individuals and families will be able to continue to receive government subsidies if they cannot afford the monthly premium.

PRIVATE INSURANCE AND ACCESSING HEALTHCARE SERVICES. How do agencies get private insurances to pay for healthcare services? Agencies (e.g., hospitals, physician offices, counseling centers) are paid via a process called billing. An agency will send a bill (i.e., a list of all the healthcare services that were provided to the client) that contains details about the type of service, the length of service, and the cost of the service. There are two major components of billing. The first is contracted costs and the second is medical coding.

Insurance companies and agencies will have what is referred to as a contract. A contract is an agreement between the agency and the insurance company that specifies how much the insurance will pay for a service. Sometimes the contracted amount (i.e., the agreed upon amount and insurance company will pay an agency) is less than what the agency charges for the service. For example, suppose that a one-hour counseling session costs $150. It might be that the contracted amount between the insurance company and the counseling center is only $90. Therefore, the counseling center will only receive $90 for the one-hour counseling session instead of the full $150.

"What about the remaining $60?" A few things might happen. First, the insurance company might require the client who has private insurance to pay the remaining $60. This $60 would be considered an out of pocket expense explained at the beginning of this chapter. Other insurance companies might require the agency to "eat the cost." "Eating the cost" is a common term used when a bill is not covered in full by the insurance company and the agency is not allowed to bill the client who is covered. Again, whether the client who has private insurance must pay the remaining balance depends on what is written into the contract between the insurance company and the agency.

The second part of billing is medical coding. Each type of healthcare service has a unique code that is entered into an electronic health record software (see Chapter 8, "Electronic Health Records). An insurance company will review the code to determine whether they will pay for services. Insurance companies look for (and will only pay for) medically necessary services. Medically necessary services are services that are needed to be provided to the person. Insurance companies will not pay for services that are not deemed medically necessary. To highlight the concept of medical necessity let's suppose that you go to your primary care physician because you have a sore throat. A medically necessary service might be running tests to determine if the person has Strep throat. A service that would not be medically necessary would be an x-ray of your wrist as an x-ray of your wrist likely has nothing to do with your sore throat. However, taking a throat culture (i.e., swabbing the person's throat) to determine if the person has Strep throat would be an example of a medically necessary service. Medically necessary services are only one aspect to receiving payment and coverage for services.

CREDENTIALING AND LICENSING. Many (if not all) insurance companies have policies that detail what qualifications a healthcare provider must have to be considered "qualified" to issue services. For a qualified healthcare professional to receive payment for providing healthcare services, the healthcare professional must be "paneled" with the insurance company. Being "paneled" means that the healthcare professional has met the credentialing requirements of the health insurance company and has registered to be a healthcare provider with the insurance company. If a healthcare professional is paneled with a certain insurance company, then he or she would be considered an "in-network" provider.

NETWORK PROVIDERS. Each insurance company has what is called "in-network" and "out-of-network" providers. "In-network" providers are healthcare providers who meet the credentialing and licensing requirements of the insurance company and are on the insurance company's panel. Out-of-network providers are not paneled with an insurance company. Each insurance company treats "out-of-network" providers differently. For example, some insurance companies will pay for healthcare services sought from an "out-of-network" provider, but the insurance company may not pay as much as with "in-network" providers. Other insurance companies may not issue any payments for healthcare services provided by an "out-of-network" healthcare professional. Being a networked provider with a health insurance company is only one factor in receiving payments for healthcare services.

PREAUTHORIZATIONS. There are times when an insurance company will require a preauthorization before payment for healthcare services are agreed to. A preauthorization means that the healthcare professional must contact the insurance company to get approval prior to issuing the healthcare services. Preauthorizations are a way that insurance companies can control how much they pay for services by making sure that the services that are being preauthorized are medically necessary. For example, suppose that a client needs residential substance abuse treatment. A healthcare provider at the substance abuse treatment facility (e.g., counselor, a member of the billing department, case manager) would contact the insurance company and detail the need for residential substance abuse treatment services. If the client meets the criteria for residential substance abuse treatment services, then the insurance company will preauthorize a certain amount of days that the agency can provide services to the client. After the preauthorized number of days has been reached, the healthcare provider would then need to determine if the client needs continued care, or if the client is ready to be discharged. If the person needs continued care, then the healthcare provider would contact the insurance company again to be preauthorized for more days to provide treatment. If the client is ready to be discharged from treatment, then the healthcare provider would contact the insurance company and provide information about the client's follow-up treatment. The example of preauthorization in a residential substance abuse treatment service is just one example of what preauthorizations look like. It is important to note that preauthorizations apply to both public and private insurance, not just private insurances. Preauthorizations occur in all areas of the health and human services, thus, it is essential that the case manager, or the healthcare professional performing case management tasks, familiarize themselves with how to conduct preauthorizations to ensure that payment is received for services provided.

SUMMARY OF PRIVATE INSURANCE

Private insurance refers to healthcare coverage for individuals and families who do not meet the criteria for public healthcare coverage (i.e., Medicaid or Medicare). There are several private insurance companies, each of which have their own levels of coverage for services, credentials that must be met to be a qualified healthcare provider, and which services need preauthorization. While many people have healthcare coverage, whether it be through public or private health insurance, there are the uninsured (people with no form of healthcare coverage). Paying out of pocket for healthcare services is expensive and many people who do not have insurance are not able to afford healthcare services on their own. However, not having insurance does not mean that the client must go without healthcare services. A client might be able to receive funding for health and human services through grants.

GRANTS

A grant is an amount of funding for health and human services that is provided by an agency to a provider so that the provider can deliver healthcare services to people who do not have health insurance. Grant funds are given to the provider and it is not expected that the provider must pay the money back to the issuing agency. To receive grant funding, the healthcare provider must apply for the grant. The application for receiving a grant is often referred to as "writing a proposal," or "writing a grant." The application process ranges in detail and complexity, depending on the issuing agency. Grants can be provided by federal, state, or local agencies. There are a variety of federal, state, and local agencies that provide grant funding.

Federal grants are funding that is provided by federal government agencies. There are several grants that can be obtained at the federal level. The Substance Abuse and Mental Health Services Administration (SAMHSA) provides several types of grant funding for health and human services. There are block grants that are offered by SAMHSA to help increase client access to substance abuse treatment services. Agencies or states can apply for the block grants and receive a set amount of money per year to help people who are uninsured access substance abuse treatment.

There are also grants that exist on the medical end of the health and human services. Many not-for-profit hospital systems can apply for grants to help cover medical services for people who are uninsured. The recipients of these grant funds are often hospital systems or primary care facilities that primarily serve individuals who are receiving public healthcare.

How does distribution of these grant funds work? The client who is uninsured can fill out a "financial hardship" application that includes information related to their insurance status, household income, number of dependents, and residential status. The client has approximately two weeks to complete and return the application to the medical provider. The medical provider will then calculate what percentage of the total bill the patient is responsible for based on the information in the application. There are times when patients can get the entire cost of the bill paid for by the grant, or times where they only pay a portion of the balance.

In primary care settings (e.g., physician, dentists), the patient can apply for financial assistance before he or she receives healthcare services. This is beneficial for increasing uninsured patients' access to care, especially if they require regular check-ups and appointments. The patient fills out an application and how much they must pay for medical services will be based upon their household size and income.

Each medical provider has a "sliding fee scale" that has different income levels. A healthcare professional will review the application information and determine into what level the patient fits. Then, the amount that the patient must pay for each appointment is determined. The patient pays his or her part and the remaining balance is covered by the grant. It is essential that the health and human service provider is aware of these grant opportunities as many people might not know that these additional supports and services are available to them.

SUMMARY OF GRANT-FUNDING

There are times when people do not meet the eligibility requirements for Medicaid or Medicare, and are not able to afford private insurance, meaning that many people remain uninsured. However, being uninsured does not mean that the client does not have access to health and human services. As was discussed in this section, there are several agencies that provide grant opportunities for health and human service agencies. Grants can be used to help fund behavioral health services, such as substance abuse service, or to cover hospital bills. In other instances, grants can help uninsured individuals reduce the cost of their healthcare by providing funds to cover a physician's bill, in part or all of it. It is important to note that not all health and human service agencies have grants to help cover healthcare costs; however, it is essential that the health and human service worker becomes knowledgeable of what healthcare facilities have grants to cover service costs and where these grants can be obtained. Knowing which agencies have grants to cover services can help to increase access to health and human services for individuals who are uninsured.

BARRIERS TO HEALTH CARE: WHY MEMBERS OF UNDERREPRESENTED GROUPS DO NOT ACCESS HEALTH CARE

When people think about healthcare, people initially think of medical care. There are certainly barriers that members of underrepresented groups face when it comes to accessing medical care, but there are also barriers that members of underrepresented groups face when it comes to accessing behavioral health care. Much of the time, these barriers are caused by lack of practitioner education and awareness about the unique issues that members of underrepresented groups face. Other times, there are systematic barriers that prevent members of underrepresented groups from accessing health care. In this section, we will examine the unique barriers that are faced by women and members of the LGBTQ community to illustrate how certain attitudes, interventions, and interactions keep members of underrepresented groups from accessing health and human services.

WOMEN

There are several barriers to healthcare that are unique to women. First barrier; it is very common for medical practitioners to minimize the severity of pain that women experience. Two scenarios will be used to illustrate this point:

> Scenario 1. *A 35-year-old male arrived for an appointment with his primary care physician. His main reason for the appointment was because he was experiencing stiffness in his neck, back, and shoulders. He also explained that he has been getting painful headaches and unable to complete tasks at work.*

Given the limited information about the male, what might you guess is going on? After you formulate your thoughts, let's look at a second scenario.

> Scenario 2. *A 32-year-old female arrived for an appointment with her primary care physician. Her main reason for the appointment was that she was having widespread muscle aches, headaches, fatigue, and difficulty concentrating.*

Given the limited information about the female, what might you guess is going on? No, there was not a typo in the two scenarios. The only difference was gender. Everything else was the same.

Results: The following are the common responses when this scenario was presented to undergraduate health care management students.

When reviewing the male's case, several students hypothesized that his symptoms were likely due to a physical injury that he acquired at work. Students also hypothesized that it might have been the case that he was injured at the gym due to not stretching or properly "warming up" before exercising.

When reviewing the female's case, students hypothesized that it was likely that she was experiencing depression or anxiety and that the depression and anxiety were causing her muscle aches, headaches, fatigue, and difficulty concentrating.

The hypotheses from the health care management students was not surprising. It is very common that when male's express symptoms such as those in the first scenario, the symptoms are initially assumed to be related to physical injury. Conversely, when similar symptoms are reported by females, the symptoms are usually assumed to be due to a mental health condition. Why is this? According to Fenton[3], researchers have shown that women who present with physical pain are often misdiagnosed as having a mental health issue, spend longer time waiting to be treated, and spend less time being seen by a physician when compared to their male counterparts. What impact might this have on women's access to healthcare? First, many women may feel that since their pain is not being validated that it is useless to access healthcare. Second, many women may believe that they are overexaggerating their symptoms and that healthcare is not needed. The general assumption that women exaggerate their pain and that much of the pain is caused by a mental health condition can have serious implications for the health and wellbeing of women.

Another barrier that is experienced by women is health and human service providers assuming that she is over-exaggerating her symptoms. There was a situation in Iowa where a woman woke her husband up in the middle of the night with severe pain.[2] The husband called the ambulance and the woman was taken to the hospital. When the woman arrived at the hospital, she explained her symptoms and was told that she would have to "wait her turn" and that she was just experiencing "a little pain." It turns out that the woman was experiencing organ failure. She had a cyst on her ovary that grew so large that it was killing her ovary. This medical condition is lethal and requires immediate surgery. However, in the woman's case, her pain was minimized, and she was told that she was overexaggerating a condition that could have led to death. Fortunately, the woman had emergency surgery to remove her ovary. However, the delay in timely medical services could have led to her death.

LGBTQ

We will examine heteronormativity and what it looks like in a health care setting. Heteronormativity refers to the assumption that all persons identify as heterosexual (i.e., attraction to the opposite sex). However, not all persons identify as heterosexual. Without awareness of one's own assumptions, the healthcare professional can cause harm and frustration to the client seeking services. An example is, a woman went to her primary care physician for an annual physical. The primary care physician asked the woman if she was on birth control. The woman stated that she was not. The primary care physician then stated, "So you're not having sex?" The woman stated, "Yes, I have sex with my girlfriend." The primary care physician then stated, "That's not really sex then" and proceeded to label the woman's sexual status as "oral only."

Situations like this are very common for members of the LGBTQ population. Overall, members of the LGBTQ community often report that it is very common for their healthcare providers to lack awareness and education on issues that are unique to members of the community. Thus, it is essential that health and human service providers work to be as knowledgeable and aware of the common experiences of members of the LGBTQ community so that culturally-sensitive care can be provided. The lack of validation and understanding of the unique experiences of the LGBTQ community can lead to members of the community not reaching out for health and human services.

CASE STUDY
LAYLA

Layla is a 22-year-old Latina who went to her local Emergency Room department because she was experiencing symptoms of a heart attack. Layla's family has a history of heart disease and so Layla became very scared. Layla's girlfriend, Maria, took Layla to the Emergency Room. Layla told the admissions coordinator that she was having pain that started in her neck and moved down to the left side of her arm. She also stated that she was having pain in her chest, sweaty palms, racing heartbeat, and blurry vision. Layla was ushered into triage (triage is where the patient receives initial screening). There were two European American registered nurses (RN) who were in the triage room when Layla got there. One RN was male, and the other RN was female. The male RN told Layla's girlfriend, Maria, that she was not permitted to be in the triage room with Layla. Layla was confused, but did not think too much about it at the time due to being scared that she was having a heart attack. The first test that the RN ran was an electrocardiogram (ECG). (An ECG is a medical test that examines the electrical impulses of the patient's heart). The results of the ECG will provide the attending Physician information about whether the heart is functioning normally, or if there are irregularities. To run an ECG, the patient must have pads placed around their heart. These pads transmit the electrical activity of the heart to the machine where the results are printed out). Layla has had ECGs performed before, so she did not feel too nervous about having another one done. However, she was uncomfortable because the male RN was the one hooking the pads up to her while the female RN sat in the corner of the room not paying attention. The male RN asked Layla to pull her shirt up so that he could attach the pads. Layla was okay with this because she was wearing a tank-top underneath that left enough room for the pads to be attached without her having to sit there in her bra. The male RN said that there was not enough room to attach the pads and asked Layla to take her tank-top off. Hesitantly, but not wanting to go against the RNs medical advice, Layla took her tank-top off and the male RN proceeded to attach the pads. However, Layla began to feel even more uncomfortable when the male RN kept saying that the one pad (which he placed on her breast) was loose. The male RN kept "adjusting" it and proceeded with the ECG. Once the ECG was done, Layla put her shirt back on as the female RN took her and Maria to the room where Layla would then see the attending physician.

Layla laid in her hospital bed and two male physicians entered the room. The two male physicians introduced themselves to Layla and Maria and proceeded to explain the procedures that they were going to perform on Layla. The first procedure was to run another ECG. The one physician stated, "Your first ECG was irregular. We can't tell if your electrical impulses are irregular or not. We are going to do another ECG to confirm." Layla was nervous due to the experience she just had with the male RN. The one attending physician checked where the pads were connected so that he could hook Layla up to the ECG machine again. The physician stated, "I don't understand why this one pad is on your breast, that is not where it is supposed to go." Layla asked if she needed to take her hospital gown down so that the pads could be adjusted. The physician said "No, it is okay. I can move it from here." The physician was very careful not to expose Layla and was able to adjust the pads without Layla having to remove her gown.

The second procedure was to take some of Layla's blood so that it could be tested to see if she had a heart attack. When a person has a heart attack, there are certain enzymes in the blood that are produced by the heart. The presence of the enzymes would confirm that Layla had a heart attack. The enzymes will also let the physician know how much damage was caused to the heart if there was a heart attack. The third procedure was to give Layla Aspirin to help thin out her blood and reduce the likelihood that she would have another heart attack.

Layla was still very nervous, but was feeling a bit calmer knowing that Maria was in the room with her and that the physician was very careful when adjusting her ECG pads. The physicians left the room and Layla waited with Maria for the results to come back. About 30 minutes later, the physicians came back into Layla's room and told her that her bloodwork looked good and that there were no enzymes present. However, the physicians wanted to confirm that the results were accurate, so they took some more of Layla's blood and sent it to the laboratory for testing. Another 30 minutes passed, and the physicians came back with the test results. It was confirmed that everything was okay, and that Layla did not have a heart attack.

The physicians suspected that what happened was that Layla had a panic attack. A panic attack happens when a person experiences very high levels of anxiety and the symptoms of a panic attack mimic that of a heart attack. Layla apologized for going to the emergency room over anxiety. The physicians told her that it was better to be safe than sorry.

Layla was discharged from the emergency room and went home with Maria. Layla was instructed to follow up with her primary care physician in one week. Layla told Maria that she felt sorry for going to the emergency room because she knows that it is going to cost a lot and she did not have insurance. Maria reassured Layla that they would *figure something out and that it is important that Layla attends her follow-up appointment.*

One week later, Layla saw her primary care physician, Ron. When Layla talked to Ron about her anxiety, Ron told Layla that he does not like to prescribe anti-anxiety medications because people become addicted to the medication. Instead, Ron told Layla just to "relax a little" and that her anxiety is "not that bad." Layla left her appointment in tears, feeling very frustrated with Ron for making it seem like Layla was over-exaggerating. When Layla got home, she checked the mail and noticed that her emergency room bill had arrived. When Layla opened it up, she saw that the amount that she owed the hospital was $8,000. The costs of her emergency room visit caused Layla to have another panic attack. However, this time, Layla made the decision to stay at home and to not seek medical services again.

CASE STUDY DISCUSSION QUESTIONS

1. What unique issues do you think Layla experienced based on her demographic variables? (e.g., based on her gender, sexual orientation, age, race, ethnicity).

2. Do you think that Layla was over-exaggerating when the male RN kept adjusting the ECG pad?

3. What reactions did you have when you learned that the male RN put the pad in the wrong place?

4. We know that to be paid for the services provided, the healthcare provider needs to list all of the services that he or she can bill for. What services did Layla receive at the emergency room that she was billed for?

5. Do you think that the repeated ECGs and bloodwork were medically necessary? Why or why not?

6. What options does Layla have to help her get her emergency room bill covered?

7. What are your thoughts about Ron's (the primary care physician) approach to treating Layla's anxiety?

CONCLUSION

There are several different types of health and human services that people can access. However, to receive health and human services, there needs to be some method of funding. Some individuals are covered by public health insurance, such as Medicaid and Medicare; others are covered by private insurance that they either purchased on the free market, or were provided coverage by their employers.

Regardless of the number of people who are covered by public and private health insurance, there are still people who remain uninsured. A client not having health insurance does not mean that the client cannot access health and human services. Individuals who are uninsured might be able to have part, or all, or their healthcare bills and services paid via grant funding. People receiving grant funding usually get some type of healthcare assistance to help cover the cost of the services they received.

While there are several types of services and funding sources for these services, certain groups of individuals experience barriers to healthcare. For example, women experience certain barriers that their male counterparts do not. As was discussed in this chapter, there is a tendency in the health and human services for women's symptoms of pain to be attributed to mental health conditions. In addition, pain reported by women often becomes minimized by health and human service providers. We examined a case where a woman's pain was minimized by medical professionals when, it turns out, she had a life-threatening condition.

We also examined how lack of culturally competent care can impact members of the LGBTQ community. We examined a case where a woman was asked if she was sexually active and she reported that, yes, she was, with her girlfriend whereby she was told that was not actual sex. Ignoring the unique experiences of members of underrepresented groups when it comes to accessing health and human services is harmful, if not deadly. Therefore, it is of the utmost importance that health and human service providers become more aware and knowledgeable about what these barriers look like and to develop culturally responsive treatment interventions.

We also looked at how stigmatizing myths create barriers and harm to members of underrepresented groups. Three main myths were examined. We looked at how current research discredits the stigmatizing myths and how these myths are still prevalent today. It is the responsibility of the health and human service provider to become more aware of existing research and how it impacts the stigma associated with certain groups of people–primarily members of underrepresented groups that are receiving public assistance.

REFERENCES

[1]Covert, B. & Israel, J. (2014). What 7 states discovered after spending more than $1 million drug testing welfare recipients. Retrieved from https://thinkprogress.org/what-7-states-discovered-after-spending-more-than-1-million-drug-testing-welfare-recipients-c346e0b4305d/

[2]Fassler, J. (2015). *How doctors take women's pain less seriously.* Retrieved from https://www.theatlantic.com/health/archives/20/15/10/emergency-room-wait-times-sexism/410515/

[3]Fenton, S. (2016). *How sexist stereotypes mean doctors ignore women's pain.* Retrieved from http://www.independent.co.uk/life-style/health-and-families/health-news/how-sexist-stereotypes-mean-doctors-ignore-womens-pain-a7157931.html

[4]Gellman, L. (1999). Poverty & prejudice: Social security at the crossroads. *EDGE: Ethics of Development in Global Environment.* Retrieved from https://web.stanford.edu/class/e297c/poverty_prejudice/soc_sec/hfemale.htm

[5]Schoenberg, S. (2015). *War on poverty: How much welfare fraud is there in Massachusetts?* Retrieved from www.masslive.com/politics/index.ssf/2015/02/war_on_poverty_how_much_welfare.html

[6]United States Census Bureau. (2015). *21.3 percent of U.S. population participates in government assistance programs each month.* Retrieved from https://www.census.gov/newsroom/press-release/2015/cb15-97.html

CHAPTER 10

REFERRALS IN CASE MANAGEMENT

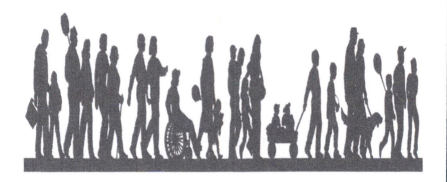

MARTHA H. CHAPIN
VANESSA M. PERRY

ABSTRACT

Referrals to other agencies will be an essential function of case management. To accomplish this task the case manager must understand clients' needs, locate referral sources, inform referral sources of the reason for the referral, follow-up with the referral sources, and be aware of confidentiality regarding information sent to and received from referral sources. This chapter will discuss how to effectively complete a referral and examine some of the challenges in making referrals.

CHAPTER HIGHLIGHTS

➤ Reasons for referral;

➤ Locating referral sources;

➤ Effective referrals;

➤ Challenges when making a referral;

➤ Following up after referrals have been made;

➤ Ethics of referrals;

➤ Underrepresented groups.

LEARNING OBJECTIVES

➤ Identify reasons for making referrals.

➤ Describe how to complete effective referrals.

➤ Identify challenges to making effective referrals.

➤ Describe ethical issues that may impact making referrals.

➤ Explain ethnic and culture issues that may need to be considered when making referrals.

The role of a case manager is to coordinate the services needed by clients to reach their end goal, which can be physiological, safety,[14] medical or mental health stability, return to work, independent or assisted living, or any number of other goals. To accomplish this task case managers should identify clients' goals and determine what information is needed to attain these goals. For this chapter, the term case manager will be used because case management job functions and titles vary. Human service professionals perform case management functions even if they do not have the title of case manager.

NEEDS IDENTIFICATION

When a new case is received by a case manager, the case manager will schedule and complete an initial assessment interview with the client. Depending upon the setting in which the case manager works, the case manager may gather physiological, safety,[14] medical, vocational, psychological, and financial information to assist in determining the client's needs and to help the client to achieve his or her goals.[10] After the initial assessment is completed, the case manager will make recommendations for services needed by the client to move the client toward goal attainment. If a client does not have food, water, shelter, or feel safe in the environment in which the client lives, other goals will not be achieved.[14] So, meeting the client's physiological and safety needs will likely be a priority for the case manager. Once the client's basic physiological and safety needs are met, the case manager can begin to address the client's remaining needs. If the case management agency is not able to provide the needed services for the client, the case manager will refer the client to another agency for receipt of these services.[6] Assuming the agency where the case manager works is not paying for these referral services, the case manager may need to justify the reason for the referral to the payer of these services to obtain approval for the referral. The case manager may also need to provide a rationale for the service requested. A rationale is a detailed explanation as to why the client needs the requested service, and how this service will help the client to achieve his or her goal. For example, if the case manager is working in a medical case management setting, the case manager may recommend to the workers' compensation insurance carrier that their client, who has bilateral carpal tunnel syndrome, received a second opinion regarding treatment from a hand specialist, particularly if the client's current treating physician is recommending a carpal tunnel release. The second opinion may support the surgery or recommend a non-invasive technique such as wrist splints or steroid injections.[1]

REASONS FOR REFERRAL

Referrals are made to other agencies when the case manager's agency is unable to provide the needed services. Referrals help the case manager to gain additional insights into his or her client and can help the client to achieve his or her goals.[5] Since case manager's function in so many different roles, this section will only discuss some of the more common reasons for referral.

MEDICAL
If a client has a debilitating diagnosis (e.g., muscular dystrophy, brain injury), a terminal illness, needs long term care, has multiple medical conditions, or medical complications, the client may need to be referred to a

long-term care or skilled nursing facility for continued medical or hospice care or for rehabilitation. [5, 16] If the client's medical condition is less severe, home health care may allow the client to have an earlier discharge from the hospital. Home health care provides nursing staff, as well as physical, occupational, and speech therapists, and personal care aides to help clients manage their medical needs and function more independently.[5] These same professionals can be accessed from private providers for clients who are not eligible for home health care services. Clients may also need to be referred to a prosthetist or orthotist, for pain management, or need durable medical equipment (e.g., wheelchair), or home modifications (e.g., ramp, railings) because of their medical condition (e.g., spinal cord injury). Clients may also be referred to a physician for specialized treatment, to obtain a second opinion, or to obtain a prescription for work hardening to help physically strengthen the client in preparation for return to work.[4] Other reasons for referrals are to gather new information, to provide the client instruction in activities of daily living, for treatment, and to improve the client's quality of life.[5, 19]

PSYCHOLOGICAL

Referral to a mental health specialist (e.g., psychiatrist, psychologist, counselor, therapist, social worker) may be necessary for treatment of mental disorders and addictions or when a client's pain needs to be managed. Further, if a client's medical or mental health condition impacts their ability to have sex, referral to a physician or sex therapist may be required.[5] Psychological evaluations can give the case manager insight into their client's intellectual, personality, and behavioral functioning, while neuropsychological assessments provide an understanding of a client's "cognitive functions as well as intelligence, verbal comprehension, verbal reasoning, memory and learning, visual and spatial abilities, and problem solving" abilities.[19, p.86]

VOCATIONAL

If a client needs vocational rehabilitation services, the case manager may refer the client to the state vocational rehabilitation services agency for assistance in job placement or independent living. When the case manager needs to know the client's physical and mental capabilities to work, the case manager may refer the client for a functional capacity evaluation or request this information from the client's treating physician.[4, 5] For guidance on career choices for clients, the case manager may refer the client for a vocational evaluation. The vocational evaluation provides information regarding the client's "abilities, aptitudes, interests, and behaviors in order to determine career development and community integration goals and the services needed to achieve them."[18, p.101]

LOCATING REFERRAL SOURCES

The Internet makes locating a referral source both easier and more complicated. The process is easier because information about referral sources is only a few clicks away. However, the volume of information available can make the actual decision-making process challenging. This section will give examples of some of the physiological, medical, mental health, substance abuse, and vocational resources available at different websites, but an all-inclusive discussion is beyond the scope of this chapter. Since not all clients have access to the Internet, the telephone can also be used to locate resources. Besides using a telephone directory, case managers and clients can dial 2-1-1, a dialing code reserved by the Federal Communications Commission (FCC) for community information and referral services. Although this service covers all 50 states, the service is not accessible in all areas of the United States.[12]

PHYSIOLOGICAL

As previously stated, physiological needs must be addressed before clients can focus on addressing other goals or consider returning to work. If clients and their families are hungry, food is their primary focus. Feeding America[11] can help case managers locate food banks in their area. If clients need assistance locating public housing or information on renting or buying a home, the U.S. Department of Housing and Urban Development[30] website can assist with locating this information. On this website is a link to the Federal Housing Administration which has information on buying a home, foreclosures, and other information of interest to home buyers and owners.[31] The U.S. Department of Housing and Urban Development[30] website also has a link to housing for Native Americans.[32]

MEDICAL

One good place to begin online medical research is the U.S. Department of Health and Human Services National Institute of Health, National Center for Complimentary and Integrative Health.[27] This website describes how to effectively evaluate online resources and provides a list of reliable online resources such as MedlinePlus[28] and healthfinder.gov.[26] MedlinePlus[28] helps case managers and clients understand medical conditions, medications, and supplements. Healthfinder.gov[26] provides similar medical information and helps case managers locate healthcare providers.

Another site that provides a comprehensive list of healthcare providers is Medicare.gov.[25] This website contains information on physician and health care providers, long term care facilities, nursing homes, inpatient rehabilitation facilities, and suppliers of medical equipment and supplies. Medicare.gov also has information on finding and comparing hospitals. An alternative way to locate both medical and mental health care professionals is to search the state licensure (e.g., Licensed Clinical Social Worker, Licensed Professional

Counselor) or certification boards (e.g., Commission on Rehabilitation
Counselor Certification, National Association of Social Workers) for the
specific professional who has the desired credentials for service provision.

MENTAL HEALTH AND ADDICTIONS

Information concerning mental health and addictions can be obtained from
the Substance Abuse and Mental Health Services Administration (SAMHSA).
Further, SAMHSA's Behavioral Health Locator[22] webpage can help case
managers find a mental health or addictions provider or substance abuse
treatment facility in the area serviced by the case manager. To learn more about
the types of mental health professionals, WebMD[38] has an article on "How to
find a therapist." MedlinePlus[28] also has resources to locate mental health
providers, but the focus is on psychologist and therapist. As previously stated,
licensure and certification boards can help case managers locate mental health
and addiction providers. If safety is the client's primary concern because of
issues with domestic violence, the case manager can visit The National
Domestic Violence[24] website to find resources in their area.

VOCATIONAL

The United States Department of Labor[33] has a wealth of employment
information. To assist clients in locating an appropriate job, the case manager
can have clients complete O*NET Interest Profiler.[34] Once a job or career is
determined, case managers and clients can research the specific job
requirements at O*NET Online.[35] To gain insight into disability and
employment issues case managers can access resources at the Office of
Disability Employment Policy.[36] State vocational rehabilitation service offices
can assist clients with job placement and independent living. Local vocational
rehabilitation offices can be found by typing into the selected search engine the
name of the state and vocational rehabilitation services.

Depending upon the environment in which the case manager works, clients
may choose who provides the needed services. Providing the client with a list
of appropriate service providers can facilitate their choice. However, client's
may offer an alternative which should be considered if the choice is a viable
option. If the client's choice is not a viable option, the client should be
informed of the case manager's reasons for this decision, and the case file
should be documented.[2]

These are only a few examples of online resources for medical, mental
health, safety, physiological, and vocational referrals. Additional information
on medical case management can be found in Chapter 4, case management and
mental health and substance abuse in Chapter 12, and case management and
vocational rehabilitation in Chapter 13.

EFFECTIVE REFERRALS

CLIENT'S PERMISSION FOR REFERRAL

Prior to initiating a referral, the case manager determines if the client is willing to meet with the referral source. Explaining the reason for the referral and how the referral will help the client achieve his or her goals can facilitate the client's willingness to be referred. The case manager should also inform the client of their desire to send information to the referral source and ask the client for permission to send this information on the client. To receive information from the referral agency, a release of information signed by the client is required.[6]

CONTACT

To make an effective referral, the case manager may contact the referral agency to confirm the appropriateness of the referral[5] if the case manager does not have previous knowledge or experience with this agency. During this initial contact, the case manager will ask about the services provided by the agency, time until an appointment can be made, the cost of the services, length of time for report receipt following the appointment, and other specific questions related to their client's needs.

APPLICATION FOR ELIGIBILITY

Once the case manager determines the appropriate referral source, the case manager will begin the referral process. The referral process varies by agency. Today many agencies have referral forms and questionnaires online for clients to complete. Depending upon the client's education and cognitive ability, the client may need assistance from the case manager to complete these online forms. If the client completes these forms independently following up with the client to insure referral form completion is recommended.

CORRESPONDENCE WITH REFERRAL SOURCE

Since case managers usually require very specific information from an agency to which they refer a client, correspondence with the agency is suggested. This correspondence can include pertinent information about the client such as the client's name, address, telephone number, reason for referral, and medical, mental health, vocational, and/or other issues that are essential for the referral source to know to effectively evaluate, treat, or assist the client.[5,6] The case manager may provide very specific questions to the referral source and should enclose a release of information.[6] So the referral source can provide the case manager with the results of the client meeting, and a written report, if desired.

CHALLENGES WHEN MAKING A REFERRAL

Although making a referral can be accomplished relatively easily, the case manager may still experience challenges. There may be long delays in scheduling or even waiting lists if an agency or the clinical staff are well respected in the community. This can result in treatment delays or the need to choose alternate referral sources, if the treatment delay may exacerbate the client's condition.

Clients may experience challenges that need to be addressed by the case manager. For example, an accessible building is essential for a person who uses a wheelchair. Further, due to limited financial resources, clients may purchase pay as you go cellular phone plans. Thus, the telephone number that worked last month to reach the client is either no longer in service or now belongs to someone else because the client could not afford to make the monthly cellular phone payments.

Transportation may also be a concern for clients. Case managers can access the bus schedule in their local area and through their local public transportation site locate paratransit for people with disabilities. Taxicabs and application (App) based transportation services may also be available in the client's geographic region. Private transportation services may be required in more rural areas.[5]

If the client requires psychological testing or a vocational evaluation, the case manager may desire a test administrator who understands the impact of culture, gender, and disability on test and evaluation results. Case managers will also want these evaluators to inform the case manager of the client's strengths and functional limitations that may affect employment or the client's ability to function effectively in their lives.[18] These are only a few examples of the challenges that clients may experience in accessing referrals made by case managers.

FOLLOWING UP AFTER REFERRALS HAVE BEEN MADE

Following up with clients and the referral agency after a referral has been made is an essential part of case management. Given the high caseloads case managers often carry, case managers may find themselves struggling to find time to make timely referrals and follow up on these referrals once they are made.[19] Without proper planning, follow up may often only take place if it is initiated by a client or an agency because a problem arose. Seasoned case managers will recognize the tremendous value follow-up contributes to case management.[19]

Following up after referrals have been made is invaluable because this process provides feedback to the referring case manager about the agency, the services provided, the client, and goodness of fit. Sometimes agencies may have untapped talents that are discovered when working with clients. Conversely, sometimes agencies may overstate their services or staff resources. The same possibilities apply to clients. Some clients may have undiscovered strengths or may be unaware of or minimize barriers or weaknesses. Without following up, the case manager may not have the opportunity to discover this information.[19]

AGENCIES

In following up with agencies, case managers may want to ask questions such as:

> ➤ How quickly did the client respond to your attempts to contact him/her?

> ➤ How would you describe the way the client interacted with staff?

> ➤ Tell me how the client's needs were met.

> ➤ Tell me about any unmet needs the client has.

> ➤ If you could change anything about the process of working with this client, what would you change?

> ➤ If you could write a summary of the client's experience with your agency, what would it say?

Asking questions such as these will provide case managers with insight on how well clients work with agencies, how well agencies provide services they advertise, and possible concerns to address with clients.

CLIENTS

In following up with clients, case managers may want to ask questions such as:

> ➤ How quickly did the agency get in touch with you?

> ➤ How would you describe the way you were treated by staff members?

> ➤ Tell me about how your needs were met.

> ➤ Tell me about any unmet needs you have.

> ➤ If you could change anything about the process of working with this agency, what would you change?

> ➤ If you could write a review for this agency, what would it say?

Asking questions such as these will provide case managers with insight on how smoothly the agency works, service gaps, and concerns to address with agencies.[19]

ETHICS OF REFERRALS

In coordinating services, case managers may encounter ethical dilemmas in dealing with confidentiality, when to decline a referral, and when to speak up. Namely, protecting client confidentiality is a challenge. Case managers will inevitably face in case management.

CONFIDENTIALITY

Given the collaborative nature of case management, case managers will undoubtedly find themselves in circumstances where they will exchange sensitive information with clients, family members, and other agencies.[15] Exchanging information also allows all human service providers to have the most comprehensive picture of clients' needs and gaps in services. With this shared knowledge, case managers can help clients make the most informed decision possible.

All case managers should abide by the Code of Professional Conduct for Case Managers,[7] or the code of ethics that pertain to their specific professional discipline. Case managers must "maintain policies that are universally respectful of the integrity and worth of each person."[3, p.28] This guiding tenet is illustrated by eight principles in the Code of Professional Conduct for Case Managers,[7] that guide and govern the profession. Additionally, case managers must adhere to the five ethical principles of beneficence, nonmaleficence, autonomy, justice, and fidelity.[7] Case managers must "[adhere] to client privacy and confidentiality mandates during all aspects of facilitation, coordination, communication, and collaboration within and outside of the client's care setting."[3, p.25-26] Confidentiality is one function of several functions that were added to the Code in 2002, reflecting the change and growth of the profession and the need to formally address confidentiality in case management.[7] Many other human service professions also share these values. This Code requires case managers to comply with federal, state, and local laws in relation to protected health information, client consent, confidentiality, and releasing information. Further, the Code refers case managers back to their disciplines professional code of ethics for ethical issues.[7] Issues regarding breach of confidentiality are important to address in case management, as respect for confidentiality is non-negotiable in many human service professions. This concern is best illustrated through the case study discussed later in this chapter.

WHEN TO DECLINE A REFERRAL

In ideal situations, case managers receive ample referrals and can meet the needs of all clients referred to them. However, situations may arise where case managers could or should decline a referral. Some examples of such situations are:

> Time: A case manager does not have sufficient time to meet the client's needs.

> Services mismatch: The services needed by a client and the services provided by an agency are not congruent.

> Dual relationship: The client and case manager have a relationship in another domain that creates a conflict of interest.

> Financial pressure: The motivation to accept a referral is primarily driven by money.

> Professional pressure: The desire to impress colleagues is the main reason for accepting a referral. For example, accepting a referral that might not be appropriate because the client was referred by a well-known colleague.

Since case management is a business, money is integral to case management practice, thus, case managers should be paid for their services. Because of this, case managers should acknowledge and reflect upon their own financial needs and not provide unneeded services to their clients. Being aware of financial needs makes case managers able to make stronger, ethical decisions.[20]

WHEN TO SPEAK UP

In an ideal world, all human service professionals act in the best interests of clients and abide by professional, ethical codes of conduct. However, this expectation is not always the case.[3] Instances may arise when case managers must advocate for their clients or perhaps file a grievance against a human service professional or agency.[21] In following up with clients, case managers may take note when clients' needs are not entirely met by agencies or, worse, misconduct occurs. In such instances, case managers must not stand by idly.[20] Case managers may need to consult with supervisors, reference their professional code of ethics, their certification body, and/or other appropriate resources to determine how to address concerns with other professionals. In instances where a violation of professional, ethical conduct is unclear, case managers should use an ethical decision-making model to formulate a plan. In the event, case managers should file a grievance against a professional or agency, case managers should use client welfare as their compass.

CASE STUDY
DONALD

A case study is used to portray an ethical dilemma case manger's may face when trying to balance confidentiality with transparency.

> *Donald is a 48-year-old Latino man with a mild intellectual disability, diabetes, and a history of substance use. He is currently working with Glenda, a Certified Rehabilitation Counselor (CRC) at a state vocational rehabilitation agency to identify barriers to maintaining employment. Glenda and Donald agree that his substance use is a significant barrier to his employment, and that addictions counseling would be valuable. Glenda referred Donald to Anchor Community Counseling, a free counseling clinic where Sandra works.*
> *In making this referral, Glenda told Donald his continued participation in vocational rehabilitation requires his sobriety. In short, he needs to remain clean and sober to continue to receive services from her agency. Sandra and Donald have begun working together to address Donald's drug use. After several weeks of working together, Donald relapses. Shortly thereafter, Glenda contacts Sandra for an update on Donald's progress. Sandra knows information about Donald's relapse may negatively impact Donald's eligibility for vocational rehabilitation services.*
> *In addition to serving as Donald's addictions counselor, Sandra is also coordinating Donald's services with Glenda. As a counselor, Sandra is obligated to respect Donald's confidentiality. She also committed to coordinating services with Glenda's agency. What should Sandra do?*

In considering this case study:

➢ How might Sandra use an ethical decision-making model to guide her decision-making process?

➢ What guidance may the Code of Professional Conduct for Case Managers provide?

➢ What guidance may other codes of ethics provide?

➢ What roles should Donald, Glenda, and Sandra play in this situation?

➢ Are there other people who should be involved?

➢ What role might culture play in this scenario?

➤ What impact will Sandra's actions have on her relationship with Donald, her relationship with Glenda, and Donald's relationship with Glenda?

➤ What other aspects require your consideration?

Sharing information between agencies is a natural component of case management. As you can see in this example, sometimes case management requires an exchange of information when the information is unsavory or information may adversely affect clients' access to services. Also, consider that in some cases, legal implications may become involved. For example, if Sandra had been coordinating with Donald's probation officer, he could have experienced legal consequences if Sandra shared information about Donald's relapse. If Donald had lost custody of his children and was working to reunify with them, Donald could have also experienced negative consequences if Sandra shared information about his relapse.

This case has no easy resolution. Honoring clients' right to confidentiality and sharing information with other agencies can be difficult to balance. Regardless of the situation, one concept may provide helpful guidance: minimal disclosure. The Code of Professional Ethics for Rehabilitation Counselors[8] discusses confidentiality at great length, and gives mention to minimal disclosure, saying, "when circumstances require the disclosure of confidential information, rehabilitation counselors clarify the nature of information being requested and make reasonable efforts to ensure only necessary information is revealed."[p.9] In bearing in mind confidentiality in the context of case management and confidentiality, consider when minimal disclosure is appropriate.[7]

UNDERREPRESENTED GROUPS

Multicultural counseling competence requires counselors to develop the awareness, knowledge, and skills to effectively function in our diverse culture. One of the multicultural counseling competencies for awareness is being "sensitive to circumstances (personal biases; stage of racial, gender, and sexual orientation identity; sociopolitical influences; etc.) that may dictate referral of clients to members of their own sociodemographic group or to different therapists in general."[23, p.71] This may include referring clients to practitioners with knowledge of different healing approaches.[13] Culture issues that may need to be considered in helping clients with their case management needs include understanding the meaning of gestures; cultural traditions, differences, and taboos; religious and spiritual beliefs, and cultural and religious conflicts within the client.[17] If clients from different racial/ethnic backgrounds need a psychological assessment, the case manager will ideally want to refer the client to a practitioner who is fluent in the client's language or who will use an interpreter during the assessment. Further, to increase the reliability and validity of the test results, the instruments need to have been measured on the racial/ethnic background of the client.[9]

There are several online health care resources that may be useful for case managers working with clients from different races, ethnicities, and cultural backgrounds. Resources and information on minority health are available from the U.S. Department of Health and Human Services Office of Minority Health, at the Office of Minority Health Resource Center.[16, 29] Information on health issues specific to African Americans, American Indians and Alaska Natives, Asian Americans, Hispanics, Native Hawaiians and Pacific Islanders[29] can be found here. Case managers may also find EthnoMED[16, 37] a valuable resource since it integrates health information with cultural beliefs. The website focuses on refugees who have fled to Seattle and the United States from war-torn countries.

DISCUSSION QUESTIONS

1. In identifying clients' needs, what types of needs should be prioritized? Why?

2. What are some ways case managers may locate resources in their local communities?

3. What are some considerations case managers should keep in mind when making an effective referral?

4. What are some challenges when making a referral?

5. What is one-way case managers can balance confidentiality with coordination of services?

REFERENCES

[1] American Society for Surgery of the Hand. (2015). *Carpal tunnel syndrome: Treatment*. Retrieved from http://www.assh.org/handcare/hand-arm-conditions/carpal-tunnel/

[2] Birmingham, J. (2008). Transitional planning. In S. K. Powell & H. A. Than (Eds.), *Case Management Society of America core curriculum for case management*. New York, NY: Wolters Kluwer|Lippincott Williams & Wilkins.

[3] Case Management Society of America. (2016). *Standards of practice for case management*. Little Rock, AR: Author. Retrieved from http://solutions.cmsa.org/acton/media/10442/standards-of-practice-for-case-management

[4] Chapin, M. H. (2005). Case management in private sector rehabilitation. In F. Chan, M. J. Leahy & J. L. Saunders (Eds.), *Case management for rehabilitation health professionals* (2nd ed., Vol. 1, pp. 304-329). Osage Beach, MO: Aspen Professional Services.

[5] Chapin, M. H. (2005). Community resources. In F. Chan, M. J. Leahy, & J. L. Saunders (Eds.), *Case management for rehabilitation health professionals* (2nd ed., Vol. 1, pp. 176-196). Osage Beach, MO: Aspen Professional Services.

[6] Chapin, M. H., Butler, M. K., & Perry, V. M. (2017). Case management. In V. Tarvydas & M. T. Hartley (Eds.), *The professional practice of rehabilitation counseling.* doi:9780826138927

[7] Commission for Case Manager Certification. (2015). *Code of professional conduct for case managers with standards, rules, procedures, and penalties.* Retrieved from https://ccmcertification.org/sites/default/files/docs/2017/code_of_professio nal_conduct.pdf

[8] Commission on Rehabilitation Counselor Certification. (2017). *Code of professional ethics for rehabilitation counselors.* Schaumburg, IL: Author.

[9] Elbulok-Charcape, M. M., Rabin, L. A., & Spadaccini, A. T. (2014). Trends in the neuropsychological assessment of ethnic/racial minorities: A survey of clinical neuropsychologists in the United States and Canada. *Cultural Diversity and Ethnic Minority Psychology, 20*(3), 353-361.

[10] Farley, R. C., & Rubin, S. E. (2006). The intake interview. In R. T. Roessler & S. E. Rubin, *Case management and rehabilitation counseling* (4th ed., pp. 51-73). Austin, TX: Pro-Ed.

[11] Feeding America. (2017). *Find your local food bank.* Retrieved from http://www.feedingamerica.org/find-your-local-foodbank/

[12] Helpline Center. (2017). *What is 211?* Retrieved from http://www.helplinecenter.org/2-1-1-community-resources/what-is-211/

[13] Hutchins, A. M. (2013). Counseling gay men. In C. C. Lee (Ed.), *Multicultural issues in counseling: New approaches to diversity* (4th ed., pp. 171-193). Alexandria, VA: American Counseling Association.

[14] Maslow, A. H. (1943). A theory of motivation. *Psychological Review*, 50(4), 370-396.

[15] Mattson, M., & Brann, M. (2002). Managed care and the paradox of patient confidentiality: A case study analysis from a communication boundary management perspective. *Communication Studies*, 53(4), 337-357. doi:10.1080/10510970209388597

[16] Mullahy, C. M. (2014). *The case manager's handbook* (5th ed.). Burlington, MA: Jones & Bartlett Learning.

[17] Powell, S. K., & Tahan, H. A. (2010). *Case Management: A practical guide for education and practice* (3rd ed.). New York, NY: Wolters Kluwer|Lippincott Williams & Wilkins.

[18] Roessler, R. T., Baker, R. J., & Williams, B. T. (2006). Vocational evaluation. In R. T. Roessler & S. E. Rubin, *Case management and rehabilitation counseling* (4th ed., pp. 101-126). Austin, TX: Pro-Ed.

[19] Roessler, R. T., & Rubin, S. E. (2006). *Case management and rehabilitation counseling: Procedures and techniques* (4th ed.). Austin, TX: Pro-Ed.

[20] Shapiro, E. L., & Ginzberg, R. (2003). To accept or not to accept: Referrals and the maintenance of boundaries. *Professional Psychology: Research and Practice, 34*(3), 258-263. doi:10.1037/0735-7028.34.3.258

[21] Sminkey, P. V., & LeDoux, J. (2016). Case management ethics: High professional standards for health care's interconnected worlds. *Professional Case Management, 21*(4), 193-198. doi:10.1097/NCM.0000000000000166

[22] Substance Abuse and Mental Health Services Administration. (n.d.). *Behavioral health treatment services locator.* Retrieved from https://findtreatment.samhsa.gov/locator/home

[23] Sue, D. W., & Sue, D. (2016). *Counseling the culturally diverse.* Hoboken, NJ: John Wiley & Sons, Inc.

[24] The National Domestic Violence Hotline. (n.d.). Retrieved from http://www.thehotline.org/

[25] U.S. Center for Medicaid and Medicare Services. (n.d.). *Medicare.gov.: Find doctors, providers, hospitals, plans & suppliers.* Retrieved from https://www.medicare.gov/index.html

[26] U.S. Department of Health and Human Services. National Health Information Center. *HealthFinder.gov.* Retrieved from https://healthfinder.gov/

[27] U.S. Department of Health and Human Services, National Institute of Health, National Center for Complimentary and Integrative. (2014, September). *Finding and evaluating online resources.* https://nccih.nih.gov/health/webresources

[28] U.S. Department of Health and Human Services, National Institute of Health, U.S. National Library of Medicine. (2017, June 8). *MedlinePlus.* Retrieved from https://medlineplus.gov/

[29] U.S. Department of Health and Human Services Office of Minority Health. (n.d.). *Office of Minority Health Resource Center.* Retrieved from https://minorityhealth.hhs.gov/omh/browse.aspx?lvl=1&lvlid=3

[30] U.S. Department of Housing and Urban Development. (2017, June 15). *HUD.GOV., U.S. Department of Housing and Urban Development.* Retrieved from https://portal.hud.gov/hudportal/HUD

[31] U.S. Department of Housing and Urban Development. (2017, June 16). *HUD.GOV., U.S. Department of Housing and Urban Development, Federal Housing Administration.* Retrieved from https://portal.hud.gov/hudportal/HUD?src=/federal_housing_administration

[32] U.S. Department of Housing and Urban Development. (2017, June 16). *HUD.GOV., U.S. Department of Housing and Urban Development, Public and Indian Housing.* Retrieved from

https://portal.hud.gov/hudportal/HUD?src=/program_offices/public_indian _housing

[33] United States Department of Labor. (n.d.). Retrieved from https://www.dol.gov/

[34] United States Department of Labor, Employment and Training Administration, National Center for O*NET Development. (2017, May 31). *My next move*. Retrieved from https://www.mynextmove.org/explore/ip

[35] United States Department of Labor, Employment and Training Administration, National Center for O*NET Development. (2017, May 31). *O*NET OnLine*. Retrieved from https://www.onetonline.org/

[36] United States Department of Labor, Office of Disability Employment Policy. (n.d.). Retrieved from https://www.dol.gov/odep/#

[37] University of Washington, Harborview Medical Center, Health Sciences Library. (1995-2017). *ethnoMed*. Retrieved from http://ethnomed.org/

[38] WebMD. (2005-2017). *How to find a therapist*. Retrieved from http://www.webmd.com/mental-health/features/how-to-find-therapist#1

CHAPTER 11

CASE MANAGEMENT: CRITICAL ISSUES IN ASSESSMENT

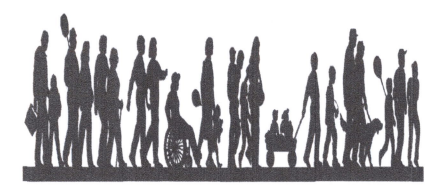

JAMES A. ATHANASOU

RALPH CRYSTAL

DENISE CATALANO

ABSTRACT

Assessment is a key phase in the management of any case. It finds its greatest application in planning for future development and resolving problems. Typically, it is associated with understanding the person as well as their context. Assessment may include physical assessments such as a manual dexterity test through to completion of an interest questionnaire, a general aptitude test battery to identify abilities, educational assessments of literacy and numeracy, quality of life, mental status assessment, community integration and even personality or temperament assessments. Sometimes assessment is mandated and at other times it involves voluntary participation. Assessment is integrated within the case management process and it is a partnership that requires the active involvement and agreement of the client to participate meaningfully, truthfully and actively. Empathy and rapport-building skills are often required prior to undertaking any formal assessment. Otherwise the validity or accuracy of the findings from assessments are questionable. An overview of fundamentals of instrument administration will be provided. Concepts that will be reviewed include reliability, validity, and norm-referenced instruments. Special attention will be given to the interpretation of the results, especially in terms of instruments that have been norm-referenced. Implications for case management practice are provided.

CHAPTER HIGHLIGHTS

- Fundamentals of standardized assessment;
- Reliability for assessments;
- Validity for assessments;
- How to use and interpret norms;
- Interpreting results.

LEARNING OBJECTIVES

The reader will be assisted to:

- Adopt assessment as a key component of effective case management;
- Evaluate the reliability and validity of assessment information;
- Interpret and report results in a professional manner.

INTRODUCTION

Assessment has always been part-and-parcel of case management[10] and is a core competence for service providers and human service workers (to simplify matters, human service and allied health professionals will all be referred to as "case managers" throughout the chapter). Assessment helps the case manager draw inferences about the characteristics of the individual and permits the construction of a client-model.

A working model of the person is then used as the basis for making clinical or service decisions. A judgement process allows case managers to formulate or test ideas that can predict accurately the behaviors of their client in a wide variety of situations.[15] The model is revised as inconsistencies appear or new information is received. The more information available to the case manager, then the more sophisticated the model becomes.

The process of assessment is a combination of both science and art. There are thousands of assessment instruments available that have been developed empirically, but interpreting the data generated by the instrument(s) accurately and appropriately, and then integrating that data with the variety of information obtained from other sources (e.g., interviews, records) requires skill, experience, and good clinical judgment.[11]

A critical challenge for case managers is to ensure that any assessment instruments used do not contain inherent sources of bias. "Bias" refers to a systematic error in which the obtained scores consistently over-estimate, or under-estimate, the true value of what is being measured for members of one group as compared with members of another group. A detailed discussion regarding test bias and test fairness is beyond the scope of a single chapter but the topic is mentioned throughout as it is relevant to a fair assessment of all clients especially those of minority groups.

Case managers should recognize it is possible for a questionnaire or test to produce inaccurate findings, such as interpretations of the scores from underrepresented populations. For example, an instrument may contain items that assumes all individuals have an equal opportunity to learn the information being assessed, or the test author assumed there is only one correct answer for an item, or the language used is one that is unfamiliar to the individual being tested. Consider how useful the scores of a personality inventory would be if your client was not fluent in the English language. As a result, any interpretation of the client's level of neuroticism, extraversion, openness, agreeableness, or conscientiousness would be fraught with difficulties. There will be more about how assessment instruments may contain cultural bias throughout the following sections

KEY ISSUES IN ASSESSMENT

WHAT IS MEANT BY ASSESSMENT?

A formal definition of assessment is "any systematic method of obtaining information from tests and other sources, used to draw inferences about characteristics of people, objects, or programs."[1, p.172] Often the term "evaluation" is a term that is used by some instead of assessment. Assessment is quite different. Assessment focuses on an individual whereas evaluation is the methodical examination of the merit or worth of an object, such as a program, a service, a policy, or an agency.

A broad range of methods exist for obtaining assessment information (i.e., data). These methods include standardized tests, rating scales, interviews, or behavioral and functional observations of the person being assessed. There is an abundance of available tests, questionnaires or inventories that can be used in an assessment process. Identifying the most appropriate questionnaire or battery of tests to use in the assessment process can be an overwhelming process for a newcomer. The case manager needs to be clear about what information is important to obtain to best understand the abilities and needs of the client. In other words, what is the question that the case manager is wanting to answer? Assessment is designed to answer questions. Clarifying the question to be answered focuses the assessment process and the type of information that needs to be gathered.

THE ROLE OF ASSESSMENT IN CASE MANAGEMENT

Case managers engage routinely in the practice of assessment to (a) identify individuals' need for services, (b) conceptualize concerns and problems, (c) develop goals and objectives, or (e) determine the intervention strategies necessary to achieve those goals.[3, 11] The assessment process begins from the moment a client indicates a need for services, is found eligible for services (i.e., becomes a client), and continues throughout the case management process. All the information gathered during the assessment process helps build the base for future decisions and plans.

The purpose of the chapter is to guide you into the world of assessment and its role in case management. One role of assessment is illustrated in the following case study and there is no better place to start our journey than with an actual case. Read the background to the case (Case study A) and note the assessments that were used by the case manager.

INTRODUCTION TO ASSESSMENT:
CASE STUDY A
ANGELA

Angela is a 57-year-old female, personal care aide who was referred originally for a mandated assessment of her potential to retrain.

Angela is now legally blind the result of a brain tumor that developed three years ago. Her brain tumor is non-cancerous but can cause several complications.

Angela's symptoms now include very poor vision, double vision, no peripheral vision, impaired mobility, diabetes and impaired activities of daily living. There are concentration problems, an effect on mood and fatigue.

The assessment comprised a structured interview of Angela's educational, vocational, psychological, social, and medical history. The structured interview was followed by formal assessments of her physical capacity (e.g., manual dexterity, grip strength, shoulder strength, pull strength, mobility), an educational assessment of her literacy, an assessment of mental competence, and a test of malingering. The test of malingering is a simple memory test that is used to see if she is exaggerating or pretending to be less competent than she really is.

The assessment resulted in the case manager and Angela deciding against the educational and training options in her region. They sought assistance through a national disability insurance scheme, a Guide Dogs association, which is a specialized service for those with vision impairments, organized the granting of a disability pension and ensured that priority was given to her social adjustment, and provided ongoing neurology and ophthalmology services.

Typically, case managers in a variety of public, private, or non-profit human service settings will work with individuals like Angela. The purpose here is to use the assessment results to help Angela to organize her life and achieve an optimal level of functioning. There is a continuous cycle of assessment, planning, and implementation[20] (see Figure 1 for a schematic representation of the cycle). Figure1 highlights the integral role of assessment in the case management process.

Assessment is an essential component of the case management process. It occurs at various levels. At a macro level, assessment informs the plan for services and guides the entire case management process. At the micro level, assessment forms the basis for determining specific services, strategies, or interventions, which include the case manager's own verbal responses to produce a desired response during a counseling session[2] Assessment is a fundamental process in case management-from application to the termination of services. Through such an assessment process, professionals in health and social services can (a) help clients identify the problem or concern, (b) generate alternative solutions for resolving the problem, (c) consider the consequences of various alternative outcomes, and (d) then identify the most appropriate treatment or services to be provided to the client.

FIGURE 1

THE CASE MANAGEMENT PROCESS FOR ANGELA

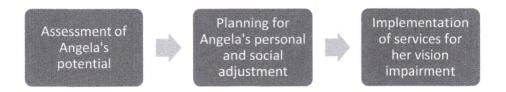

Social workers, counselors, psychologists, and other professionals will assess not only the individual, but also the individual within the context of the situation and his or her environment to determine the most efficient and effective treatments or services. A broader and all-encompassing aspect is highlighted by a systems framework[11] which adopts a holistic perspective across time. A systems framework considers the various influences in someone's life. Individual and intrapersonal influences include: personality, gender, abilities, or age. Context variables relate to influences such as the family, school, peers, workplace, geographical location, or even the media. The random influences that affect any life are also considered. The reciprocal interaction between these three sets of influences (individual, context and randomness) can be mapped at any point in time–in the past, at present, or even in the future.

Applying the holistic model to Angela means the case manager will view her situation in terms of its past and present and future context. The influence of factors such as her disability, together with other factors such as her age, gender, aptitudes, or values will be considered. Her geographical locations and its limitations on access to services is considered; the availability of community services is taken in to account; and the limited family support and the reliance on friends and acquaintances will also be relevant. For a comprehensive assessment, attention should be paid to an assessment of both the individual and his or her environment, with an equal emphasis on understanding his/her strengths (assets). Comprehensive means occurring at both the individual level (person), and the environmental level (i.e., an equal balance of positives and negatives).[16]

TABLE 1

COMMON ASSESSMENTS FOR USE BY PROVIDERS AND HUMAN SERVICE WORKERS

Domain	Common methods of assessment
Medical	Purdue Pegboard
	Grip strength dynamometer
	Shoulder strength dynamometer
	Back-leg pull strength dynamometer
Intelligence	Wechsler Abbreviated Scale of Intelligence
	Wonderlic Personnel Test
	Test of General Reasoning Ability
	Mini-Mental State Examination
Personal adjustment	NEO Personality Inventory-3
	Visual Analog Moods Scale
Social skills	Interview
	Inventory of Altered Self-Capacities
	Measures of Psychosocial Development
	Brief International Functional Capacity Assessment
Family information	Interview
	Personal History Checklist for Adults
Abilities	Wide-Range Achievement Test 4
	Test of Adult Basic Education, 9 and 10
Interests	O*NET Interest Explorer
	Reading-Free Vocational Interest Inventory:2
Aptitudes	General Aptitude Test Battery
	Wiesen Test of Mechanical Aptitude
	Differential Aptitude Test Battery
Work values	O*NET Work Importance Locator
Career development	Self-Directed Search
	Working Styles Assessment
Vocational maturity	Career Thoughts Inventory
Spiritual	Interview
	FACIT-Sp
	Spiritual Well-Being Scale

Most importantly, assessment should be viewed as a continual process in case management requiring a sophisticated integration of information using multiple methods, from multiple sources of assessment information.[11] Case managers must be prepared to re-evaluate their clients throughout the case management process to determine if progress is being made, or more information is needed, so appropriate adjustments can be made to treatment or services. By implementing a continuous evaluation process of the client, the case manager is more likely to recognize in a timely manner when the client is achieving success toward his or her goal, or when the client's progress has temporarily been halted perhaps due to an unanticipated barrier or deficiency. It is important for case managers to know when additional supports or services are needed by a client so that he or she can continue making progress toward the treatment or service goal. By involving the client in the continuous assessment process, the case manager is also modeling for the client an effective problem-solving strategy which the client can learn to use when other barriers occur.

DOMAINS OF POTENTIAL ASSESSMENT INFORMATION

Some examples of information that will be important for the provider to obtain include:

➢ Medical-physical (e.g., nature of impairment or disability, information about functioning, dexterity, grip strength);

➢ Psychological (e.g., intelligence, personal adjustment);

➢ Social skills (e.g., appropriateness, ability to form relationships);

➢ Family information (e.g., availability of support, nature of relationships)

➢ Educational-vocational (e.g., abilities, aptitudes, interests, work values, career development);

➢ Spiritual (e.g., hope, beliefs, values); and

➢ Environment (e.g., accessibility, assistive technology needs).

Each domain area of information can be assessed using multiple methods, such as standardized tests, rating scales, interviews, or observations. Some relevant assessments for these areas are listed in Table 1.

THE INTERVIEW AS AN ASSESSMENT TOOL

You will note that the interview features as an assessment method are provided in the list outlined in Table 1. The interview that a case manager conducts with the client is the most frequent form of assessment in the case management process. The interview provides key sources of information about the client in an efficient and effective way. Case managers have several different formats that can be used for conducting an interview: unstructured, structured, and semi-structured.

An unstructured interview consists of open-ended questions that allow the case manager the flexibility to respond to a client's response. Structured interviews are guided by a specific set of questions asked in a specific sequence. The structure or organization of the interviews is helpful in improving the consistency of the interview as an assessment method, but it reduces the flexibility of the case manager to further explore client responses. The semi-structured interview combines both the structured and unstructured interview methods by starting with a set of questions, but allows the interviewer to follow up on responses and ask additional questions. The structured clinical interview for making a psychological diagnosis is an example of a semi-structured interview.

Interviews, however, do have limitations as an assessment tool. A client may be a poor historian or present a distorted perspective of an experience. A client may also lack the necessary cognitive insight to provide useful information, or may be highly defensive and provide only partial or filtered information. Self-reported information can be influenced by a client's desire to present him or herself in a more socially appropriate way, or exaggerate symptoms and conditions. Additional methods of assessment can help identify discrepancies, or provide support for the client's self-assessment.

The case manager may also be vulnerable to sources of error while synthesizing and interpreting information. For example:

➤ service providers and human service workers may ask questions in a manner that influences the client's response (e.g., asking about what difficulties are experienced when they may not exist);

➤ observations made during the interview are situation-specific and may not generalize to other situations (e.g., a client may present appropriately in an interview but be more aggressive at home);

➤ a previous experience by the case manager may exert undue influence on inferences about a client who describes a similar experience (e.g., previous dealings with drug addicts may create stereotypical views in a case manager);

➤ individuals who share one characteristic with persons known to the case manager may lead to assumptions that other characteristics are shared (e.g., the scholastic aptitude of a high school dropout might be underestimated); and

➤ initial impressions may exert undue influence on the case manager's impressions of the client (e.g., dishevelled dress or appearance may belie a person's true character).

The challenge with biases formed during the case management process is that prejudices may be resistant to change. Information inconsistent with the case manager's initial impressions may be ignored or discounted, while information that is consistent is given more weight. It is impossible to completely avoid making judgment errors based on biases, but psychologists, social workers, counselors, and others have an ethical responsibility to be aware of them, attempt to minimize their occurrence, and to determine if clinical interpretations are based on the available evidence. A more comprehensive approach is to supplement the interview with information obtained from standardized tests, rating scales, and observations.

THE IMPORTANCE OF ASSESSMENT IN THE DECISION-MAKING PROCESS

The role of assessment is to provide the information necessary for making decisions throughout the case management process. Assessment can also provide important feedback regarding the effectiveness of interventions, and identify new issues needing to be addressed. In the case management process, assessment can specifically be used for:

- ➢ describing a client's current functioning,
- ➢ determining eligibility for services or benefits,
- ➢ confirming, refuting, or modifying impressions formed by the case manager,
- ➢ identifying therapeutic needs and recommending forms of interventions,
- ➢ providing information for diagnoses of emotional, behavioral, and cognitive disorders,
- ➢ monitoring treatment over time to evaluate the success of interventions, or identifying new issues to be addressed,
- ➢ managing risk and identifying treatment reactions, and
- ➢ providing feedback to the client as a therapeutic intervention.[11]

IMPLICATIONS FOR CASE MANAGEMENT PRACTICES
The goal of assessment is to assist service providers in the construction of a model of their client. When conducting an assessment:[11]

- ➢ clarify the purpose to select assessments that will provide appropriate results;
- ➢ include the client as a collaborator to increase the value and utility of the assessment process;

➢ consider the reliability and validity of the results – there should be sufficient evidence to choose an assessment;

➢ assess with different approaches to corroborate information, such as the findings from an interview with test results or reports;

➢ use a holistic approach that offers a "big picture" of the client;

➢ recognize there may be multiple problems the client is experiencing, such as depression and substance misuse – a comprehensive assessment would be necessary for providing information relevant to both disorders;

➢ treat all results as tentative – they offer hypotheses that need validation;

➢ consider the influence of other factors, such as age, gender, race, and culture on test results; and

➢ use the assessment results to provide therapeutic feedback to the client, to assist with improving the client's self-awareness and self-understanding potentially leading to positive changes and outcomes.

Case managers who incorporate the above principles into their practice of assessment, and who remain vigilant about sources of bias in their clinical judgments, may have an advantage in creating more accurate conceptualizations of their client's characteristics and problems. A more accurate model is likely to lead to more effective and efficient treatment and service decisions.

FUNDAMENTAL CONCEPTS IN ASSESSMENT

Accurate identification of a client's concerns and problems, and effective and efficient decision-making requires case managers have an adequate understanding of fundamental concepts of assessment devices and practices. Assessment has its own set of specific terms and it is helpful to have a working knowledge of them. The fundamental concepts to be covered include:

➢ understanding the term "test;"

➢ observational and functional assessments.

➢ differentiating among assessments of maximum or typical performance;

➢ reliability and validity;

➢ methods of assessment that produce quantitative or qualitative data; and

> ➤   characteristics of standardized tests

TESTS

Fundamental to assessment practice is the utilization of tests. A test is defined as "a systematic procedure for observing behavior and describing it with the aid of numerical scales or fixed categories."[5,p.32] Tests can be used to provide an objective measure of a sample of behavior that focuses on hypothetical traits presumed to be possessed by an individual in different degrees (e.g., anxiety, intelligence).[2] Predictions about an individual's behavior in other situations of interest (e.g., performance in school) can be based on the results of tests. Tests also allow the case manager to determine if any changes have occurred in the client's behavior because of the treatment or services provided or, given no changes occurred, if alternative treatment approaches or services should be considered. Tests are a fundamental tool in the assessment process–how effective the test is as a tool depends on the purpose for which it is used.

OBSERVATION AND FUNCTIONAL ASSESSMENTS

The common view of a test is merely that of a paper-and-pencil measure but this is a very limited conception. Tests can include standardized observations that occur within an interview (e.g., appearance, manner, thinking, communication). They can include behavioral observations that give a case manager an idea about someone's performance in real work and living tasks. Tests can include work samples that are simulations of tasks in a job. Tests also encompass ecological assessments that emphasize the use of real environments for observing the behavior of a client, such as in judgment or decision-making. Functional assessment of strength or dexterity or mobility or communication are also tests that describe an individual in terms of his or her skills and current behavior.

MAXIMUM AND TYPICAL PERFORMANCE

There are two types of determinations that can be made with tests – we can describe an individual's maximum performance or behavior, or we can describe an individual's typical performance or behavior.[5] Maximum performance relates to skills, abilities, achievements, or aptitudes. The level of performance is very helpful in initial conceptualizations of the client and most often helps in the establishment of goals, such as for education or careers. Maximum performance behaviors include general mental ability (i.e., intelligence), current skills resulting from past learning (i.e., achievement), and capacity or potential for performing specific skills (i.e., aptitude). Assessing indicators of maximum performance provides an evaluation of the best possible performance of the client. Typical performance refers to how a person tends to behave. Interests, attitudes, or values helps to help to predict the satisfaction a person might have in different life situations. Personality characteristics such as extraversion or neuroticism also provide information regarding typical behaviors.

A multitude of tests exist for assessing a client's abilities, aptitudes, personality characteristics, or interests. Independent reviews of available instruments and tests can be found from sources, such as the *Buros Mental Measurement Yearbooks* (http://buros.org/test-reviews-information). Note that test publishers have formal requirements for the purchase of commercially available assessments of maximum and typical performance. A pre-requisite is special training in the administration and interpretation of results. A critical component of assessment interpretation is to understand how applicable the tests are when assessing characteristics of a member of an underrepresented population. Assessments developed for a middle class, English speaking population may discriminate against minority groups due to language, cultural content, or the way they are presented. As discussed previously, the potential for a test to contain bias is not to be underestimated and thus those who administer and interpret assessment information must be well trained in multicultural assessment practices and develop multicultural awareness and sensitivity into their personal perspective.

QUANTITATIVE AND QUALITATIVE DATA

Tests can provide quantitative or qualitative information. Quantitative data is typically obtained from the results of tests with numerical scores, rankings, or ratings. Qualitative information is descriptive in nature.

Quantitative results are designed to provide relatively objective or reliable indexes of individual attributes and can allow for a large amount of information to be collected in a short time. Test scores, rating scales, or behavioral observations for which the frequency and intensity of a behavior has been recorded are all considered forms of quantitative data. For instance, the *Visual Analog Mood Scale* is reported as a profile of eight scores. The eight scores are an example of quantitative data.

Qualitative information, on the other hand, is usually gathered through the interview process. Qualitative information, for instance, can come from an interview, where feelings of sadness, of being overwhelmed, where isolated thinking and thoughts of worthlessness might be reported by a client. An interview is not only the first face-to-face contact with client but is used throughout the case management process. It is the most widely used of all assessment methods. Qualitative information is important as it complements the results from standardized tests.

STANDARDIZED ASSESSMENT

A standardized assessment has two meanings. The first is that an assessment such as a test requires that detailed rules such as timing or the words used to introduce a task are followed strictly. If a different set of word are used to introduce a test, then the task may be presented as slightly differently to a client. A simple example is on a multiple-choice quiz where someone is advised that if they are not sure they should guess compared with wrong answers will be penalized. Formal or commercial assessment instruments have user manuals or instruction with the procedures for the administration, observation, and scoring.[4]

Standardized assessment also has a second meaning. Standardized refers to the findings or results from measures that have been administered to one or more large groups of individuals (referred to as the standardization or normative sample). For instance, many educational or intelligence tests are standardized on a representative sample of the population, so that a person's ability can be compared with their age. That way, the reading level or intelligence quotient (IQ) or career development of a young person will not be compared with that of a mature adult but with his/her peers. The assessment is standardized because the testing and reporting are prepared according to a specific set of rules so that the performance of other examinees, (when administering the instrument according to the same specific set of rules) can be compared to the performance of the normative sample. Only when the standardized procedures have been strictly applied can an examinee's performance be measured in comparison to the performance of the normative sample (i.e., others who have similar demographic characteristics).

One limitation for standardized assessments is when the normative sample does not accurately represent the test taker. An example would be determining whether the mechanical interests of a young male with a learning disability were high or low in comparison with others. If the instrument was only standardized on community college students, office employees or those with developmental disability then any comparison is fraught with difficulties. A normative sample may underrepresent sex, ethnic, or racial groups and introduce a form of bias that discriminates. The better standardized instruments provide users with a detailed test manual describing the characteristics of the normative samples. A test manual or user's manual should be reviewed carefully by the person conducting the assessment to determine if it is an appropriate instrument to use with specific clients, such as those who are members of an underrepresented population.

IMPLICATIONS FOR CASE MANAGEMENT PRACTICE

Case managers and professionals in the health and human services are typically working under an ethical code that provides standards of practice designed to protect the public and that defines the profession. For those who conduct assessments, attention must be paid to those sections in their ethical code that address ethical behavior regarding appropriate assessment practices. Professionals adhere to those ethical codes specific to their profession, and although some professionals may adhere to multiple professional ethical codes, there are some common issues that all professionals who conduct assessments as well as refer their clients for an assessment, must consider. Some of these issues include:

> Who is the client? The client can be the person being assessed or the referral source. There is always a responsibility to act ethically to both the person being assessed and the referral source;

> Has the client provided informed consent for the assessment? The purpose of the assessment needs to be clearly stated and the person being assessed has the right to know how the information will be used. Some details about the nature of the assessment, the questions the assessment is designed to answer, and the goals of the assessment can be explained in language the examinee understands;

> Has the person administering and scoring the assessment instruments or procedures been appropriately trained and is he or she competent and qualified to administer, score, and interpret the assessment results?

> Have the appropriate instrument(s) been selected for the assessment? Are the results reliable and valid for an examinee according to his or her age, race, culture, sex, language, or other relevant characteristics?

Case managers or other professionals conducting an assessment must be fully aware of their ethical responsibilities regarding the assessment process and interpretation of assessment results (e.g., awareness of the potential for test bias). Given the importance of assessment in the case management process, the improvement of a case manager's assessment procedures should be a high priority to effectively assist their clients in overcoming barriers, accomplish their goals, and maximize their quality of life. The next section of the chapter examines the reliability and validity of assessment results.

UTILIZING TEST RESULTS

Assessments should provide information that is not known or could not readily be obtained. They are tools to assist a case manager. The results can inform decisions about personal, educational, or social adjustment. In many respects having accurate information regarding a person's interests, temperament, aptitudes, intellectual potential, academic level of functioning, social and personal adjustment is a foundation for the case management process. For instance, test results are utilized in a psychiatric care setting to help people achieve their recovery goals or plan a path to achieving those goals. Of necessity, the case manager operationalizes a concept such as depression or anxiety, so that it can be assessed or measured or applied to a person's situation. In the following section a basic understanding of concepts such as personality or intelligence will be outlined. There will be a critique of using measures of ability and functioning.

TEST RELIABILITY

Reliability is synonymous with the consistency of the findings from a test, survey, observation, or other measuring device. To use an example, a valid scale will give the correct weight; a reliable scale will produce the same results for the same object time and time again. Note that it is possible for a scale to be reliable but invalid; but a scale that is valid is always reliable. The same analogy applies to test scores.

A reliability coefficient is often the statistic of choice in determining the reliability of a test. Typically, reliability is reported a correlation, which measures the intensity and direction of a relationship between two or more variables. Correlations are important and often cited in the test manuals or user guides for assessment instruments. Correlations are statistical indexes that show whether the pattern of scores in two groups is similar. A positive correlation means that results from two sources are directly related, so that high scores on one are matched largely by high scores on the second source. A negative correlation occurs when high scores on one source are reflected in low scores from the second source. The chart in Figure 2, provides a guide to interpreting the size of the correlation coefficient that is reported in a set of results or in a user's guide for an assessment.

FIGURE 2

A GUIDE TO INTERPRETING THE MAGNITUDE OF A CORRELATION

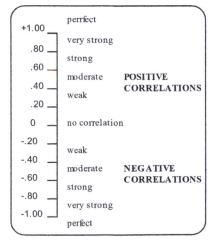

Reprinted with permission[9]

Test-retest reliability is fundamental. Reliability refers to the test's consistency among different administrations of the test. To determine the coefficient for test-retest reliability, the same test is given to a group of subjects on at least two separate occasions. If the test results are reliable, the general ordering of results from the first administration should be similar to the results from the second. It is expected that the relationship between the first and second administration to be a high positive correlation (see Figure 2) because the results are fairly stable over time. Those who scored highly on the first occasion tended to score high on the second; those who scored lowly on the first occasion tended to score low on the second occasion.[8]

There are other types of reliability indicators. These include (a) parallel forms or equivalent reliability where there are two versions of an assessment; (b) split-half reliability measures evaluate whether one-half of an assessment gives results similar to the other half (normally the results for the odd and even numbered questions are compared); and (c) internal consistency reliability is a statistical evaluation of the homogeneity of the items and it evaluates whether all the questions or items are assessing the same phenomenon (it is often reported as a coefficient alpha or Cronbach alpha or sometime a Kuder-Richardson 21 coefficient – both can be interpreted in the same way as the correlations in Figure 2).

TEST VALIDITY

Validity is probably the most important concept in the behavioral sciences. It implies truth and accuracy. In assessment, validity refers to the degree in which a test result is a true indicator of what we intended to measure. Validity itself cannot be measured in the way that reliability can be measured but it is a matter of gathering evidence in support of validity or verifying the truth of its claims. There are basic types of validity evidence and they fall into some neat groupings.

CONSTRUCT VALIDITY. Construct validity is the most theoretical of the validity evidence categories. Construct validity is the extent to which a test result reflects a theoretical concept (e.g., personality, intelligence) accurately.[8] For many psychological constructs (i.e., concepts) such as personality, that are artificial or difficult to measure, the notion of validity becomes complex. Anxiety, for instance, is intensely individual and comprises a range of physiological responses or individual symptoms and it can be generalized or specific, as well as chronic or acute. It overlaps with aspects of phobia, panic attack, or post-traumatic stress. As a simple example, "1 + 1 = _____ " would represent basic addition, but does the question also represent the construct of intelligence? If we have a difficult time defining the construct, we are going to have an even more difficulty measuring it. Test user manuals should report construct validity evidence that involves seeing whether the results from the assessment are theoretically consistent with other measures. For instance, we might check the extent to which the results overlap with other constructs such as depression or stress, whether the results are reflected in expected anxious behaviors or consistent with physiological indictors of anxiety.

CONTENT VALIDITY. Content validity is concerned with a test's ability to include or represent all the content of a construct. To use the same example as previously, a question like "1 + 1 = ___ " may be a valid basic addition question but would it represent all the content that makes up the study of mathematics? It may be included on a scale of intelligence, but does it represent all of intelligence? The answer to these questions is no. To develop a valid assessment of intelligence, not only must there be questions on math, but also questions on verbal reasoning, analytical ability, and every other aspect of the construct we call intelligence. There is no easy way to determine content validity aside from subject matter experts.[8] Expert opinions can differ depending on the theoretical orientation of the expert.

CONCURRENT VALIDITY. Concurrent validity is a type of criterion validity. For something to be true there needs to be a criterion or benchmark of some sort. Concurrent validity refers to the extent to which the results correlate directly with another measure of the same construct (or even indirectly with a measure of an opposite construct). Concurrent validity can also be demonstrated by comparing the results from an assessment with another already valid measurement. A new test of adult intelligence, for example, would have concurrent validity if it had a high positive correlation with the *Wechsler Adult Intelligence Scale* since the Wechsler is an accepted measure of the construct we call intelligence.[8]

PREDICTIVE VALIDITY. Predictive validity is another type of criterion validity. For an assessment to be of any real use it must tell us something that we do not know or tell us about the future. It must have predictive accuracy. Assessment results that do not predict are insignificant in the real world of case management. As an example, the *Scholastic Aptitude Test* (SAT) is used by college screening committees as one way to predict college grades. The *Graduate Management Admission Test* is used to predict success in business school. The main concern with these, and many other predictive measures is predictive validity because without it, they would be worthless. Predictive validity is determined by computing a correlational coefficient comparing SAT scores and college grades. If they are directly related, then we can make a prediction regarding college grades based on SAT score. We can show that students who score high on the SAT would be expected to receive high grades in college.[8]

OTHER TYPES OF VALIDITY. There are other types of validity evidence, such as consequential validity of the results (i.e., the personal and social implications of an assessment). As a newer category of validity evidence, it quite rightly considers the far-reaching repercussions of any assessment process. Some reports will also mention face validity. Face validity is not a psychometric validity but reflects the extent to which the content of the assessment instrument appears at face value that is by inspection and consideration of the semantic content of the items, to assess what it is designed to measure. In other words, whether an assessment of numeracy contains mathematics questions, or a disability assessment contains questions about functional ability.[14]

FACTORS AFFECTING VALIDITY

Tests generally used by case managers have typically been assessed for and meet accepted standards for reliability and validity. However, any modification in testing procedure needs to be indicated as such changes may render the test result invalid. Nevertheless, the interpretation of the test results even when modifications are made can be useful by the case manager who knows the client and knows how jobs in the real world are performed and can be modified. Knowing the medications [e.g., stimulant for Attention-deficit/hyperactivity disorder (ADHD) or anticonvulsant for epilepsy] an individual is taking and how these may influence performance is necessary for the case manager. A medication may cause drowsiness or increase attentiveness and mental alertness.

Validity can be affected by the length of time that a person has been out of school and when taking a test can impact performance. A 20-year-old person who has recently been in school and has taken tests recently may score better than a 40-year-old person who has not taken a test in over 20 years, all other factors being equal. The results for an older person may be adversely affected when the norms or table of results used for educational comparison are based on say high school students rather than other adults. Nevertheless, tests are a means to an end and not an end in themselves. The case manager uses test results as one piece of a total picture. Other pieces may include current or prior employment, educational attainment, family and significant other support, interests, motivation, and secondary gain. Thus, cut off scores often reported for entrance into an occupational training area can be negated by the presence of a strong support network, motivation, and interests.

Another example of when test interpretation is at the discretion of the case manager is based on cultural and individual factors. Dexterity tests measure speed and accuracy. However, when told by the test administrator to work as fast as possible, some individuals by their nature work fast and accuracy suffers. Others work slowly and have high levels of accuracy. Understanding these factors is important in the use and interpretation of the test.

Test administration and the rapport between the evaluator especially for some sections of intelligence and achievement tests can make a difference in how the individual scores. Some evaluators give credit for answers that other evaluators would discount. The test taker is more likely to do his or her best if there is good rapport between the test taker and the case manager. A case manager administering a reading proficiency test to a person whose primary language is not English may rate the individual as having a lower proficiency or achievement level because the individual did not understand the meaning of certain terms. However, other factors as noted may compensate for lower test scores.

The professional who is utilizing tests for career planning or occupational placement uses his/her clinical skills and judgment when doing counseling. Each test utilized has different criteria for determining reliability and validity. For example, the reliability of an interest inventory may not be as important as the validity of an intelligence test.

Reliability of interests may vary if a person's interests change dramatically when the person is presented with information or even allowed to observe different occupations. A client may have certain foundational interests, such as working with people but the context such as the specific job may change with seeing the work environment, nature of the work, working conditions, and potential wages. Whereas with intelligence, unless there has been a traumatic accident or injury, intelligence remains relatively stable over time. Reliable (and valid) measures of intelligence will reflect that stability across different test administrations.

With validity, we also want to make sure that an intelligence test correlates with actual mental abilities. Thus, we may have results from other tests that measure intelligence which the individual has taken and with which we can compare the current result. As an example, validity can be established by comparing the individual's prior or current educational or employment functioning with the test results obtained with the intelligence test we are using. Establishing validity for an interest inventory can be done by comparing interest test results from individuals successfully performing different occupations with the results from the interest inventory we are using regarding facilitating career choices.

INTERPRETING AND UTILIZING TEST RESULTS

Utilizing tests results in case management is an individual, one-on-one process. It is unlike the large-scale group tests used for college and university admissions decisions. In case management we use assessment results across a wide spectrum of human service and allied health professional contexts. The use of assessment could range from probation and parole settings, drug and alcohol clinics, family services, disability agencies, psychiatric units, aged care, rehabilitation providers, or hospitals, through to schools and workplaces. It includes individuals with problems of personal or social adjustment, individuals with developmental disabilities transitioning from school to work, persons who have chronic illness, individuals with a sudden onset of disability, patients or institutional clients. The applications and use of assessment results are countless and it is difficult to generalize. In the following section reference is made only to assessment in vocational rehabilitation. It is merely a generic example, but the assessment ideas and principles are readily transferable to other fields of personal and social assessment in case management.

In case management for vocational rehabilitation, a person's assessment results are used to assist them make wise choices based on education, geographic location, age, personal considerations, and interests. For this reason, consideration is given to the individual's age, prior employment, education, support system, self-concept, as well as socio-economic factors such as prior or anticipated earnings.

To round off this discussion an assessment case study of a client is presented. Background demographic, education, employment, and disability information as well as test results are given.

Some results are reported in stanines. These are not complex to interpret and to assist in understanding: a stanine converts raw test scores to a 9-point scale with a 5th stanine being at the 50% percentile or median. In the case study, the raw score obtained on the achievement test is the actual score of the person then the stanine, percentile, or a grade equivalent are provided.

In practice, the case manager might take the results from these tests and in combination with the past education, employment, and disability levels assist the client determine occupational areas that would be a good fit considering their support system and environmental factors.

CASE STUDY B
JAMES

BACKGROUND INFORMATION

Age:	40 years of age
Education:	High School graduate
Marital Status:	Married

INJURY

James was involved in a motor vehicle accident while at work. He suffered an injury to his right ankle, right knee, low back, and neck. He broke several ribs and bruised his kidneys. He did not require surgery. James reports having pain in his right ankle and knee, low back, neck, and in his chest. He reported having depression and anxiety, which causes him to have panic attacks. James states that he has periodic crying spells and feels frustrated and aggravated since being injured because of being unable to work and support his family. James reported that he has gained weight since being injured. He does not use a brace, cane, crutch, or nerve stimulation unit. He reported having pain in his back, right knee and right ankle. James is not working currently. He said that he is unable to play sports, jog, fish, walk in the woods, preach, go to church, or work since being injured. He reported the ability to take care of his personal needs, but his wife helps him with bathing. He can do dishes and laundry. He reported that he has not driven since being injured due to the pain in his back, right ankle and right knee. He is right-hand dominant.

EDUCATION

James graduated from high school. He does not have any formal vocational training. However, he is certified to operate over the road vehicles. He learned his job duties through on the job training and experience. He reported that he can read and understand a newspaper and general interest magazines. He can count change at a store. He can write a list and a message without difficulty.

EMPLOYMENT

At the time of the injury James was employed with a tree service when he was told that he could no longer work because of having to wear a foot boot and take medication. When he last worked, he was paid $16.85 per hour. He started employment with this company as a grounds man and cut brush and trees for right of ways. He lifted over 100 pounds and did this work for about 2½ years. He then got a job climbing trees to clear power lines which he did for about three months. He was promoted to being an as needed foreman and did this for about three years. Promotion to a working foreman followed. He operated a bucket truck and climbed and cut trees and oversaw up to three workers. James gave out and oversaw work assignments. He did not hire or fire. He kept records.

James was promoted to general foreman. This did not entail physical work. He oversaw about 25 employees and made sure the work was done properly. He was a general foreman for about 17 months. He was off for about two weeks and then returned to his general foreman job but did not do the physical work. His doctor had given him a boot and told him that he needed the boot and medication to be able to work. However, the company told him that he could not perform the work because of the boot and having to take medication. His position was terminated.

PHYSICAL AND PSYCHOLOGICAL FUNCTIONING

The information provided below represents a summary, as best could be determined of the critical medical information as it relates to James's ability to function and perform gainful activity.

PHYSICAL

James's restrictions are that he cannot lift, handle, or carry objects greater than 25 pounds and that he would not be able to engage in activity that requires recurrent bending, squatting, or stooping.

PSYCHOLOGICAL

James was diagnosed with a Major Depressive Disorder, Single Episode, Moderate, Anxiety Disorder, not otherwise specified, and pain disorder associated with both psychological factors and a general medical condition. It was recommended that James should only perform lower stress work.

VOCATIONAL TESTING

James was administered the Differential Aptitude Test Battery for the assessment of aptitudes. An aptitude is the potential to learn in a specific area. The aptitudes cover the following skill areas: verbal, numerical, and abstract reasoning; mechanical reasoning, space relations, spelling, and language usage. He scored as follows:

James was also administered the Kaufman Intelligence Test. His measured intelligence quotient is in the below average range of intellectual functioning. This is broken down into a verbal intelligence, a non-verbal intelligence and a full-scale or composite intelligence. The results are noted below in terms of IQ, percentile, and a verbal description:

Aptitude	Stanine	Percentile
Verbal reasoning:	6th	70th
Numerical ability:	5th	50th
Abstract reasoning:	4th	30th
Mechanical reasoning:	7th	85th
Spatial Relations:	4th	35th
Spelling:	5th	50th
Language Usage:	4th	25th

Reasoning ability	IQ	Percentile	Description
Verbal	IQ=82	12th	Below Average
Nonverbal	IQ=84	14th	Below Average
Composite	IQ=83	13th	Below Average

James was given a test of academic achievement, the Wide Range Achievement Test (WRAT-4). This covers reading, sentence comprehension, spelling, and arithmetic. The results are listed below as a raw score, a percentile, and a grade equivalent. This highlights the various ways in which results from an assessment can be presented and interpreted.

Achievement	Raw score	Percentile	Grade equivalent
Reading	52	18	9.8
Sentence Comprehension	40	12	9.2
Spelling	36	14	7.3
Arithmetic	37	25	7.3

The results of the WRAT-4 indicate that James has a reading level that would enable him to read and understand a newspaper and general interest magazines; and read and follow information needed for being able to read and understand technical and complex information and instructions. He would not have trouble reading and understanding information and reports as might be required for a cashier, service, counter clerk, or counter sales job.

With his level of spelling, James would be able to write information and instructions, and write orders in an inventory clerk, or cashier job. He can write reports, notes, messages, and instructions.

His arithmetic level indicates that he can perform basic arithmetic functions such as adding, subtracting, multiplying, and dividing and would not have difficulty with fractions, decimals, ratios, and percentages.

A 5th-6th grade level is generally viewed as the threshold for being able to function in society. James is literate and would not have difficulty being able to perform jobs that required the application of academic abilities. A 10th-11th grade level is needed for formal education and training at a technical or community college.

James was also administered an interest inventory, the Self-Directed Search. This assesses six different interest types: realistic, investigative, social, enterprising, and conventional. He demonstrated high interests in jobs related to manual labor, managerial, and supervisory work activities (i.e., realistic).

This case study highlights a complex program of assessment that was applied at the outset in the case management of an individual. Not every case manager will utilize such a wide range of assessments but in this instance the professional decided that it was important to first obtain a detailed educational and employment history. Then there were gaps in the information that needed to be addressed. For this reason, the potential to learn was explored through aptitude tests. A surprising clinical finding is that people often have more potential than they have demonstrated in their life. So, test results are intended as a means of equal opportunity and affirmative action in case management. They are not the restrictive process that is often assumed by many laypersons.

Standardized assessments have the potential to provide information that is not otherwise readily available to the case manager. Far too often, their value as indicators of unrecognized human potential has been overlooked.

Vocational and educational assessments are just one factor that case managers might use to assist the individual make an informed choice and proceed with case management services. Test results might suggest that the individual will be successful in an educational endeavor, but because of financial and family considerations choose an on-the-job training program. The individual may not want to relocate and thus the case manager may need to help them explore options for employment in the local community.

Educational and vocational assessments are only a means to an end and not an end in and of themselves, with the end being career choice and successful job placement. As such the professional needs to look at assessment not to be used to screen people out because of not achieving a certain score but to screen people in for services and to use test results to identify through career counseling the best and most appropriate training and employment fit for the individual.

A study conducted by Crystal[6] examined skilled industrial, trade, and equipment operation workers who incurred a work injury and were unable to perform their past work because of the injury. The sample just included individuals who learned their past work through on the job training and experience. A battery of vocational and educational tests was administered. It was found that if these individuals had been given these tests when they were in high school they would not have met the aptitude and intellectual requirements for the occupations that they had successfully performed for many years. The investigator questioned the validity of the tests regarding predicting occupational success. More importantly, it was recommended that in future a variety of factors regarding the individual including motivation and support systems be considered when making career choices.[9]

CONCLUSION

In prior years, the question was: are we as case managers or other human service professionals merely "jacks of all trades?" That argument is being settled as we now have requirements for certification and in some instances, there is a movement towards licensure of professions. We operate in a holistic environment in which assessments are part of the case manager's toolbox in the context of evidence based practice and our knowledge of clients including their motivation, support systems, and background (age, education, disability, geographic location) among other factors. The principles of evidence-based practice are useful for considering when using assessments to case management. The ideology of evidence-based practice is derived from the field of public health and is defined as "the conscientious, explicit and judicious use of current best evidence in making decisions about the care of the individual patient. It means integrating individual clinical expertise with the best available external clinical evidence from systematic research" ("Evidence based medicine: what it is and what it isn't," paragraph 2).[13]

In health, an evidence-based approach is the integration of clinical expertise, patient values, and the best research evidence into the decision-making process for patient care. Clinical expertise refers to the clinician's cumulated experience, education, and clinical skills. The patient brings to the encounter his or her own personal preferences and unique concerns, expectations, and values. The best research evidence is usually found in clinically relevant research that has been conducted using sound methodology.[13] Evidence-based practice has been applied to assessment in case management. For instance, Fleming, Del Valle, Kim, and Leahy[7] indicated that counselors are under increased pressure to adopt and pursue such evidenced-based practices, and the professional literature has been criticized for a lack of empirical work providing support for individual-level interventions. They reviewed 25 years of research with specific attention to empirical studies related to active employment-focused interventions and present models of best practices. Studies were classified into categories based on interagency collaboration, counselor education and customer outcomes, services to a targeted group, supported employment and evidence-based practice, empowerment and customer self-concept, essential elements of service delivery, and miscellaneous vocational rehabilitation services and outcomes. They concluded that there was a need for evidence-based practice.

The application of evidence based to assessment for practitioners speaks to the utilization of all available information to assist the client identify and achieve his/her vocational and career goals. This includes using valid and reliable educational and vocational test results, obtaining input from the client and significant others regarding occupational aspirations, using existing information when available, and understanding the work environment in which the person will enter. Combining this information using professional counseling techniques will lead to successful client outcomes. Utilizing these factors in a holistic way and applying our theories and techniques will facilitate educational, vocational, and social planning. The appropriate use of tests within case management helps to ensure client success.

This chapter has emphasized how formal, standardized assessments offer a unique opportunity to enhance the value of case management. Assessment allows the case manager to gain new knowledge about a person. It allows one to focus on a person's strengths, talents, or aptitudes. At all times, the potential of the person being assessed is paramount. The client/applicant is not merely the object of the assessment but hopefully a willing participant in a collaborative process. Assessment is always subject to a strict code of professional ethics. In particular, the confidentiality and privacy of the person must be observed. In short, the goal in case management is not necessarily the assessment of a person but rather the use of assessment for a person. As case managers, we are fortunate that so many well-established approaches to assessment are available to us in our goal of promoting the potential of each client.

DISCUSSION QUESTIONS

1. What are the components of assessment in case management?

2. What are the advantages and disadvantages of the interview as a method of assessment?

3. What is the purpose of assessment in case management?

4. How can case managers ensure that the client benefits from assessments?

5. What technical aspects are key issues in formal, standardized assessments?

6. To what extent do scores provide realistic information about a client?

7. Outline some ethical considerations associated with assessment in case management.

REFERENCES

[1] American Educational Research Association, American Psychological Association, & National Council on Measurement in Education (1999). *Standards for educational and psychological testing*. Washington, DC: American Educational Research Association.

[2] Anastasi, A., & Urbina, S. (1997). *Psychological testing* (7th ed.). Upper Saddle River, NJ: Prentice Hall.

[3] Bervin, N. L. & Drout, M. O. (2012). Assessment. In D. R. Maki & V. Tarvydas (Eds.), *The professional practice of rehabilitation counseling* (pp. 213-240). New York, NY: Springer Publishing Company.

[4] Bolton, B. F., & Parker, R. M. (2008). *Handbook of measurement and evaluation in rehabilitation* (4th ed.). Austin, TX: PRO-ED, Inc.

[5] Cronbach, L. J. (1990). *Essentials of psychological testing* (5th ed.). New York, NY: Harper Collins.

[6] Crystal, R. M. (2000) The relationship between education, abilities, and prior employment of persons with work injuries and employment. *Rehabilitation Professional, 8*(2), 35-39.

[7] Fleming, A. R., Del Valle, R., Kim, M., Leahy, M. J. (2013). Best practice models of effective vocational rehabilitation service delivery in the public rehabilitation program: A review and synthesis of the empirical literature. *Rehabilitation Counseling Bulletin, 56*(3), 146-159.

[8]Heffner, C. L. (2017). Test validity and reliability. Retrieved from
https://allpsych.com/research methods/validityreliability/

[9]Lamprianou, I., & Athanasou, J. A. (2009). *A teacher's guide to educational
assessment*. Rotterdam, Netherlands: Sense Publishers.

[10]Linz, M. H., McAnally, P., & Wieck, C. (Eds.) (1989). *Case management:
Historical, current and future perspectives*. Cambridge, MA: Brookline
Books.

[11]Meyer, G. J., Finn, S. E., Eyde, L. D., Kay, G. G., Moreland, K. L., Dies, R.
R., Eisman, E. J., et al. (2001). Psychological testing and psychological
assessment: A review of evidence and issues. *American Psychologist, 56*(2),
128–165.

[12]Patton, W., & McMahon, M. (2006). *Career development and systems theory.
Connecting theory and practice* (2nd edition). Rotterdam, Netherlands: Sense
Publishers.

[13]Sackett, D. L., Rosenberg, W., Muir Gray, J., Haynes, R. B., & Richardson,
W. S. (1996). Evidence based medicine: What it is and what it isn't? *British
Medical Journal, 312*. doi: https://doi.org/10.1136/bmj.312.7023.71

[14]Segen, J. C. (2005). *Concise dictionary of modern medicine*. Baltimore, MD:
Johns Hopkins University Press.

[15]Woodside, M., & McClam, T. (2018). *Generalist case management: A
method of human service delivery* (5th ed.). Boston, MA: Cengage Learning.

[16]Wright, B. A., & Lopez, S. J. (2005). Widening the diagnostic focus: A case
for including human strengths and environmental resources. In C. R. Snyder
& S. J. Lopez (Eds.), *Handbook of positive psychology* (pp. 26- 44). New
York, NY: Oxford University Press.

PART II: CASE MANAGEMENT IN ACTION

Navigating Various Case Management service settings

CHAPTER 12

CASE MANAGEMENT, MENTAL HEALTH, AND SUBSTANCE ABUSE

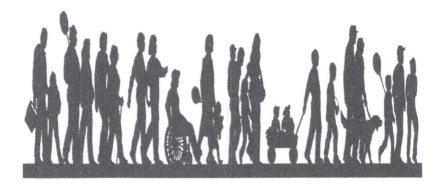

CARRIE L. ACKLIN

ABSTRACT

As can be noted so far in the book, a variety of service providers deliver case management services to a diverse set of clients. In this chapter, we will look at what case management services look like in the mental health and substance abuse field. When a person is referred for mental health or substance abuse treatment (in some cases a person is referred to both), he or she will have a level of care assessment completed. The purpose of the level of care assessment is to determine if mental health and substance abuse services are appropriate for the client and, if so, what type of treatment is the most appropriate for the client. We will also examine the multidimensional approach to mental health and substance abuse services, discuss the concept of least restrictive level of care, examine the various types of mental health and substance abuse services, and discuss how ignoring multicultural considerations can lead to misdiagnoses and invalidation. It must be noted that the interventions highlighted in this chapter can be used to facilitate services for ALL populations, including those who might be part of underrepresented groups in the United States.

CHAPTER HIGHLIGHTS

➤ The processes involved in accessing mental health and substance abuse treatment;

➤ The various types of mental health and substance abuse treatment services;

➤ Multicultural considerations in mental health and substance abuse treatment services.

LEARNING OBJECTIVES

➤ Identify the six dimensions in the multidimensional approach to determining the appropriate level of care.

➤ Describe and explain the concept of the least restrictive level of care.

➤ Examine the various types of inpatient and outpatient mental health and substance abuse treatment services.

➤ Identify and examine how ignoring multicultural considerations in mental health and substance abuse can cause harm to the client.

FROM THE BEGINNING: WHAT ARE MENTAL HEALTH AND SUBSTANCE ABUSE TREATMENT SERVICES?

Mental health and substance abuse treatment services are services that help clients learn ways to improve their overall health and wellbeing. There are several types of mental health and substance abuse services (which we will discuss later), but first, it is important for the healthcare practitioner to understand the systems and structure of mental health and substance abuse services as these systems and structures guide the types of treatment services that an agency can provide. In order for an agency to provide mental health and substance abuse services, the agency must be accredited. Accreditation refers to a set of rules, policies, and guidelines that the agency must follow to be considered "qualified" to provide services. These sets of rules, policies, and guidelines are referred to as accreditation standards.

The agency that creates the accreditation standards is often referred to as an accreditation body. For example, the Commission on Accreditation of Rehabilitation Facilities (often referred to as CARF) is an international accreditation body for aging services, behavioral health (i.e., mental health and substance abuse services), children and youth services, employment and community services, and medical rehabilitation.

The purpose of accreditation is to help agencies improve their quality of services. An agency is also regulated by federal and state laws. For example, there are laws that regulate the credentials that a healthcare provider must have to provide services. With reference to credentialed mental health and substance abuse providers, it is often the case that the healthcare practitioner is required to have at least a bachelor's degree and, in many cases, a master's degree. In the mental health and substance abuse field, practitioners are often required to also have a license to practice. Each state has their own set of qualifications (e.g., coursework, practical field experience) that a practitioner has to meet to become licensed.

Laws also regulate how treatment services are provided. For example, (as we will see later in the chapter) there are laws that detail how many hours of a given treatment service a client must have and how often the client's treatment plan is reviewed and updated. It is imperative that the healthcare practitioner is knowledgeable about the laws that regulate treatment services to ensure that the client's rights are not violated; and to be compliant with the regulations. Not following treatment laws can lead to negative consequences for an agency. The consequences can range from mild (e.g., receiving a written warning) to severe (e.g., closure of the agency).

To make matters more complicated, there are laws that are specific to mental health treatment services and laws that are specific to substance abuse treatment services. Therefore, in many states, the mental health system functions separately from the substance abuse system. Why is this important to know? Knowledge about the laws regulating mental health and substance abuse treatment services is important as each system has their own regulations.

Since the mental health system has separate regulating bodies from substance abuse treatment services, clients often become frustrated and, oftentimes, confused. The reason for client frustration and confusion is that if the client needs both mental health and substance abuse services, they often have separate intake assessments and will likely see one counselor for mental health services and another counselor for substance abuse treatment services. Seeing two counselors can be counterproductive for the client. Why? It might be the case that the client is addressing the same issues in both types of counseling. The redundancy of addressing the same issues with two different counselors can also lead to client confusion, especially if each counselor has their own counseling techniques and interventions. The client might feel that one counselor is guiding in one direction while the other counselor is guiding in a different direction.

While it seems to make sense that the quality of services for the client can be improved by addressing both mental health and substance abuse in one treatment setting, the fragmented systems makes it so that being able to provide both services in one setting difficult. The reason it is difficult to provide services for clients with co-occurring disorders (i.e., clients who have both mental health and substance abuse issues) is because of the regulations that must be followed under each system (as previously discussed). Let's look at what providing services to clients with co-occurring disorders looks like in a practical setting.

Each state has their own mental health administration and substance abuse administration where the rules and regulations of providing each service is determined. While each state has similar rules and regulations, the rules and regulations vary from state to state. To illustrate the impact of having two systems, the systems in the state of Illinois will be used as an example (with the understanding that other states will be similar to Illinois, yet different).

The Illinois Department of Human Services houses the agencies that regulate mental health services and substance abuse services. The Division of Mental Health Services is the regulating body of mental health treatment services in Illinois. Specifically, the Division of Mental Health Services is responsible for ensuring that all mental health providers in the state follow what is called Rule 132. Rule 132 is a piece of legislation that details requirements for each type of service that is provided (e.g., staff to client ratio, how many hours of treatment the client should have, minimum credentials of the provider); how often a client needs to have an assessment done; and how often the client's treatment plan needs to be reviewed.

Rule 132 also details administrative processes for delivering mental health services. For example, Rule 132 requires that in order to provide counseling services, a provider must be (at a minimum) a qualified mental health professional (QMHP). To be a QMHP in Illinois, the provider must possess a master's degree in a counseling-related field (e.g., rehabilitation, clinical mental health, psychology, social work). A provider who possesses a bachelor's degree in a counseling-related field can also provide services, however, the bachelor's level practitioner is considered a Mental Health Practitioner (MHP). What this means is that the MHP cannot provide counseling services, but can provide other services such as case management and community based support.

A third qualification that will allow a practitioner to provide mental health services is what is referred to as a Licensed Practitioner of the Healing Arts (LPHA). A LPHA is eligible to assume higher positions in an agency, such as a supervisor, a quality assurance team member, or an administrator. To become a LPHA in Illinois, the provider must be licensed–which means that he or she has met certain educational, training, and supervisory standards. Another aspect of Rule 132 is how often a client' assessment and treatment plan need to be updated. A client's assessment needs to be updated at least once a year and the client's treatment plan must be updated and reviewed every six months for outpatient treatment services. (We will discuss other types of services later in this chapter).

Why are accreditation standards, licensure requirements, local, state, and federal laws important to know? First, it is to ensure that appropriate services are being provided and to monitor the client's progress in treatment. Second, if the provider does not meet the review dates (e.g., once per year for assessments and every six months for treatment plans), the agency will not get paid for any services that are provided until the assessment or treatment plan are updated and reviewed. Many health and human service providers are not taught in their higher education training about the nuances of providing services and, therefore, struggle when they enter the field.

The Department of Alcoholism and Substance Abuse (DASA) is the agency that regulates substance abuse treatment services in Illinois. DASA's regulating law is referred to as Rule 2060. Much like Rule 132 on the mental health end of services, Rule 2060 details:

➢ agency and provider qualifications and credentials;

➢ what each type of substance abuse treatment service must include;

➢ staff to client ratio; and

➢ how often treatment plans and assessments need to be reviewed.

For example, to provide substance abuse services in Illinois, the practitioner must be eligible to obtain their Certified Alcohol and Drug Certification (CADC) within two years of their start date. There are several ways that a provider can become a CADC with a combination of education and experience. That is, a person with a high school diploma can become a CADC if he or she has two years of paid experience, 150 hours of clinical supervision, and 225 hours of addiction counseling specific education. If a person has a bachelor's degree or higher, the degree can substitute for the work experience requirements.

Much like Rule 132, Rule 2060 dictates how often a client's treatment plan needs to be updated. For example, for outpatient counseling, the client's treatment plan must be reviewed every 60 days or after 9 hours of treatment have been provided (one or the other, not both). Therefore, an agency must determine if they want to review the treatment plan after 60 days, or after 9 hours of treatment.

An additional component of Rule 2060 is that the provider must provide education to the client about communicable diseases such as tuberculosis, HIV/AIDS, and Hepatitis C. The reason the educational component is required is because communicable diseases tend to be higher in the substance abuse population when compared to people who do not abuse substances. Therefore, providing this education to clients can help the client become more aware of how to reduce any high-risk behaviors that can lead them to contract or transmit communicable diseases.

A third component of Rule 2060 is that all treatment plans must be reviewed and signed off on by a Medical Doctor (MD). The MD will review the treatment plan to determine if additional medical services need to be recommended to the client. A treatment plan is not considered to be valid unless it has an MD signature within 72 hours.

Many health and human services providers express that they do not learn about the rules and regulations in their higher education courses. One reason for this might be because each state has their own sets of rules and regulations. Nonetheless, the information related to rules in Illinois was presented to help you get a basic understanding of what goes on "behind the scenes" in mental health and substance abuse treatment services.

HOW DO CLIENTS ACCESS MENTAL HEALTH AND SUBSTANCE ABUSE TREATMENT SERVICES?

It has already been established in chapter 3 what occurs during the initial intake interview. There are also intake interviews when a person is seeking mental health and substance abuse treatment services. For this chapter, the initial intake interview will be referred to as a level of care (LOC) assessment. The reason that the intake interview is referred to as a LOC assessment is because the primary purpose is to determine what type(s) of mental health and/or substance abuse treatment services are the most appropriate for the client.

The LOC assessment is a comprehensive interview that covers the client's background which includes (but is not limited to) referral source, family history, previous or current medical and mental health diagnoses, previous or current substance abuse, previous or current medications, legal history, household size and income, and living situation. During the LOC assessment, the provider gathers this information to determine if mental health or substance abuse service s are appropriate and, if so, what type of treatment is the most appropriate for the client.

After the LOC is determined, the provider will make a referral to the appropriate type of treatment. We will see shortly that there are a variety of mental health and substance abuse services and each service has its own eligibility criteria. Therefore, the provider must be knowledgeable about the various types of treatment and the eligibility criteria so that it can be ensured that client is referred to the right type of treatment. Not being in the right type of treatment can have a negative impact on the client. For example, (*to take things out of the context of mental health and substance abuse for a moment*), suppose you went to your Primary Care Physician (PCP) because you think you broke your leg. Suppose that the PCP prescribed you cough medicine for your broken leg and sends you on your way. Obviously, nothing was done to fix your broken leg because the right type of treatment was not being used. It is the same with mental health and substance abuse services–administering the wrong type of treatment will not help the client become better.

One important point to note is that there are times when a client is referred to a certain type of treatment, but never receives the treatment. There are a few reasons for why this might happen: First, the client has the right to choose what type of treatment he or she is willing to participate in. There are times when a client refuses a referral to a certain type of treatment and expresses that he or she wants to be in a different type of treatment. As human service providers, we need to be sensitive to the client's right to choose his or her treatment, but also help the client to understand the benefits of receiving the appropriate treatment type.

Another time when a client might not access the appropriate treatment service is when the service is not available. For example, suppose that a client needs hospitalization for mental health issues, there are several instances (especially in rural areas) when the hospital is full and cannot admit any more clients. When the service type is full, it is often said that "the agency has no beds" or "all of the beds were full". When an agency's beds are full, the health and human service provider can put the client on the agency's waiting list, look for other agencies that provide similar treatment services, or make a referral to a lower level of care. The concept of "level of care" is discussed next.

WHAT IS MEANT BY LEVELS OF CARE?

A "level of care" refers to the characteristics of the service. Characteristics of services include:

➤ treatment setting;

➤ treatment length (i.e., how many hours of service the client receives each week); and

➤ treatment duration (i.e., how long the client is involved in services).

In mental health and substance abuse services, there are several levels of care. Services that are provided in a controlled environment (e.g., in a hospital setting or rehabilitation center) are said to be "higher levels of care" when compared to services such as outpatient treatment (e.g., services where the client goes to an agency for a number of sessions each week). The concept of levels of care is directly related to the concept of restrictiveness.

Restrictiveness refers to how much structure the treatment setting includes. For example, a client who is in a hospital-based treatment setting would be considered more restricted than a client receiving community based services in their home. The reason the hospital-based treatment setting is more restricted is because (when compared to the community based services) there are agency rules and policies that generally dictate when the client receives treatment services such as individual or group therapy, what the client can and cannot have (e.g., not permitted to have razors, perfume, caffeine), when the client eats (e.g., breakfast, lunch, dinner), when family members can visit, and what time is "lights out" (i.e., when the client goes to bed). Generally, the more structured a treatment service, the more restricted it is. Why is it important to understand what restrictiveness is? The answer lies at the core philosophy of making treatment referrals: The philosophy is referred to as "least restrictive level of care."

When referring to the least restrictive level of care, it is the provider's responsibility to determine what type of treatment can best meet the client's need for the lowest level of restrictiveness as possible. Why is this important? To answer that question, let's look at what deinstitutionalization is. Deinstitutionalization was a movement in the 1960s and 1970s that was geared toward moving clients out of hospitals (i.e., institutions) and re-integrating them into the community. With the advent of psychotropic medication, it was being found that several clients who were institutionalized did not need the intense structure of a hospital-based institution. Further, what was discovered was that several clients (especially clients with psychiatric disorders) were being "mass institutionalized." This mass institutionalization created treatment settings that health and human service providers could not keep up with. Further, there was a shortage of qualified health and human service providers to deliver services. Thus, the quality of services that clients were receiving was declining. Currently, the concept of deinstitutionalization is emphasized for providers to deliver mental health and substance abuse services in the least restricted level of care. For example, a person wants services to help them learn how to manage their money. It would not make sense to refer the client to a hospital to develop money management skills. Instead, helping the client develop money management skills can be provided in an outpatient setting where the client is seen once a week. So, when determining the appropriate level of care, the provider must take into consideration the level that the client's needs can best be met.

Understanding least restrictive level of care is also important when helping the client access follow up services. For example, a client might initially be referred to a rehabilitation facility where he or she receives services for two to three weeks, but will need additional supports and services after completion of the treatment at the rehabilitation facility. The provider would decide what lower level of care would best meet the client's needs. The movement through the different levels of care (in this case from a higher level of care to a lower level of care) is referred to as the continuum of care.

CONTINUUM OF CARE

The continuum of care refers to the different types of services that range in level of restrictiveness. It is the provider's responsibility to help facilitate the client's movement through the continuum of care to coordinate effective service delivery. The continuum of care often includes making referrals to lower levels of care and following up to confirm that the client was able to access the lower level of care. The continuum of care in mental health and substance abuse treatment ranges from inpatient (i.e., residential) treatment to outpatient treatment.

It is important to note that not all clients start at a high level of care and move to a lower level of care. Some clients might enter in a lower level of care and have their needs met while other clients might start at a low level of care and need a higher level of care. Suppose a client (who will be called Joe) had a LOC assessment completed and was referred to outpatient substance abuse counseling services to help him address his alcohol use. Joe was initially referred to receive counseling services one a week. After three sessions, Joe told his counselor that his drinking increased to daily alcohol use and that he feels that he cannot manage his drinking any longer. The counselor could continue to see Joe on a weekly basis, but the current level of care that Joe is receiving (outpatient) does not appear to be helping him reduce his alcohol use. The counselor would need to re-assess Joe's alcohol use and make a referral to a higher level of care (perhaps residential rehabilitation). Joe's example displays how clients might start out in a low level of care (in this example, outpatient) and require a higher level of care (e.g., residential rehabilitation).

The continuum of care is similar between mental health and substance abuse treatment services, even though these services are often provided separately. The next section details the various types of treatment services in mental health and substance abuse. However, it is important to understand that the names and characteristics of each service can vary by state. The following is to be used as a general guideline for understanding the various types of treatment services. There are two main categories of services: Inpatient and Outpatient.

INPATIENT TREATMENT SERVICES

Inpatient treatment services (often referred to as residential services) are used when the client stays overnight at an agency until he or she has completed services. The amount of time that a client receives inpatient treatment services depends on his or her needs and varies for each client. The reason that the amount of time varies for each client is because each client presents with his or her own unique needs and there is a treatment philosophy that mental health and substance abuse services are individualized.

Individualization of services means that each client's treatment plan is unique to his or her needs and that no one approach to providing services is appropriate for all clients. Below are descriptions of the various types of residential mental health and substance abuse treatment services. As a general rule, unless specifically stated, the descriptions of the treatment types can be generalized to both the mental health and the substance abuse field.

DETOXIFICATION. Detoxification (commonly referred to as detox) is a medical substance abuse treatment service that helps the client safely come off of substances that he or she has been abusing. This LOC is reserved for clients who would experience withdrawal symptoms if they did not receive medical treatment. When a client uses a substance for an extended period of time in a consistent manner (e.g., drinking alcohol daily for six months), the client is at risk of withdrawing if he or she would suddenly discontinue the substance use.

Withdrawal from certain substances can be life-threatening if the client does not receive detoxification treatment. For example, a client presented to the LOC assessment and stated that he or she had been drinking alcohol for the past six months on a daily basis. The client would likely be at risk of serious withdrawal symptoms if he or she stopped drinking alcohol without medical treatment. Alcohol withdrawal is life-threatening and should be taken seriously. Early signs of withdrawal from alcohol can be sweating, shakiness, goosebumps, nausea, diarrhea to more serious symptoms such as seizures, delirium tremens (i.e., the "DTs" which are a series of hallucinations and delusions), and major organ failure.

A second substance that has life-threatening withdrawal symptoms are benzodiazepines (often referred to as "benzos"). Benzos are a category of prescription medications (e.g., Xanax, Ativan, Valium) that are used to treat anxiety disorders. Benzodiazepine withdrawal is very similar to alcohol withdrawal in that the client may experience symptoms of sweating, shakiness, nausea, and seizures.

Withdrawal from opioids (i.e., heroin and prescription medications such as Vicodin, Norco, Oxycodone, Oxycontin, Percocet, Fentanyl, Morphine) can mimic withdrawal symptoms from alcohol and benzodiazepines, however, withdrawal from opioids is not life-threatening. Although the range of withdrawal symptoms vary based on the substance that the client is withdrawing from, the most common substances of abuse that are seen in detoxification services are alcohol, benzodiazepines, and opioids.

CRISIS STABILIZATION. Crisis stabilization is primarily a residential mental health treatment service that has an average length of stay from three to five days. Crisis stabilization services differ from traditional hospital-based mental health services (to be discussed below). The purpose of the crisis stabilization unit is to provide therapeutic and psychiatric support for individuals who present with suicidal or homicidal ideation. Suicidal ideation is when an individual has thoughts or plans to harm themselves. Some individuals who access crisis stabilization may present with suicidal thoughts with no plan or means in place to carry out the thoughts of harm. Other individuals may present to the crisis stabilization unit with either an active plan to harm themselves with the means to do so, or they may have attempted to harm themselves.

Homicidal ideation, in contrast to suicidal ideation, is when an individual has thoughts or a plan to harm someone else. Much like suicidal ideation, individuals with homicidal ideation may present with only thoughts, but no active plan, to harm someone, or an individual may present with thoughts, an active plan, and the means necessary to harm another person.

It is crucial when a human service professional is working with a client that the professional assess for suicidal or homicidal ideation. The primary focus is on the safety of the client and the safety of others. Therefore, the human service professional must be knowledgeable of the agency policies and procedures that he or she is working with regarding clients who may present with suicidal or homicidal ideation. It is also important to understand that when a client presents with suicidal or homicidal ideation, confidentiality takes a "back seat" to ensuring the safety of the client and others. Therefore, in many situations, the human service professional does not have to go through the steps of obtaining client consent to release personal identifying information. Further, in the case of homicidal ideation with an active plan, an identified person to harm, and the means to carry out the harm, the human service professional has a duty to warn the targeted person of the client's intent and the means to harm them. These steps should be taken as soon as possible and a referral for crisis stabilization treatment should be prioritized.

MEDICALLY-MONITORED RESIDENTIAL SERVICES. Medically monitored residential services are treatment services that take place at an agency and are staffed by medical professionals (e.g., nurses, physicians) and clinicians (e.g., counselors, case managers). Some states differentiate between the different types of medically-monitored residential services. For example, in Pennsylvania, there is a distinction between medically-monitored short-term residential treatment (i.e., a length of stay shorter than 30 days) and medically-monitored long-term residential treatment (i.e., a length of stay of about 90 days). The key term here is "medically-monitored" regardless of whether the residential service is considered short-term or long-term. This means that the treatment service has access to medical practitioners 24 hours a day, 7 days a week (also referred to as "24-7"), but there is not an attending physician on site 24-7.

In medically-monitored short-term residential treatment, the primary focus is on client rehabilitation, (i.e., helping the client to re-integrate skills and tools that he or she needs to function optimally in their home setting). This might include implementing healthy coping skills (e.g., deep breathing to help reduce anxiety, or perhaps using social skills to help build a healthy support network), or it could also include re-establishing certain vocational skills (e.g., organization, time management, resumé writing).

Long-term medically-monitored residential treatment services tend to focus more on habilitation of the client. As was previously mentioned, habilitation includes helping the client develop the skills and tools that are needed to function optimally in their home setting. Habilitation may include the development of interpersonal skills to develop a healthy support network, money and time management skills, vocational skills, or relapse prevention skills (i.e., a set of skills that are used to prevent symptoms from reoccurring).

MEDICALLY-MANAGED RESIDENTIAL TREATMENT SERVICES. Medically-managed residential treatment services are very similar to medically-monitored residential treatment services, but the service setting and staff is slightly different. The key distinction between the two types of residential treatment services is that in medically-managed residential treatment, there must be a physician on staff 24-7. Medically-managed residential treatment services are typically provided in a hospital-based setting. Clients who seek these services typically present with a mental health or substance use disorder or both; and a medical condition that can only be safely treated and monitored in a medical setting. For example, a client would likely be appropriate for this LOC if he or she presented with depression, anxiety, an alcohol use disorder, and cirrhosis (i.e., inflammation of the liver usually caused by alcohol that impairs the liver's ability to filter out toxins in the body). The primary aim of this LOC is to not only to stabilize the client's mental health or substance use disorders, but to also gain medical stabilization for his or her medical condition.

SUMMARY OF RESIDENTIAL TREATMENT SERVICES

There are several types of residential treatment services. Detoxification is a substance abuse treatment service that helps the individual safely come off of substances. Crisis stabilization is a service for individuals that present with suicidal or homicidal ideation with the primary goal of helping the individual to phase out of the crisis.

Medically-monitored short-term residential treatment involves 24-hour medical supervision with the goal of rehabilitation, but does not have an attending physician on-site 24-7. Medically-monitored long-term residential is very similar to short-term residential in terms of treatment setting and professional staffing, however, the focus tends to be on habilitation instead of rehabilitation and involves a longer length of stay.

Medically-managed residential treatment services are often in a hospital-based setting where there is an attending physician on staff 24-7. Not every client will begin in a residential treatment setting after a LOC is completed, but some do. After the client is discharged from residential treatment services, he or she is typically referred to a lower LOC that is outpatient rather than residential. Much like residential treatment services, there are several different types of outpatient treatment services that vary in terms of service setting, length of stay, and intensity (i.e., how many hours per week the client is receiving treatment services). The human service professional that is providing case management services plays a key role in the client's movement through the various LOCs.

OUTPATIENT TREATMENT SERVICES

Outpatient treatment refers to counseling services that are provided at the agency, but do not involve the client staying overnight. The number of hours that the client receives services depends on the type of outpatient treatment. The types of outpatient treatment services that will be discussed in this section are:

➢ Medically monitored non-residential services;

➢ Halfway houses;

➢ Partial hospitalization;

➢ Intensive outpatient; and

➢ Outpatient.

MEDICALLY MONITORED NON-RESIDENTIAL SERVICES. Medically monitored non-residential services are often provided in the community to provide support for the client in his or her home setting. One of the most common medically monitored non-residential service that is provided is called Assertive Community Treatment (ACT). ACT is an evidence-based comprehensive treatment program that was developed to help provide community support for individuals with psychiatric disorders who were transitioning out of a hospital-based treatment program.[8] ACT is a team-oriented approach of 10-12 practitioners that can include counselors, psychiatrists, psychologists, and nursing staff. The ACT team works with clients in their home and community setting to help them move toward their recovery. There is no maximum length of stay in ACT services. In other words, a client can be involved in ACT for as long as it is appropriate for this level of care. The team-approach in ACT services means that each practitioner (whether it be a case manager or a therapist) does not have his or her own caseload. In other types of treatment, it is common that the practitioner has a list of clients that is "assigned" to him or her. In ACT, the team shares the caseload and rotates which clients they see and when.

The primary purpose of ACT services is to help clients function optimally in their home setting with a goal of preventing re-hospitalization. The scope of services provided in ACT can range from individual mental health and substance abuse therapy, assistance going out in the community (e.g., grocery shopping, job hunting, or to medical appointments), psychiatric services, or help with developing and becoming involved in community services.

HALFWAY HOUSES. Halfway houses are houses within the community that enable clients to re-integrate into the community with therapeutic support. Halfway houses are not typically advertised in the community as halfway houses in order to help reduce the stigmatization associated with receiving this type of service. Clients who are involved in a halfway house typically receive both individual and group therapy with involvement in community services, like self-help groups (e.g., alcoholics anonymous, referred to as "AA" or narcotics anonymous often referred to as "NA").

The primary purpose of the halfway house is for the client to continue to build his or her social and interpersonal skills to function optimally in a community-based setting. The length of stay at a halfway house can vary based on the client's needs. A client may be involved in halfway house services for one month up to one year (again, depending on his or her needs). When involved in halfway house services, the client lives at the house as though it was his or her own home, but lives with other clients and works toward becoming employed. The client can go out in the community as he or she wishes, but will generally have a curfew to abide by.

The philosophy behind many halfway houses is to provide an atmosphere where the client can work on several aspects of his or her life (e.g., returning to work, returning to school, family relationships) in a mutually supportive atmosphere that fosters collaboration among fellow halfway house clients. The treatment team is usually comprised of psychiatrists, psychologists, counselors, and other support professionals (e.g., those that help administer medications, provide supervision and guidance within the agency as well as in the community).

PARTIAL HOSPITALIZATION. Partial hospitalization (often referred to as a day program) is a less restrictive level of treatment service. The client goes to an agency for services and stays there throughout the day, but goes home at the end of the day. The client can be involved in partial hospitalization for three to six months, but the length of stay depends upon the needs of the client. For example, a client's needs might be met with three months of partial hospitalization services but it might also be the case that a client needs more than three months of services.

The primary purpose of partial hospitalization is to help the client implement activities of daily living while reducing the likelihood that the client would need residential treatment services. The human service professionals that provide partial hospitalization services typically include psychiatrists, psychologists, counselors, case managers, and other support professionals (e.g., people who help administer medications or supervise activities both within and outside of the agency). The types of treatment that clients receive in partial hospitalization are vast. They could include activities such as implementing activities of daily living (e.g., cooking, cleaning, laundry), engaging in social activities (e.g., fundraising, dances, support groups, group therapy, or individual therapy). The client attends services for approximately 20 hours per week for at least three days.

INTENSIVE OUTPATIENT. A common "step-down" from partial hospitalization is a client who is involved in intensive outpatient treatment (IOP). The client typically receives at least 9 hours of individual and group therapy per week. The client attends services approximately three days out of the week, but attendance can vary based on agency and state regulations. IOP helps the client address issues such as using healthy coping skills that do not involve the use of substances, addressing co-occurring disorders (e.g., addiction, anxiety, and depression), and implementing healthy activities of daily living when they leave treatment. The client is involved in both individual therapy and group therapy. Some topics addressed during group therapy can include (but is not limited to) relapse prevention (i.e., preventing a return of symptoms or substance use), parenting, anger management, building healthy social supports, time management, and money management. Once an individual completes intensive outpatient treatment, he or she is typically referred to outpatient treatment which is less intensive than intensive outpatient treatment.

OUTPATIENT. Outpatient treatment is one of the lowest levels of care. A client who is involved in outpatient treatment can typically receive up to (but usually not exceeding) 8 hours of care per week. The client can be involved in both individual and group therapy. The number of hours that a client is seen in outpatient treatment is based on his or her individual needs. It might be that a client is only involved in individual therapy and is seen for one hour a week, or it could be that the client is involved in both individual and group therapy and is seen weekly for individual therapy and goes to group twice per week. Outpatient is like IOP except the hours of care the client receives is different. Much like IOP, the client can address multiple issues in outpatient treatment which may include (but is not limited to) relapse prevention, anger management, healthy coping, developing healthy supports, family relationships, money management, time management, etc. The primary purpose of outpatient treatment is to provide therapeutic support while the client works on his or her recovery.

SUMMARY OF OUTPATIENT TREATMENT SERVICES

The variety of the different types of mental health and substance abuse outpatient treatment services is vast. These outpatient services can range from highly intensive (e.g., medically-monitored non-residential services and partial hospitalization) to less intensive (e.g., intensive outpatient and outpatient treatment). The treatment teams in each type of outpatient service setting tend to be very similar (e.g., psychiatrist, psychologist, counselors, case managers, other support staff), but the philosophy and purpose of each type of outpatient treatment can vary. Nonetheless, it may be that a client is transitioning from residential care to outpatient treatment, but it may also be that the client only needs outpatient treatment service. Remember, a guiding philosophy on determining which LOC is the most appropriate for the client is the least restrictive level of care that can adequately meet the client's needs. You might be asking yourself how the appropriate LOC is determined. We will look at the different assessment tools that are used to help the healthcare practitioner determine the appropriate LOC.

AFTER THE LOC ASSESSMENT: DETERMINING THE APPROPRIATE LEVEL OF CARE

There is no standard set of criteria in the U.S. that is used to determine which LOC is the most appropriate. The criteria that is used to determine LOC varies from state to state and is usually guided by state law. While the criteria vary from state to state, there are very common similarities that can be found in each state. One similarity is using the criteria to examine a multidimensional approach to determining LOC. The multidimensional approach includes criteria that assesses multiple aspects of the client's life, (e.g., acute intoxication and withdrawal; biomedical conditions; mental health symptoms; willingness to participate in treatment and treatment engagement; relapse potential; and recovery environmental support). Below, we will look at each of these dimensions and the general criteria that is examined under each dimension. It is important to note that these criteria are subjective, meaning that they are up to the interpretation of the human service practitioner. When determining LOC, there is a lot of interpretation and assessment from the human service practitioner to arrive at what services would be most appropriate for the client. The case study at the end of this section will provide an illustration of what assessment might look like in a clinical setting.

THE MULTIDIMENSIONAL APPROACH TO DETERMINING LOC IN MENTAL HEALTH AND SUBSTANCE ABUSE TREATMENT

As mentioned in the beginning of this section, there is no universal standard set of criteria in the U.S. that is used to determine which LOC is the most appropriate for a client. Some states may use a set of criteria (i.e., the American Society for Addictions Medicine [ASAM]).[5] The ASAM provides multidimensional criteria for each level of care for both adults and adolescents. Another common set of criteria that some states use is called the Level of Care Utilization System (LOCUS).[2] The LOCUS is also a multidimensional approach for determining the appropriate LOC for adults and adolescents with mental health or substance abuse problems.

Please keep in mind that the ASAM and LOCUS may not be used in each state while we work on discussing the different types of criteria. There may be cases where a certain state develops its own criteria (e.g., the state of Pennsylvania uses their own multidimensional criteria called the Pennsylvania Client Placement Criteria[3]). The following description of the multidimensional criteria should be used as a guide to familiarize yourself with the general aspects of LOC placement criteria.

DIMENSION 1: ACUTE INTOXICATION AND WITHDRAWAL. The first dimension (acute intoxication and withdrawal) examines whether the client presented to his or her LOC assessment either under the influence of substances, at risk for, or currently in, withdrawal from substances. As was previously mentioned in this chapter, it is important to assess a client's risk of withdrawal. If the client is currently experiencing, or is at risk of withdrawal, the human service professional must be sure to make a referral for detoxification treatment as soon as possible. The reason for this is that a client who is withdrawing from substances of abuse will not be able to focus on any other treatment goals until detoxification treatment is completed. However, the client could be at risk for withdrawal, but is currently under medically supervised treatment to suppress the withdrawal symptoms.

An example of risk for withdrawal is a client who is involved in medication management treatment for opioid addiction. Medication management is a treatment service where the client receives certain medications to prevent withdrawal symptoms from happening. In opioid treatment, two common medications that are used are suboxone and methadone. Both suboxone and methadone are opioids that last longer than common opioids of abuse (e.g., prescription pain killers, heroin) and, therefore, can help the client stop abusing opioids. Suboxone works by combining the effects of opioids with a medication that blocks the effects of feeling "high" from opioids. Ideally, suboxone treatment is short-term (e.g., less than 12 months) for a person who had been abusing opioids.

Methadone is like suboxone only that it does not contain the additional medications that block the effects of the opioids. Individuals who are on methadone maintenance tend to be involved in treatment longer than those who are in a suboxone program. If the client would suddenly stop taking his or her suboxone or methadone, they would start to feel the effects of withdrawal. However, if the client is taking his or her medications as prescribed and not abusing them, then it may be that his or her risk of withdrawal is low. This certainly impacts the human service practitioner's assessment of whether the client would need detoxification services.

DIMENSION 2: BIOMEDICAL CONDITIONS. The second dimension, biomedical conditions, looks at what medical conditions the client presents with and whether these medical conditions are being adequately treated. For example, it may be that the client has type II diabetes, but it is being adequately treated through the client's primary care physician. In this case, the provider may assess that although there is a biomedical condition present it is being adequately treated. In another case, a client has a long history of alcohol abuse and was recently tested for liver disease, but is not yet receiving any type of medical care for the liver disease. In this case, the human service practitioner may assess that the client needs hospital-based residential services to help address both the alcohol use disorder as well as the liver disease.

DIMENSION 3: MENTAL HEALTH SYMPTOMS. As in any intake interview or assessment, it is essential for the human service practitioner to assess whether there are any mental health symptoms present and, if so, determine the potential causes of the symptoms, the severity of the symptoms, the symptoms impact on the client's ability to engage in his or her activities of daily living, and whether the symptoms are being adequately treated and managed. For example, a client might present with symptoms of depression (e.g., lack of energy, feeling sad and hopeless, inability to concentrate, over or under eating, over or under sleeping). However, it might also be determined that there is co-occurring substance use as well. Therefore, the human service practitioner would want to assess how long the depressive symptoms have been happening and whether the depressive symptoms occurred before, during, or after the substance use. Some substances of abuse (e.g., alcohol, cocaine) can make depressive symptoms worse. It might also be that the depressive symptoms occurred before any substance use and the substance use is a catalyst for self-medicating for the depressive symptoms.

Of course, this is just one of the many examples of mental health symptoms that clients can present with. Risk of harm to self or others is also taken into consideration under the mental health dimension. The human service practitioner must be able to assess whether there is a threat of harm to self or others and determine the extent to which the client and others' safety is at risk. It is essential that the human service practitioner gathers comprehensive information regarding the symptoms, current or past treatment, and current or past medications that the client is or was on.

DIMENSION 4: WILLINGNESS TO PARTICIPATE IN TREATMENT. It is important for the human service practitioner to understand that not all clients are self-referred to treatment. Self-referral means that the client expressed a desire on their own terms to access mental health or substance abuse treatment services. There are times when the client is referred by external sources such as physicians, probation or parole officers, friends, or family members. In mental health and substance abuse treatment, the human service practitioner assesses the client's willingness to participate and engage in treatment by using the transtheoretical model of the stages of change.[6] The transtheoretical model of stages of change consists of six levels:

- precontemplation;
- contemplation;
- preparation;
- action;
- maintenance; and
- relapse.

PRECONTEMPLATION. Clients who are in the precontemplation stage of change tend to believe that there is no problem or interference of their symptoms on their daily living. Clients who are in the precontemplation stage are often referred to treatment by an external source such as a family member, a friend, a probation, or parole officer. Signs that a client is in the precontemplation stage of change can be:

- minimizing the severity of symptoms;
- denial of symptoms; or
- rationalization or justification of why the symptoms are not problematic.

A client who minimizes the severity of symptoms tends to take a situation that, to others, is problematic and make it seem like it is not a big deal. An example of rationalizing is if a client says "my depression is not as bad as people will say it is. I mean, sure I get a little sad, but it is not a big deal." A client who justifies his or her symptoms provides excuses for why the symptoms are present or why there is a certain behavior. With reference to substance use as an example, a client may say "Even though my family says I have a drinking problem, I only drink because they are the ones who are stressing me out." These are both examples of what a person who is in the precontemplation stage of change may say or do.

CONTEMPLATION. A person who is in the contemplation stage of change begins to consider the possibility that there is a problem or that something needs to change. A person who is in the contemplation stage of change often experiences ambivalence. Ambivalence means that the person might recognize the need for change, but is hesitant to follow through with the change. An example of what it might look like in a clinical setting: A client may express, "Well, I suppose that my depression is worse than I thought, but I don't really know if I am ready to change things about the people that I hang around or change wanting to be alone all of the time." There are certain interventions and strategies that can be used to help someone reduce their ambivalence about moving forward with change and to help them move toward the preparation stage.

PREPARATION. The preparation stage of change is characterized by the person preparing the needed resources and tools to act on making the change happen. For an individual who may need residential treatment, this might include preparation by informing family and friends of the decision to enter residential treatment or by packing clothing that will be needed during their stay. An individual in the preparation stage of change has made the commitment to making the change and is working toward engaging in behaviors that will allow the person to make the change.

ACTION. This stage of change is characterized by the person committing to making a change and implementing the skills, tools, and strategies that are needed to carry out the change. In the example of the individual who may decide to engage in residential treatment, this may involve actively going to the treatment center or actively calling a family member or a friend to take him or her to the treatment center.

While in treatment, the individual will work toward building skills and tools that are needed to reduce his or her overall symptoms with a goal to increasing the individual's ability to function as independently as possible. Once these skills and tools are learned and the individual has learned how to implement the skills and tools, he or she would then move into the maintenance stage of change.

MAINTENANCE. The maintenance stage of change is characterized by the individual's ability to maintain the skills and tools that he or she has learned and implemented in his or her daily living. The key feature of the maintenance stage of change is that the person no longer requires intensive therapeutic assistance in implementing skills and tools on a routine basis. However, this is not to say that an individual in the maintenance stage of change is no longer in need of therapeutic supports and services, it simply means that the person is able to carry out his or her activities of daily living (e.g., money management, time management, bathing, working, cooking, etc.). However, if the individual starts to show signs or symptoms that could be problematic, he or she may move into the relapse stage of change.

RELAPSE. Relapse is a return to the distressing behaviors or symptoms that brought the client to treatment to begin with. Please keep in mind that not all providers adhere to this definition of relapse. To some providers, relapse can occur when the client starts to exhibit maladaptive thinking patterns that can, ultimately, lead to the distressing behaviors and symptoms that brought the client to treatment.

A client who is in the relapse stage of change might exhibit signs of denial (e.g., believing that their behaviors, thoughts, and actions are not problematic), minimization (e.g., "downplaying" the severity of a problem), or justification (e.g., providing excuses for one's behavior). A client who is in the relapse stage of change is no longer maintaining the positive changes that they may have previously made. The stages of change model provide a general guideline of how people go through changes in their lives. This movement through the stage of change is not always a linear process, discussed next.

A person may not follow the sequence of starting out in the precontemplation stage then moving to contemplation, then to preparation, then action, maintenance, and relapse. The progression through the stages of change is a fluid and dynamic process that can involve skipping stages (e.g., moving from precontemplation to action or moving from contemplation to relapse), or moving back and forth through the stages (e.g., moving back and forth between precontemplation and contemplation or back and forth between relapse and maintenance). The reason this is important to understand is that humans are complex beings and it is difficult to implement concrete "rules" of human behavior. The stages of change model are simply used to gauge where the person is in terms of readiness to change and willingness to engage in treatment. After this has been determined, the human services professional can look at the fifth dimension of the multidimensional approach: relapse potential.

DIMENSION 5: RELAPSE POTENTIAL. The relapse potential dimension examines the client's risk factors that could lead to a relapse. Recall that relapse can be defined as either the return of symptoms that were the source of distress (e.g., anxiety, depression, strained relationships, hallucinations, delusions), return to substance use, or a return to thoughts, feelings, and behaviors that lead to a return of distressing symptoms or substance use. Risk factors can be defined as people, places, and things that can increase the likelihood of symptoms recurring, or people, places, and things, that increase the likelihood of the person returning to substance use. It is important to understand that relapse potential does not relate only to either a return of symptoms or a return to substance use. Relapse potential can include both the presence of symptoms in addition to a return to substance use. Often, there are distressing symptoms that a person has difficulty coping (i.e., dealing) with and will use substances to help alleviate the distressing symptoms. If the person is currently in a state of distress or is currently using substances, the human services practitioner will assess what factors are contributing to the continuation of distressing symptoms, substance use, or both.

DIMENSION 6: RECOVERY ENVIRONMENT SUPPORT. The recovery environment support dimension takes into consideration factors such as the client's living situation (e.g., living with friends, family, independently, homeless) as well as the client's natural supports. Natural supports refer to any person, organization, or agency that the client is involved with that provides the client with physical or mental support. Physical support may include helping the client engage in their activities of daily living (e.g., bathing, dressing, or washing clothing, etc.). Mental support may include providing love, affection, and stability (e.g., financial, emotional, or housing stability) for the client.

Researchers have shown that natural supports are an integral part of a person's recovery.[4] Determining the extent to which the client has natural supports is critical to helping the client enter recovery. If the client does not have a natural support system, the practitioner can help the client access supports such as self-help groups, (e.g., community-based groups comprised of community members who share a similar interest). A classic example of a self-help group is Alcoholics Anonymous (commonly referred to as "AA"). Members of AA come together to talk about their lives and any issues they may be having (e.g., cravings that include thoughts and urges to drink or use substances, relationship difficulties) and to provide support to one another (e.g., emotional support, encouragement, socialization). The six dimensions in the multidimensional approach to determining the appropriate level of care helps to provide a framework for the practitioner to assess if services are needed and, if so, at what level. However, determining the appropriate LOC is not always straightforward.

IMPLEMENTING THE MULTIDIMENSIONAL APPROACH TO DETERMINE APPROPRIATE LOC

Now that the various levels of mental health and substance abuse treatment have been discussed and the multidimensional approach to determining the appropriate LOC has been introduced, let's look at how determining the appropriate LOC looks like in a practical setting. Keep in mind that each health and human services agency will have similar, yet varying, criteria to guide the provider in determining what type of mental health or substance abuse treatment (or both) is the most appropriate for the client. Although each agency will have varying criteria for determining the appropriate LOC, there are unique issues that members of underrepresented groups experience in mental health and substance abuse treatment. A theme that cannot be dismissed when examining the outcomes of many of the following underrepresented groups is discrimination, be it unintentional or not. Here, we will explore the unique issues experienced by women, people with disabilities, and people of color, (to name a few).

WOMEN IN MENTAL HEALTH AND SUBSTANCE ABUSE TREATMENT

According to SAMHSA,[9] women have a higher rate of mental health and substance use disorders when compared to their male counterparts. More specifically, women tend to have higher rates of depression, anxiety disorders, eating disorders, bipolar disorders, and schizophrenic-related disorders than males. Further, SAMHSA[9] asserted that the presence of a mental health disorder increases the likelihood that there is a co-occurring substance use disorder. *Why is the presence of mental health symptoms more common in women when compared to men?* The answer is fairly straight forward. In the U.S., there is a general expectation that women are to be the "caretakers" of the household (e.g., making sure the household is clean, taking care of the children, assuring laundry is done). However, what is oftentimes overlooked is that the number of women who are working is increasing. Thus, there is a paradigm shift from women being the "housekeepers" to being members of the workforce. This paradigm shift creates a conflict when it comes to an assumption about the roles of women in the U.S. Further, women experience higher levels of stress when compared to men. This stress is experienced both inside the home and in the workplace. An example, it is well known that women are paid less than men for performing the same job. Thus, women are expected to perform equally, if not better, than men for less pay. Factors such as higher stress and low pay contribute to the higher rates of co-occurring disorders in women. Understanding the unique issues faced by women can help the case manager use effective interventions, such as validating the life experiences of women.

PEOPLE WITH DISABILITIES

The presence of a disability can impact the person's overall health and wellbeing. But, there is a debate whether having a disability increases the likelihood of a mental health or a substance use disorder. What is not debatable is that people with disabilities experience unique stressors compared to people without disabilities. Stressors such as chronic pain, financial hardship, low socioeconomic status, and limited education (to name a few) can increase the likelihood that a person with a disability uses substances as a coping mechanism.

Another issue faced by many people with disabilities when it comes to accessing mental health and substance abuse treatment services is that not all facilities are fully accessible. Many outpatient and residential treatment agencies require that a person is fully ambulatory (e.g., able to get around from place to place independently). Agencies that lack ramps, wide hallways, and wide doorways would not be accessible to a person who uses a wheelchair. Another way an agency might not be fully accessible is if the agency lacked materials that were translated to Braille (e.g., pamphlets, treatment plans). The lack of materials in alternate media formats (e.g., Braille) would be a barrier to a person who was blind or low-vision.

Last, an agency that does not provide interpreter services (i.e., a person who can translate spoken language to sign language) would be a barrier for a person who is Deaf or hard of hearing. It is important that the case manager is aware of the unique barriers faced by people with disabilities so that resources can be coordinated to facilitate the treatment process and reduce the barriers that create unequal access for people with disabilities.

PEOPLE OF COLOR

The number of people with color (e.g., African Americans, Latino Americans) who are diagnosed with a mental health disorder is disproportionate to the number of European-Americans with mental health disorders. According to Schwartz and Blankenship,[7] African Americans are three to four times more likely than their European-American counterparts to be diagnosed with a psychiatric disorder while Latino Americans/Hispanics are three times as likely to be diagnosed with a psychiatric disorder when compared to European Americans.

There are several factors associated with the overrepresentation of mental health disorders in people of color. First, there is a lack of culturally competent care for people of color in the mental health and substance abuse field. A lack of awareness and understanding of unique issues that people of color face can lead to misdiagnoses. As an example, African American males are diagnosed with schizophrenia-related disorders five times more than their European American male counterparts.[7]

Often, providers do not investigate the accuracy of such diagnoses and assume that the diagnosis is correct. This can lead the case manager to make erroneous assumptions about the client, which can cause harm in several ways. First, there is stigma associated with certain diagnoses. By not understanding how the client was diagnosed, the associated symptoms, and who provided the diagnosis, the case manager may further stigmatize the client.

Another way that the case manager may cause harm is by invalidating the client's lived experiences. For example, people of color tend to report that they do not feel like they are heard, believed, or understood by providers. This invalidation can discourage the client from engaging in, or returning to, services.[1] Acklin and Wilson[1] define validation as providing truth to one's story. When a client feels that he or she has been validated, the quality and effectiveness of services increases when compared to clients who are not validated by the provider. Therefore, it is essential that the case manager has a working knowledge, awareness, and understanding of the unique issues experienced by people of color and the impact that these unique issues have on service quality and engagement.

PUTTING IT ALL TOGETHER: CASE STUDY CARTER

Carter is a 38-year-old African American male who was referred by his parole officer to have an assessment completed. Carter was incarcerated for two years for possession of marijuana and was recently released on parole two months ago. When Carter was asked if it was a mental health or substance abuse assessment, he replied

254

"Well, I don't know. I was in jail for the past two years because I was caught with a controlled substance. My parole officer said that she thought I needed both mental health and substance abuse treatment because I have been feeling really depressed and anxious lately." The healthcare practitioner continued with the LOC assessment and learned that Carter had a previous diagnosis of schizoaffective disorder. Upon further assessment, Carter explained that he and his ex-wife got into an argument about his ex-wife's new boyfriend. He explained that his ex-wife's new boyfriend would follow him around town and threaten him. Carter talked about how he felt threatened, but that the local police department would not press any charges since there were no restraining orders on his ex-wife's boyfriend. Carter explained to the practitioner that his ex-wife's boyfriend pointed a gun at him and threatened him if he tried to see his two sons. Carter talked about how his ex-wife's boyfriend reported Carter to the local police department for trespassing on his property. The practitioner talked with Carter more about the situation and Carter stated that he was arrested for trespassing and was court-ordered to have a mental health evaluation. Carter explained that it was during the previous evaluation that he was given the diagnosis of schizoaffective disorder because "the psychologist felt that I was over-exaggerating when I told her that I was being followed around town by my ex-wife's boyfriend. She said that I was experiencing a high degree of paranoia and made a referral for inpatient mental health treatment where I was locked up for a month."

When asked about his past substance use, Carter stated that he had been smoking marijuana daily for the past three years until he was incarcerated for possession of marijuana with intent to distribute. Carter stated that he has not used since he was released from prison, but that he has been thinking about smoking weed a lot to help his anxiety and depression. Carter stated that he has never been in substance abuse treatment before. Carter reported a history of alcohol use between the ages of 18 to 22 and that he "never really drank more than a pint of vodka, it just wasn't my thing." Carter denied any other current or past substance use.

As the LOC assessment progressed, the practitioner learned that Carter's natural support system was limited. Carter was homeless at the time of the assessment. When asked about his living situation, Carter indicated that he had been "bouncing" from house to house, but that it is not a stable environment. When asked about the "friends" that Carter was living with, he indicated that they all use drugs and alcohol. Further, Carter stated that his family are heavy marijuana users. With reference to managing his health, Carter stated that he did not have a primary care physician and has not been in for a check-up for over four years (when he was sent to the inpatient mental health treatment center). Carter stated that, to the best of his knowledge, he does not have any medical conditions that he needs to attend to.

The provider that was completing Carter's LOC assessment was a European American female in her late 50s named Karen. Throughout the assessment, Karen was having a difficult time determining what type of treatment would be the most appropriate for Carter. She also felt uncomfortable talking about Carter's situation with his ex-wife's boyfriend as she could not tell if Carter was telling the truth or exaggerating. Carter noticed that Karen was uncomfortable during the LOC assessment, which made him feel as though he should stop talking because he was worried that Karen (much like his past counselor) would make him go to inpatient mental health treatment. As the LOC assessment progressed, Carter told Karen "You know, everything is fine. I am sure that I am just misunderstanding the situation with my ex-wife's boyfriend. I shouldn't have even brought it up." To which Karen responded, "It is okay to bring it up, I am just concerned about your perception of the situation and possible delusions that you might be having that we might want to look into getting treated." Further, Karen was unsure about Carter's honesty about his current marijuana use. Karen believed that it is unlikely that people only use marijuana, and no other substances, therefore, she determined that she cannot rule out the possibility that Carter is underreporting his use. She expressed to Carter "I know that it is sometimes difficult to disclose personal information, especially to someone that you just met, but it is very important for me to know all of the details of your substance use so that I can make sure that you can get the help that you need." Carter started to feel even more guarded and replied, "What use do I have to come in here and lie to you, especially since my probation officer drug screens me all of the time?" Karen stated "Carter, I am going to need you to not be so defensive. I am just trying to help." Karen proceeded with the LOC assessment, but found it increasingly difficult to get Carter to disclose the information that she was seeking.

CASE STUDY
DISCUSSION QUESTIONS

1. What is the primary presenting issue in Carter's case?

2. What are your thoughts about Carter's diagnosis of schizoaffective disorder?

3. Do you think that Carter needs services? If so, mental health, substance abuse, both?

4. What are your thoughts about Carter's overall reaction to Karen?

5. What are your thoughts about Karen's reactions to Carter?

CONCLUSION

Many clients present with symptoms of both mental health and substance abuse. Since the mental health and substance abuse service system is fragmented, many clients may feel confused about what type of service they need. To determine what type of treatment is most appropriate for the client, they will have a LOC assessment completed. The LOC assessment assists the practitioner in determining whether services are needed, and what type of services are the most appropriate. A common approach to determining the appropriate LOC is the multidimensional approach that examines the client's risk of withdrawal, biomedical complications, mental health symptoms, willingness to engage in treatment, recovery environment support, and relapse potential. While the LOC assessment and multidimensional approach are comprehensive, complications in determining the appropriate LOC arise when the practitioner lacks awareness, knowledge, and skills for attending to multicultural considerations. As we saw in this chapter, ignoring multicultural considerations can lead to misdiagnosis and invalidation–two factors that can be very harmful to the client. Human service practitioners must have a working knowledge of how to apply multicultural considerations to prevent harm to ALL of the clients they serve, including people who may be part of underrepresented groups in the United States.

REFERENCES

[1]Acklin, C. L., & Wilson, K. B. (2017). Barriers to substance abuse treatment: Why validation plays a crucial role. *SciFed Journal of Addiction Therapy, 1*(1), 1-7.

[2]American Association of Community Psychiatrists. (2000). *Level of care utilization system for psychiatric and addiction services: Adult version 2000.* Pittsburgh, PA: Author.

[3]Bureau of Drug and Alcohol Programs. (2000). *The Pennsylvania client placement criteria.*

[4]Laudet, A. B., Morgen, K., & White, W. L. (2006). The role of social supports, spirituality, religiousness, life meaning, and affiliation with 12-step fellowships in quality of life satisfaction among individuals in recovery from alcohol and drug problems. *Alcohol Treatment Quarterly, 24*(1-2), 33-73.

[5]Mee-Lee, D. E. (2013). *The ASAM criteria: Treatment criteria for addictive, substance-related, and co-occurring conditions.* Rockville, MD: American Society of Addiction Medicine.

[6]Prochaska, J., & DiClemente, C. C. (1984). *The transtheoretical approach: Crossing traditional boundaries of therapy.* Homewood, IL: Dow Jones-Irwin.

[7]Schwartz, R. C., & Blankenship, D. M. (2014). Racial disparities in psychotic disorder diagnosis: A review of empirical literature. *World Journal of Psychiatry, 4*(4), 133-140.

[8]Substance Abuse and Mental Health Services Administration. (2008). *Assertive community treatment: Building your program.* DHHS Pub. No. SMA-08-4344. Rockville, MD: Center for Mental Health Services, Substance Abuse and Mental Health Services Administration, U.S. Department of Health and Human Services.

[9]Substance Abuse and Mental Health Services Administration. (2015). *Women matter!* Retrieved from https://www.samhsa.gov/women-children-families/trainings/women-matter

CHAPTER 13

CASE MANAGEMENT AND VOCATIONAL REHABILITATION

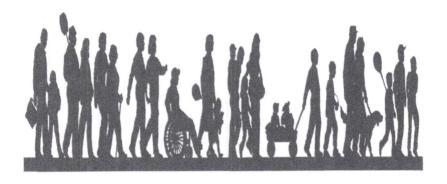

BRYAN O. GERE

YASMIN GAY

ABSTRACT

The primary goal of vocational rehabilitation services is to empower persons with disabilities to become gainfully employed, economically independent, and live in their own communities. Case management is the cornerstone in the delivery of comprehensive and cost effective vocational rehabilitation services. Case management services are needed in the vocational rehabilitation process to facilitate access to medical-restorative, evaluative, and support services to meet the clients' comprehensive vocational or employment needs. This chapter will provide a framework for working with clients in the vocational rehabilitation system. Specific topics will include types of services offered in vocational rehabilitation, funding for services, service outcomes, and common barriers experienced by all clients in the vocational rehabilitation system. The peculiar challenges faced by underrepresented groups in the vocational process are highlighted through a case study and discussed to increase understanding of diversity related concerns.

CHAPTER HIGHLIGHTS

- ➢ Understanding Disability and Vocational Rehabilitation;
- ➢ Case Management Framework in Vocational Rehabilitation;
- ➢ Case Management Process in Public and Private Rehabilitation Agencies;
- ➢ Funding for Vocational Rehabilitation Services;
- ➢ Case Management, Vocational Rehabilitation, and Underrepresented Groups.

LEARNING OBJECTIVES

- ➢ Understand the Case Management framework that is used in working with clients in the vocational rehabilitation system.
- ➢ Identify the types of Case Management services that are offered in vocational rehabilitation.
- ➢ Identify funding sources for individuals that receive vocational rehabilitation services from public and private agencies.
- ➢ Know the types of vocational rehabilitation outcomes in both public and private agencies.
- ➢ Understand how the characteristics and experiences of underrepresented populations adversely disadvantage them in the

260

vocational rehabilitation process leading to poor or undesirable outcomes and how such outcomes can be enhanced through case management.

UNDERSTANDING DISABILITY AND VOCATIONAL REHABILITATION

The presence of a disability significantly impacts the employment and career development of persons with disabilities. There is a consensus that the provision of individualized vocational rehabilitation services can facilitate the employment or career development of persons with disabilities.[2,6] Vocational rehabilitation (VR) services focus on assisting individuals with physical, mental or developmental disability to acquire work-related skills, abilities, and attitudes to overcome the barriers related to accessing, obtaining, and maintaining a job. Additionally, vocational rehabilitation services also assist persons with disrupted employment to be retrained to return to work. Thus, vocational rehabilitation services are beneficial to persons with either congenital or acquired disabilities to become gainfully employed, live independently and contribute to society. A congenital disability is any physical or mental impairment that is present at the time of birth of an individual whereas, acquired disability is any physical or mental impairment that is not present at birth but occurs at any other time during an individual's lifetime.

In the U.S., vocational services are offered by the state-federal agencies, private for non-profit, and for-profit agencies (through insurance companies or workers compensation). In the next section, we will examine in detail the diverse types of vocational rehabilitation systems in the U.S. to provide an understanding of the types of client populations served, and the services that are provided.

PUBLIC SECTOR VOCATIONAL REHABILITATION

Public sector vocational rehabilitation services also known as the VR program emerged in the early 20th century in response to the employment needs of veterans and industrial workers with disabilities.[11] The goal of the VR program is to provide individuals with disabilities with an array of medical, restorative, vocational, and support services that facilitate employment, community integration, independence, and overall quality of life. The VR program also aims at reducing dependence on government assistance, increasing earning capacity, and enabling beneficiaries to contribute to society through taxes.

Today, there are three main public sector vocational rehabilitation programs in the U.S., namely the VR program, Veterans' Rehabilitation or Vocational Rehabilitation and Employment program, and federal/state workers compensation programs. The focus of the VR program is to provide comprehensive services to civilians with disabilities to achieve employment and independence. The VR program is available in each of the 52 states of the U.S., although some states have a second state VR agency that primarily caters to persons that are visually impaired. However, VR programs largely serve civilians with disabilities, veterans, active duty service members, and those transitioning from military to civilian life are serviced in the Vocational Rehabilitation and Employment program.[17]

The Vocational Rehabilitation and Employment program, also referred to as the VR&E program, focus on assisting veterans, and service members who are in the process of transitioning from military to civilian employment to address employment barriers, and transition to civilian employment or living. Persons served in the VR&E program are active duty members of the armed forces with severe injury or illness expected to receive an honorable separation from active duty, veterans with service-related disabilities with an honorable discharge, as well as service members transitioning from military to civilian life. The VR&E is administered under the U.S. Department of Veterans Affairs, with several offices located within each state of the country.

For many active duty service men and women as well as veterans, making that transition to civilian life often require seeking out careers and obtaining the right training and support to become gainfully employed. This is because the skills and knowledge of service men and veterans may not be compatible with those that are required for jobs in civilian work settings. Further, due to service related disabilities, many veterans may require significant retraining and support to facilitate their employment needs. Thus, vocational rehabilitation services are important in facilitating employment and related service outcomes for veterans with various types of disabilities.

Federal/State workers compensation programs also provide vocational rehabilitation to federal or state employees who are injured or acquire an occupational illness. The goal of federal/state workers compensation programs is to minimize the impact of the disability and assist injured workers to return to gainful employment.[4] Federal employees are typically covered under the Federal Employees' Compensation Act (FECA), whereas workers at the state and local level are covered under special laws or state regulations applying to workers employed by private employers.[14] Although the public VR system serves many individuals with disabilities, a reasonable number of persons with disabilities requiring vocational rehabilitation services are served by private sector vocational rehabilitation agencies.

PRIVATE SECTOR VOCATIONAL REHABILITATION

Private sector rehabilitation programs refer to vocational rehabilitation agencies that are privately owned and operated on a for-profit or non-profit basis. For-profit vocational rehabilitation services are operated as private profit seeking business. Thus, a defining characteristic of a private for-profit vocational rehabilitation program is fee for service. In private sector for-profit vocational rehabilitation programs, the focus is on providing services to individuals with work-related disabilities to return to a prior or related level of vocational, physical and mental functioning, and reduce economic losses to the workers and employers. Private for-profit vocational rehabilitation practice encompasses workers compensation, medical case management and forensic rehabilitation. In workers' compensation, a vocational counselor facilitates or coordinates services in the areas of vocational evaluation, assessment, career development, vocational counseling, job analysis, job placement and job development.[4,18] Additionally, vocational counselors in workers compensation provide case monitoring and follow-up, labor market surveys, ergonomic and workplace accessibility consulting, disability management, and medical case management. Medical case management is focused on the provision and coordination of appropriate medical care to someone that is injured or a person with a disability.

In forensic settings, vocational counselors coordinate services that assist in litigation, social security disability insurance, vocational expert testimony, job restructuring consultation, consultation on the Americans with Disabilities Act (ADA), job seeking skills training, and employee assistance program (EAP).[11] Litigation cases may involve workers' compensation, personal injury, life care planning, divorce or dissolution of marriage, employment discrimination, medical/professional malpractice, product liability, and others. You can find additional information on forensic case management in Chapter 15, "*Case Management in Forensic Environments.*"

Private non-profit vocational rehabilitation programs began as community or sponsored programs that catered to the poor or the visually impaired. Over time, two types of private nonprofit vocational programs emerged; vocational workshops that provide vocational evaluation, work adjustment and placement services, and medical-oriented programs that focus on physical therapy, speech therapy, and related services. Currently, vocational workshops which are community-based programs provide a supportive environment for individuals with physical, mental, and developmental disabilities that enable them to acquire job skills and experiences to move into the labor market or become permanently employed in these facilities. Supportive environments are environments that provide access to resources, supports, and services that enable individuals with disabilities to learn and develop the necessary vocational and independent living competences.

Previously called *sheltered workshops,* and presently referred to as vocational workshops, affirmative industries, or industrial workshops, vocational workshops provide services to private contractors, government agencies, and Medicaid providers in the areas of vocational training and employment of individuals with disabilities.[7] A vocational workshop is a work setting that exclusively provides employment to persons with disabilities. Affirmative industries are community-based rehabilitation facilities that provide employment to both disabled and nondisabled individuals. In vocational workshops, disabled individuals are paid below the customary wage, in affirmative industries, persons with disabilities receive the same customary wage and benefits as colleagues without disability in the same job position.

CASE MANAGEMENT FRAMEWORK IN THE VOCATIONAL REHABILITATION

As in many human and allied health services organizations, case management is the cornerstone of vocational rehabilitation services. Regardless of the practice setting, case managers in human services spend a significant amount of their time in facilitating training and employment services for the client populations they serve.

The case management framework is typically client-centered, strength-based, logical, collaborative, systemic, holistic, culturally responsive, and are outcomes driven. Relative to the vocational rehabilitation process, case management involves working collaboratively, and with each client to identify vocational needs, develop a vocational plan, coordinate services to provide training and other necessary support, placement, and employment follow-up services to meet the client's comprehensive vocational or employment needs. Case management also includes working with the clients' family or support system, other professionals, and community or government agencies to obtain vital resources that facilitate the vocational rehabilitation process. Furthermore, the case management framework requires vocational counselors to adopt a holistic and culturally responsive approach that takes into consideration clients' broader physical, psychological, socioeconomic realities, and respect for clients' cultural identity. Consideration of the broader physical, psychological, socioeconomic factors is important because they are likely to intervene in the ability of clients to benefit from services and the interactions between the counselor and the client and ultimately on the employment outcomes.

Although the case management process varies across health and human service agencies and settings, there are some commonalities. Specifically, each practice setting typically adapts the process to fit its objectives and the needs of the clients. Relative to the case management process in the VR program, Roessler and Rubin[10] outlined the following steps:

➢ Screening/Eligibility Determination;

➢ Assessment and Rehabilitation Plan Development;

➢ Implementing (Care Coordination);

➢ Placement and Support Services;

➢ Monitoring;

➢ Evaluation.

CASE MANAGEMENT PROCESS IN PUBLIC AND PRIVATE REHABILITATION AGENCIES

SCREENING/ELIGIBILITY DETERMINATION (INTAKE SERVICES)

When clients are referred for vocational rehabilitation services, their general service needs, and specific vocational goals are often not known. It is therefore incumbent on the vocational counselor, as part of the case management process, to engage the clients and identify their needs so that an appropriate response can be made. Client engagement is the most crucial factor in intake because it initiates a professional relationship and the case management process. It is therefore important for vocational counselors and other service providers to create a welcoming environment that facilitates the engagement process.

Through intake services, vocational counselors are afforded the opportunity to intimately know the client as they identify clients' situations and perceived needs relative to vocational rehabilitation. Vocational counselors should also develop a plan for interaction and delineate the goals that he/she wants to achieve via the intake interview.[10]

During intake, counselors also collect vital information about the client and use the collected information as the basis for determining eligibility and service needs. Eligibility determination is an important aspect of the case management process in both public and private vocational rehabilitation agencies. To receive services in the VR program, an individual must meet three eligibility criteria; (1) the individual must have a disability that causes an impediment to employment, (2) it is assumed that the individual can work, and (3) the individual requires vocational rehabilitation services to become employed.[3,7] As previously stated relative to VR&E services, eligibility is tied to having a severe injury that prevents continued military service, a service-connected disability, and be determined to need rehabilitation services for employment. Also, the individuals should expect to receive, must have received, or will receive an honorable or other than dishonorable discharge from service. Eligibility for VR&E services is within a 12-year period commencing on the date of separation from active duty or the date of notification of disability status.[17]

In private for-profit programs, an individual that presents for vocational rehabilitation services must have a work-related injury or an injury covered by an insurance policy. Whereas in public programs, all eligible persons are entitled to an evaluation and other services.[11] For individuals to be eligible for services in private nonprofit programs, they should have an acceptable diagnosis (medical condition that qualifies for a disability), must be at or above 22 years of age, and meet the financial criteria (low income or earn below a stipulated amount) for acceptance.[17]

ASSESSMENT AND EMPLOYMENT PLAN DEVELOPMENT

Based on the collected information during the intake interview the service provider may sometimes secure medical, psychological, and vocational assessment services from other agencies to obtain a greater understanding of the client's situation. According to Roessler and Rubin,[10] the purpose of the medical, psychological, and vocational assessments is to (1) determine clients' physical and mental capacities and limitations, (2) determine the ability of clients to demonstrate the appropriate behaviors in work or social settings, and successfully fulfill the demands of either roles.

Some examples of appropriate work behaviors include punctuality and cooperating with others on tasks. When making the referrals for assessments, vocational counselors should endeavor, with the client's permission, to share relevant synopsis of client's prior medical, social, educational, and vocational history. Such information will enable the professionals conducting the assessment to focus on the assessment and to obtain specific information that will be useful for the development of the client's Individualized Plan for Employment (IPE).

An IPE is a document that outlines the rehabilitation goals for a client and the services and resources that will be utilized for the client's employment or independent living goals. It is the responsibility of the vocational counselor to review with the client all the information obtained from the assessments to identify the vocational or independent living needs and strengths including service or support requirements that can facilitate the development of the rehabilitation plan.

Vocational counselors are typically required during the assessment and plan development period to have face to face meetings with the client, their friends, families, or another support system to identify focal areas for service and to agree on specific services that should be provided to the client. Obtaining the client's feedback on the assessments provides the vocational counselor with a good understanding of the client's values, choices, and concerns. It is also important for vocational counselors to document clients' feedback and to have accurate case notes on all the discussions and resolutions reached.[9]

Working in collaboration with the client, the counselor then draws up a vocational rehabilitation plan that reflects the assessment of client's situation, their needs, supports, strengths, goals (immediate, short and long-term), and a plan of action to achieve the developed goals.

PLAN IMPLEMENTATION

The implementation of the IEP is a deliberate and purposeful activity that involves the vocational counselor working with the client, family members, and employment placement specialists to deliver on the tasks that are outlined in the case plan (i.e., the IEP action plan). During this time, vocational counselors are expected to make the necessary referrals for services and to advocate on behalf of the client for resources and access to the necessary services. For instance, case managers may need to plan with outside agencies for short or long-term involvement or engagement of the client in some type of service or activity.

Advocacy for access to services and resources or direct purchase of services is arranged to facilitate the implementation of the plan. It is expected that vocational counselors build good relationships with a network of service providers through open and regular communication, and shared understanding of the outcomes. An important task for vocational counselors during this phase is to coordinate services and address the tasks that are outlined in the plan, document the activities that are undertaken, as well as the responses of the IEP team and the client.

PLACEMENT AND SUPPORT

Clients that have completed their training are often assisted with becoming gainfully employed through job matching and placement. The vocational counselor or placement specialist should assess for placement readiness and ensure that clients get the best placement based on assessment results, training, and services received.[10] Support and follow-up services should be provided to the client to ensure job retention, expose or re-introduce clients to new workforce programs and services, and to inform them of new job openings within their communities.

MONITORING

Vocational counselors are responsible for initiating a case monitoring process that reviews a client's progress and update and refine goals in line with the progress made. Case monitoring helps to identify gaps and barriers and enables the vocational counselor to implement creative ways to address client needs. In addition, in the event of the occurrence of unforeseen crises, counselors are better able to decisively resolve these contingencies, without much loss of time or resources. More importantly, monitoring allows the counselor to assess the client's progress and to prioritize the next steps to be taken to successfully actualize the rehabilitation plan. After the client has successfully been trained and successfully placed, the case manager should continue to maintain the relationship with both the client, family, friends, and other support systems to ensure a smooth transition from the service setting to their employment in the community.

EVALUATING VOCATIONAL REHABILITATION OUTCOMES

Outcome evaluation is the final stage of the case management process. Although not directly related to each program participant, outcome evaluation assists program administrators in assessing the effectiveness of the case management process and more importantly, the vocational rehabilitation process. For instance, to evaluate program outcomes, the Rehabilitation Services Administration (RSA) collects and reports summary data on case outcomes in (RSA-911). RSA is the federal agency that oversees the provision of vocational rehabilitation services to persons with disabilities. Outcomes are evaluated by determining whether clients achieved a successful closure (Status 26). Status 26 is a case status code in the VR program. The status system is a federally mandated system that tracks a client's progress through the VR process.

MANAGEMENT IN PRIVATE SECTOR REHABILITATION

In private sector or forensic rehabilitation, there are several focal areas for case management. These include workers compensation, social security determination, marriage dissolution, medical malpractice, employment discrimination, personal injury litigation, life care planning, disability management, and employee assistance programs (EAP) related to substance abuse counseling.[10]

In workers compensation, case management is focused on coordinating services that facilitate the return to work of injured employees to a better level of functioning and to their original work or employment position. In other focal areas (e.g., social security determination, marriage dissolution) case managers act as unbiased experts to testify concerning the full extent to which the client can engage in substantial gainful activity.[10] Someone applying for social security benefits is a claimant.

Case managers in private rehabilitation provide expert knowledge on disability trajectory and ways to enhance the quality of life of persons with chronic illness or catastrophic illnesses (as in the case of life care planning). They facilitate services that proactively minimize the risk of injury, chronic medical conditions or disability (disability management). They provide substance abuse and wellness counseling (employee assistance programs) and advice employers on the implementation of the Americans with Disabilities Act of 1990.

FUNDING FOR VOCATIONAL REHABILITATION SERVICES

An important aspect of case management in the vocational rehabilitation process is to understand the type of funding that is available and the sources of such funding. In the U.S., vocational rehabilitation programs are traditionally funded from three sources; federal grants, state grants, and private insurance. The VR program is funded through federal and state grants. At the inception of the VR program, funding for the program was provided on a 50-50 matching basis between the federal government and the states.[5] This funding formula continued until the 1954 Vocational Rehabilitation Act, that increased the federal share of funding from 50-50 to $3 federal dollars for every $2 of state dollars. With the Rehabilitation Act 1965, the match rose to 60/40.[8] Federal-state funds also changed to a 75-25 ratio because of the 1965 Vocational Rehabilitation Act.[5] Per the provisions of the vocational rehabilitation act amendments, 1968 and 1975, the federal ratio further changed to 80/20. However, federal funding has declined marginally over the decades due to funds paucity. Currently, based on the Rehabilitation Act Amendment, 1998, federal grants fund 78.7 percent (based on the state population and per capita income), whereas, state's fund 21.3 percent of the total program cost.[16] States provide the required match and have the option to contribute funds beyond their required match. States that are unable to provide their full match receive reduced federal grants and the funds are allocated to other states.

The VR&E is also federally funded through grants that are administered under the Veterans Administration program. Approximately 60,000 veterans are served per year in the U.S. in the 138 field offices across the country.[17]

Employers fund federal and state workers compensation programs. Each government agency pays for the cost of coverage or benefits to their employees. Federal employees are covered by the Federal Employees Compensation Act (FECA) program, which is administered by the Department of Labor (DOL).[15] Similarly, state workers compensation programs are funded through payments made by an employer; whether it is a government agency or private business organizations.

Private for-profit vocational rehabilitation programs are funded through payments by insurance companies. Private nonprofit vocational programs are funded by federal, state, and local governments as well as private organizations. Some of these include Medicaid, Medicare, Social Security Disability insurance, RSA Title 1 grants, Workforce Innovation and Opportunity Act, Ability One Program, and from the contractual arrangement with private businesses.[18] Please refer to Chapter 9 *"Funding Sources"* to obtain additional information on sources of funding.

CASE MANAGEMENT, VOCATIONAL REHABILITATION, AND UNDERREPRESENTED GROUPS

Clients from underrepresented backgrounds (e.g., gender, race, ethnicity, and sexual orientation) are likely to have certain characteristics and experiences that adversely impact them in the vocational rehabilitation process leading to poor or undesirable outcomes. Due to discrimination, many underrepresented populations lack access to basic infrastructure, housing, and employment opportunities. For instance, due to the socioeconomic disparities, underrepresented populations that present for services are more likely to have severe disabilities compared to their White/European American counterparts.[17] Additionally, the following are also some specific characteristics that adversely impact underrepresented groups:

> ➤ Negative perceptions about the client and their potential;

> ➤ Language proficiency;

> ➤ Distrust of formal authorities; and

> ➤ Support System.

NEGATIVE PERCEPTIONS ABOUT THE CLIENT AND THEIR POTENTIAL. Negative perceptions about the client and their potential constitute a significant barrier in the vocational rehabilitation process[14] Racial bias has contributed to vocational counselors providing fewer and qualitatively lower services, training, and placements to minorities compared to whites.[12] Failure to acknowledge diversity and the unique needs of underrepresented groups and people of color often results in service underutilization and early termination of services.[6] Also, underrepresented, racial, and ethnic minorities are sometimes socialized to associate certain jobs or occupations as inaccessible. Individuals with disability may therefore focus on low-level positions and unskilled occupations because persons with similar disability characteristics are over-represented in such occupations and because they believe that such jobs are readily accessible to them.[1] For instance, in a study examining whether people with stuttering experienced role entrapment based on stereotypes, Gabel et al. reported that respondents in the study indicated that 23 careers that required more communication and public communication skills were less appropriate for persons that stuttered compared to those who did not stutter.[6]

When these opinions are repeatedly shared and internalized by indivduals who stutter, they are likely to accept a position that requires little or no speaking. However, there are a significant number of individuals who stutter who are working in occupations that require a lot of public speaking. For instance, two of Hollywoods greatest, Samuel L Jackson, and James Earl Jones, are both stutterers.

Similarly, for Lesbians, Gays, Bisexuals, Transsexuals, Queer/Questioning, Intersex, and Allies (LGBTQIA) with disabilities, restriction in occupational choice is often influenced by anticipation of employer attitudes and the overall discrimination in the workplace.[12] As with persons without disability, many lesbian and gay people with disability are concerned about the extent to which they can successfully hide their sexual orientation to be accepted and become successful in their jobs. In a national study using 534 gay men and lesbians, 12% of the study participants reported that they have not disclosed their sexual orientation to anyone at their workplace.[9] Gays and lesbians also struggle with how they can daily navigate their work environments with their multiple identities.

LEVEL OF LANGUAGE PROFICIENCY. Another important consideration for vocational counselors when working with underrepresented client populations is the level of language proficiency. In the VR system, the emphasis is placed on the use of English language as the dominant communication language. However, many client groups are proficient in non-verbal communication expressed through body language (e.g., eye contact, posture, voice tone, and attention).

DISTRUST OF FORMAL AUTHORITIES. Clients from racial and ethnic groups of color also tend to distrust formal institutions and the individuals that represent them due to historical factors such as systemic racism and oppression.[14] A case in point is the infamous Tuskegee Syphilis Study involving 600 African American men (399 of these men had syphilis and 201 did not have the disease). The participants were deceived, given placebos, and were refused treatment even when penicillin became readily available to treat the condition. As a result, over a hundred participants died from the condition and related complications.

This distrust constitutes a barrier to developing a good working alliance that fosters positive rehabilitation outcomes. When counselors reinforce the distrust by failing to listen to client interests or concerns, act unprofessionally toward clients, deliver services in a confusing manner, and engage in discriminatory practices, it is likely that clients will not cooperate or trust the process, leading to poor program outcomes.[14] A counselor's bias may inappropriately influence the rehabilitation process and its outcomes.

Negative perceptions about the client and their potential constitute a significant barrier in the vocational rehabilitation process.[1] Minorities and especially blacks are more likely to be found ineligible for VR services compared to whites. As a result, fewer minorities are accepted into the VR program compared to whites.[13]

SUPPORT SYSTEM. Another important consideration when working with underrepresented groups is the different nature and type of support systems available. In general, persons with disabilities tend to be isolated and have fewer social supports than persons without disabilities.[13] However, successful vocational rehabilitation requires support and assistance from family, friends, and significant individuals in the community (e.g., clergy) in several areas such as finances, religious and emotional support, and transportation. This support assists the individual in carrying out activities of daily living, cope with disability-related stressors, plan and establish vocational rehabilitation goals, build on acquired or learned skills, and facilitates access to necessary community resources through advocacy. Whereas, African Americans and Hispanic/Latinos consider their immediate family members as a support system, LGBT clients may not have a family support group due to rejection or familial conflicts about their sexual orientation.[9] It is important within the case management process to assist clients to strengthen their existing supports, while also collaboratively identifying ways to develop new relationships and support for their overall process.

CASE STUDY
MARISA

Marisa is a 37-year-old Hispanic male to female transgender that acquired a spinal cord injury 3 years ago and is in a wheelchair. Marisa has not changed her name legally, therefore her legal name is Marion. Marisa is currently working with Michael her case manager at Lennox Rehabilitation Services in helping her locate employment. Marisa has a degree in accounting, 4 years of experience as a junior accountant, and recently passed her certification exam. Michael encouraged Marisa to apply at an area accounting firm for an account executive position. Marisa applied online and was granted an interview.

Marisa came into the Lennox office for her scheduled appointment with Michael and expressed feeling depressed and hopeless. She shared with Michael that the interview went well and she was very excited about all the opportunities the company offered. She noted that she felt good about the interview and the opportunity overall. Marisa then noted that she received a call from human resource (HR) and they extended the job offer to her, with the condition that she presented to work as Marion, not Marisa. She noted that the company felt this would be best and would prevent confusion. Marisa noted that she needed the job and is considering the offer.

CASE STUDY
DISCUSSION QUESTIONS

1. What can Michael do to increase his understanding of Marisa's experience, while also continuing to provide effective case management services?

2. Discuss the occupational challenges and barriers Marisa and other individuals with disabilities from underrepresented groups encounter.

3. What are some cultural considerations Michael should consider as he continues to work with Marisa and other individuals with disabilities from underrepresented groups.

4. What type of support or resources should Michael consider for Marisa?

CONCLUSION

Case management is a vital aspect of the vocational rehabilitation process. In both public and private vocational rehabilitation settings, case management services provided by vocational rehabilitation counselors facilitate the provision of services for individuals to return to work following a work-related injury or prepare persons with disabilities with the necessary work experience to become gainfully employed. The vocational counselor must collaborate with the client and their immediate or extended support systems in the community to identify and address the client's physical, medical, emotional, psychosocial, financial, behavioral, and other needs, as well as those of their support systems.

From a broader perspective, case managers are expected to work in collaboration with professionals from across several health and human service practice settings which may include physiatrists, internists, psychologists, physical therapists, occupational therapists, speech-language pathologists, rehabilitation specialists, and social workers. Sound case management practices are needed to address personal and environmental barriers that hinder clients, especially underrepresent populations from achieving successful vocational rehabilitation outcomes.

Most case management efforts tend to focus more on the coordination of services to facilitate the training and placement effort. However, the application of case management practices should take clients' unique personal and environmental factors into consideration which may lead to better employment outcomes across client populations. Discontinuation of services, client attrition, and poor outcomes will continue to be prevalent among underrepresented populations unless vocational counselors are able to better identify and address their client's unique issues and needs.

REFERENCES

[1]Byars-Winston, A. M., & Fouad, N. A. (2006). Metacognition and multicultural competence: Expanding the culturally appropriate career counseling model. *The Career Development Quarterly, 54*(3), 187-201.

[2]Beveridge, S., & Fabian, E. (2007). Vocational rehabilitation outcomes: Relationship between individualized plan for employment goals and employment outcomes. *Rehabilitation Counseling Bulletin, 50*(4), 238-246.

[3]Boden, L. I. (2005). The adequacy of workers' compensation cash benefits. In K. Roberts, J. F. Burton Jr. & M. M. Bodah (Eds.), *Workplace injuries and diseases: Prevention and compensation* (pp. 37–69). Kalamazoo, MI: W. E. Upjohn Institute for Employment Research.

[4]da Silva Cardoso, E., Romero, M. G., Chan, F., Dutta, A., & Rahimi, M. (2007). Disparities in vocational rehabilitation services and outcomes for Hispanic clients with traumatic brain injury: do they exist? *The Journal of Head Trauma Rehabilitation, 22*(2), 85-94.

[5]Elliott, T., & Leung, P. (2005). Vocational rehabilitation: History and practice. *Handbook of vocational psychology, 3,* 319-343.

[6]Gabel, R. M., Blood, G. W., Tellis, G., & Althouse, M. T. (2004). Measuring role entrapment of people who stutter. *Journal of Fluency Disorders, 29,* 27–49.

[7]Migliore, A., Grossi, T., Mank, D., & Rogan, P. (2008). Why do adults with intellectual disabilities work in sheltered workshops? *Journal of Vocational Rehabilitation, 28*(1), 29-40.

[8]Pruett, S.R., Rosenthal, D.A., Swett, E. A., Lee, G.K., & Chan, F. (2008). Empirical evidence supporting the effectiveness of vocational rehabilitation. *Journal of Rehabilitation, 74,* 56-63

[9]Ragins, B. R., & Cornwall, J. M. 2001b. Walking the line: Fear and disclosure of sexual orientation in the workplace. Paper presented at the annual meeting of the Academy of Management, Washington, DC

[10]Roessler, R. T., & Rubin, S. E. (2006). *Case management and rehabilitation counseling: Procedures and techniques.* Austin, TX: PRO-ED.

[11]Rubin, S. E., & Roessler, R. (2008). Foundations of the vocational rehabilitation process, Austin, TX: Pro-Ed.

[12]Schneider, M. S., & Dimito, A. (2010). Factors influencing the career and academic choices of lesbian, gay, bisexual, and transgender people. *Journal of Homosexuality, 57*(10), 1355-1369.

[13]Shavers, V. L. (2007). Measurement of socioeconomic status in health disparities research. *Journal of the National Medical Association, 99*(9), 1013.

[14]Sue, D. W., & Sue, D. (2016). *Counseling the culturally diverse. Theory and Practice.* (7th ed.). Hoboken, NJ: Wiley & Sons Inc.

[15]Szymendera, S. (2012). The Federal Employees' Compensation Act (FECA): Workers' Compensation for Federal Employees.

[16]United States Department of Education (2015). Vocational rehabilitation state grants. https://www2.ed.gov/programs/rsabvrs/index.html

[17]Veteran Affairs (2017). Vocational rehabilitation and Employment. Retrieved from http://www.benefits.va.gov/vocrehab/eligibility_and_entitlement.asp

[18]Weed, R. O., & Berens, D. E. (2010). Private sector rehabilitation. *International encyclopedia of rehabilitation. Retrieved from http://cirrie. buffalo. edu/encyclopedia/en/article/11.*

CHAPTER 14

ALLIED HEALTH CASE MANAGEMENT

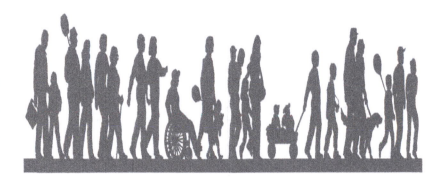

SHALINI MATHEW

AMBER KHAN

YASMIN GAY

SHIRLENE SMITH AUGUSTINE

TYRA TURNER WHITTAKER

ABSTRACT

Health care is an increasingly diverse field where many specialties interact to provide optimal client care. Using a multidisciplinary team approach, each team member functions in a specific role consistent with his/her professional expertise. This chapter provides an overview of case management in a variety of medical disciplines. Information on the different types of medical services including inpatient and outpatient services, Allied Health case management services, funding for services, and common barriers encountered by clients in the medical case management system are presented in this chapter.

CHAPTER HIGHLIGHTS

➤ An overview of case management in allied health;

➤ Allied health case management;

➤ Allied health case management and medical services;

➤ Funding services for allied health care;

➤ Barriers encountered by consumers in allied health case management systems.

LEARNING OBJECTIVES

➤ To understand what Allied Health case management is.

➤ To Identify the types of medical services.

➤ To explore the different levels of case management services in Allied Health.

➤ To identify common barriers faced by clients in Allied Health case management systems.

OVERVIEW OF CASE MANAGEMENT IN ALLIED HEALTH

Allied Health refers to the domain of medical practices that support physicians and nurses. To ensure this support, Allied Health professionals work as a team to evaluate, support, and provide treatment to a variety of injuries and diseases. Therefore, the Association of Schools of Allied Health Professions[17] defines Allied Health as a segment of the workforce that includes a diverse group of professionals who deliver services involved in the identification, evaluation, and prevention of diseases and disorders, dietary and nutrition services, and rehabilitation and health systems management.[17] Therefore, various professionals such as dental hygienists, mental health counselors, diagnostic medical sonographers, dietitians, social workers, medical technologists, substance abuse counselors, occupational therapists, physical therapists, lactation consultants, radiographers, and speech-language pathologists as well as other professionals are all considered members of the Allied Health profession. This chapter reviews how each of these professionals contribute to the Allied Health care team.

As previously mentioned, many professions come under the Allied Health umbrella. We will briefly name and give a succinct description of several of these professional areas of expertise. According to the Bureau of Labor Statistics,[15] a dietician is a member of the Allied Healthcare team who evaluates the client's nutritional and health care needs and provides information to manage food and nutritional intake.[15] A social worker helps people by identifying and treating various day to day problems.[15] Substance abuse counselors identify and treat issues such as problematic drug and alcohol use and other behavioral problems such as eating disorders.[15] Occupational therapists help the person with a disability get back to normal daily life activities.[15] A physical therapist works with individuals with physical challenges to improve movement and reduce pain.[15] A lactation consultant is a health professional specialized in the clinical management of breastfeeding. A medical sonographer is a health professional specialized in producing images of internal structures, using ultrasound imaging. Though there are different professionals involved in Allied Health case management, the goal is to ensure the best outcome for the clients.

WHAT IS ALLIED HEALTH CASE MANAGEMENT?

As the need for health care continues to increase, professionals are welcoming the interdisciplinary team approach as a measure to expand services, integrate diverse perspectives and interventions, while coordinating care to address multiple issues, concerns, and needs of the client. The interdisciplinary team approach to service delivery embodies the construct of case management in which client's individual needs are assessed and subsequently addressed. The Allied Health case management integrative team approach allows for a more comprehensive and practical approach to meeting the client's complex needs. Often, clients have multiple issues that require additional support services, treatments, or both. As such, clients often receive fragmented services, that increase the likelihood that some of the client's needs and issues will not be adequately addressed. For example, a newly diagnosed HIV positive, unemployed, pregnant woman with two children and a substance abuse history requires the coordination of multiple services. In this example, several social and medical issues need to be addressed to ensure a successful outcome. The most noticeable issues are the HIV positive diagnosis, pregnancy status, substance abuse history, minor children, and unemployment. At a minimum, medical personnel (e.g., doctors, nurses) will be involved in her treatment. The medical services received are likely to be supported by the following Allied Health professionals: an addictions counselor, a social worker, a mental health counselor, a dietician, and possibly a lactation specialist. The Allied Health team will consult with the medical personnel to develop a comprehensive treatment plan. Focusing solely on the HIV positive status, to the exclusion of the other current concerns, will likely result in outcomes that do not holistically address the multiple intersecting needs of this client. For instance, failure to address the substance abuse issue can result in medication mismanagement, potential problems with her pregnancy (e.g., miscarriage, premature birth, low-birth weight), and high-risk behaviors. Therefore, addressing all salient client issues is paramount in the case management process. The diverse needs of the client are achieved through an interdisciplinary treatment team approach among the health care professionals, which is the foundation of case management in Allied Health.

Although medical and Allied Health professionals embrace the practice of case management, some view Allied Health case management as merely linking clients to services or service providers while others view Allied Health case management as purely coordinating client care. Moxely[10] affirmed the difference in perception by defining case management as a client-level (depending on individual client's needs) strategy for promoting the coordination of human services.[10] Allied Health case management takes a holistic approach while considering the needs of the client to guarantee that the specific services and treatment needs are met. Lamb[7] noted that the absence of a clear picture of case management is not surprising because the practice of case management has expanded very rapidly in just a few years in response to intense pressures to identify new methods of care delivery that will improve the quality of client care as well as saving the cost of care.[7] The process of Allied Health case management serves as a measure to address specific needs and expand service delivery through assessment, planning, linking, and monitoring services that clients may receive.

The case manager's assessment of the client is vital and should be comprehensive. Additionally, assessment should include information that is relevant and significant. Assessment can be enabled by addressing elements such as the client's background, history of the problem or need, strengths and supports, as well as the case manager's observations and perceptions of the client. Hence, the information gathered from the assessment assists case managers in developing a comprehensive, individualized plan to address the needs and problems discovered during the assessment. The plan should illustrate progression towards the expected outcome (i.e., the needs and problems of the client are addressed). Therefore, it is imperative that case managers become aware of the services, resources, supports, and educational forums in the community.

The last phase of the case management process is the monitoring phase, which includes keeping account of the client's progress as it relates to the respective goals. Monitoring requires collaboration with other health professionals to ensure that the client's needs and concerns are addressed so that adjustments to the plan can be made, if desirable. Utilizing a comprehensive approach to Allied Health case management ensures that each element of the client's needs, along with the available resources, is considered to ensure an optimal outcome for all clients.

LEVELS OF CASE MANAGEMENT IN THE ALLIED HEALTH PROFESSION

Case management is organized into three levels: administrative, intensive, and blended (targeted) case management. Case management functions differ across Allied Health professions. For example, nutritional care may not include an administrative role, whereas in vocational rehabilitation, all three levels of case management are present. Although the functions may differ across the profession, the goal of improving client outcomes is embraced by all Allied Health professionals. The three levels of case management are discussed in the following paragraphs.

ADMINISTRATIVE LEVEL OF CASE MANAGEMENT. The administrative level of case management occurs when working with individuals who function independently, and mostly utilize services when issues (e.g., new diagnosis, unemployment) occur. Clients who function independently may need additional support, guidance, and assistance navigating systems and resources to address the client's needs and issues. Case management at the administrative level requires that the Allied Health team is equipped with relevant knowledge about the resources and services that clients can access. The Allied Health team functions at a macro level coordinating the identification and delivery of services to the clients at an administrative level. For instance, a person with a disability may need assistance with securing employment. An administrative function of the Allied Health case manager may involve connecting the client to an agency or counselor who assists explicitly with job development and placement services. Helping the client navigate resources to obtain gainful employment captures the nature of the administrative level of case management. In cases where the client has more extensive needs, a more in-depth or intensive level of case management may be warranted.

INTENSIVE LEVEL OF CASE MANAGEMENT. The intensive level of case management occurs when working with individuals who require more time and attention regarding supervision, support, and assistance. Intensive level of case management has a smaller caseload compared to the administrative level and blended levels of case management. Intensive level of case management focuses on the severely ill and the terminally ill clients. Therefore, the intensive level of case management is rigorous and may require 24-hour availability from the Allied Health case manager. Intensive case management is often seen when working with individuals with severe mental illnesses such as schizophrenia. Allied Health case managers providing intensive case management services may contact the client frequently as they monitor the client's behavior, coordinate medication delivery, conduct frequent home visits, and possibly arrange for transportation to services with health care providers. The Allied Health case manager may also provide 24-hour weekly emergency crisis intervention coverage if needed. The added monitoring and supervision provided in intensive case management allows for a more personalized approach to case management, which should result in greater management of the condition over time.

TARGETED/BLENDED CASE MANAGEMENT. The targeted or blended case management level has a different element than that of administrative and intensive. The targeted level of case management focuses on a targeted group of people in a specific geographic location, or a group of people with a common diagnosis. The targeted or blended level of case management occurs as the same case manager provides the client continuous care. This level of case management helps build client rapport. Targeted case management is illustrated when providing substance abuse interventions in rural Appalachia. For example, a coal miner residing in rural Appalachia and on Medicaid requires case management services to address his addiction to codeine, which resulted from a work-related accident. Medical, behavioral health, social, and educational services, along with familial support, may be coordinated to address his addiction. In short, targeted case management allows the client to obtain optimal care and wellness more quickly through providing a customized approach to service delivery, which is one of the goals of this level of case management.

ALLIED HEALTH CASE MANAGEMENT AND MEDICAL SERVICES

As previously stated, Allied Health is comprised of many different facets including home health counselors (health care services that are provided at home (e.g., palliative care, nutrition), social workers, nutritional services, and other professionals who work to meet the physical, emotional, and psychological needs of the client. While the notion of case management is diversely defined and practiced, the primary goal is to help clients improve and effectively manage their quality of life. As an interdisciplinary approach, Allied Health case management increases the likelihood of meeting the client's needs and advocating on the client's behalf within the healthcare system.

Advocacy and service coordination are essential elements used in the Allied Health case management process since persistence is sometimes needed to ensure that the client receives efficient health care services. As a client advocate, the Allied Health case manager looks at a variety of paths, solicits the most appropriate plan, and coordinates the support and expertise of other professionals, agencies, vendors, and family members.[9] For example, in home health settings, many individuals who are discharged from inpatient facilities are returning home to receive services that were historically provided in a hospital setting. As such, the case manager coordinates care among a range of Allied Health professionals. Through the provision of case coordination and advocacy services, the client can achieve the goals outlined in the treatment plan.

To be an effective client advocate, the Allied Health case manager must also be aware of the unique dynamics present when working with special populations. The distinct functions of the Allied Health case manager are viewed in the next section by exploring three unique populations in Allied Health-HIV/AIDS, substance abuse and co-occurring disorders, and geriatric populations.

ALLIED HEALTH AND SPECIAL POPULATIONS

PEOPLE LIVING WITH HIV/AIDS. Human immunodeficiency virus (HIV) is a progressive disease that compromises the immune system making it difficult for the individual to fight infections. If left untreated, the infections will worsen and may lead to death in the advanced stages. Late-stage HIV (i.e., the most severe) is referred to as Acquired Immunodeficiency Syndrome (AIDS). AIDS represents a cluster of symptoms which may include pneumonia, respiratory tract infections, and cancer.[18]

The Allied Health team is an essential component of HIV/AIDS primary care. The Allied Health team ensures that the client, who is HIV positive, receives every aspect of health services such as pharmacological intervention, nutritional assessments, psychological support, substance abuse treatment if present, education to prevent and avoid the transmission and training for healthy and safe sex. The goal of Allied Health case management with the HIV/AIDS population is to educate, strengthen and improve the client's quality of life. This goal is achieved through the mutual partnership between the client and the case manager, referrals to a specialist when needed, health education, and counseling support.

Case managers also help clients apply for insurance benefits, get housing, or find mental health or substance abuse services.[18] Services are not limited to the client with HIV/AIDS, but to his/her family and immediate social support system. The interdisciplinary approach utilized by the Allied Health team ensures that the HIV positive client's needs are addressed holistically.

SUBSTANCE ABUSE AND CO-OCCURRING DISORDERS. Substance abuse case management services have many unique considerations. The process should be client-centered, since every client will need something different. The Allied Health professionals must act as an interdisciplinary team to meet the individual needs of clients who may have substance abuse and or co-occurring disorders. For example, a client who has an alcohol use disorder, diabetes, and visual impairment requires collaboration between a substance abuse counselor, pharmacy technician, and a vocational rehabilitation counselor to address mental and physical health, and employment needs. The case manager must dissect the needs of the person and work with the team to address each area concerning the client. Another aspect of the case management role is to advocate on behalf of the client and to educate the client on available resources.

The Allied Health case manager's role is visible in inpatient behavioral health facilities for chronic substance abuse and mental health disorders. In the behavioral health setting, the goal of case management is to return the client to the highest level of functioning while simultaneously working to improve the client's overall well-being.[14] Additionally, in the behavioral health setting, the case manager must have individualized knowledge related to the client, develop a plan, and coordinate an interdisciplinary team that may include a psychiatrist, social worker, substance abuse professional, and family member with whom the client lives. Summers[14] noted that because individuals with chronic mental health disorders and substance abuse problems do not live as long as the general population. This may be due to a variety of factors such as failure to seek help, co-existing medical issues, access to quality care, financial barriers, systemic challenges, and cultural notions, because the stigma is often attached to substance abuse and mental health. Case managers are urged to integrate the client's physical health, substance abuse, and mental health needs to facilitate a longer and healthier lifespan.[14]

GERIATRIC POPULATION. Aging is an inevitable process in the life of human beings. Aging increases the need for care and wellbeing and providing case management services for the elderly can be challenging if it is not approached from the unique needs of the client. The elderly client's physical, cognitive, social, and emotional health must be assessed to determine needed resources and services. As the client ages, there may be progressive deterioration in physical and emotional health. This means that, the Allied Health team must critically examine all domains of health with the goal of providing optimal care. For example, an elderly client with Alzheimer's, diabetes, and limited mobility due to age, requires a more comprehensive approach to Allied Health case management. Upon considering the complex needs of the client, the Allied Health case manager may partner with a physician, nurse, nutritionist, physical therapist, and counselor to address goals outlined in the treatment plan. While the composition of the Allied Health team may differ based on the unique needs of the geriatric client, the goal of promoting optimal health remains the same.

FUNDING SERVICES FOR
ALLIED HEALTH CARE

This section provides a "snapshot" of the types of funding services for Allied Health care. See Chapter 9, *Funding Sources*, that focuses specifically on funding services. Health care is an expensive entity in the United States. Several government-supported programs exist to address health care (i.e., Medicaid and Medicare). Another form of funding in health care is from private health insurance plans. Some health care agencies provide services on a "sliding scale" that is based on the client's income. Additional health care organizations have "charity care" that utilizes grant funds to cover the cost of health care services for eligible clients. Additionally, clients not receiving these benefits may have to use their funds to cover health care costs. Thus, the primary funding sources are Medicaid, Medicare, private health insurance, "charity care," and an individual's finances.

The most extensive government programs in the United States are Medicare and Medicaid. Medicare provides health care funds for the elderly, persons with disabilities, and people receiving long-term treatment (e.g., dialysis). Medicaid provides health care funds for certain individuals living below the poverty level and persons with disabilities. Private insurance can be purchased from insurance companies. Corporations purchase most private insurance as a benefit for employees. Other programs provide resources for individuals with certain medical diagnoses (e.g., Ryan White HIV/AIDS Program, St. Jude's Children's Research Hospital). The Ryan White HIV/AIDS Program[1] provides funding in areas such as medication, support services, and education for persons living with HIV/AIDS. St. Jude's Children's Research Hospital provides services for children diagnosed with cancer and cancer related conditions. Ultimately, funding from governmental or private sources are used to provide the services identified during the case management process.

BARRIERS ENCOUNTERED BY
CONSUMERS IN THE ALLIED HEALTH
CASE MANAGEMENT SYSTEM

Service outcomes determine the purpose and success of the treatment provided to clients in Allied Health organizations. Simply stated, service outcomes reflect the results of receiving treatment. Moreover, service outcomes also largely determine if the client who is receiving treatment will continue to access the services provided. If the service outcome is favorable, the client has a greater chance of accessing services when needed. Alternatively, if there are unmet health needs and the client did not receive a satisfactory service outcome, the chance to access services and have positive outcomes are likely to decrease for the client. It is critical that Allied Health case managers explore individual and systemic barriers that may impact the outcome of case management services.

ALLIED HEALTH CASE MANAGER BARRIERS

Literature supports the fact that clients who come from underrepresented groups may feel a lack of connection with service providers. This is a risk factor for early termination or client "drop-out" from Allied Health services.[13] Allied Health case managers need to address the factors that affect service outcome to ensure that treatment goals are met for all clients receiving services.

Case managers need to be aware of their own biases and be prepared to work with underrepresented groups. Why? Because a case manager's bias against underrepresented groups can and have often acted as a barrier to service delivery, many times service delivery is impacted negatively.[2] Preparing case managers to work with individuals from diverse backgrounds will help to ensure the best outcome for all clients.

The barriers faced by clients in the Allied Health case management system can be unique to the individual or group (e.g., financial barriers, individual characteristics of the client, and systemic barriers.). Furthermore, the barriers encountered by clients in Allied Health case management can have an impact on service outcomes and can depend upon the unique situation of the client, the health care facility, and the services provided in the individual areas where clients may be seeking medical attention. Indeed, barriers can hinder the ability to access service. For example, if the Allied Health case manager does not have adequate cultural competence, the client may feel insecure in the treatment process because of the lack of cultural competence from the service provider. The insecurity in the client, due to lack of cultural consideration from the service provider can be a barrier to access services for the client.

The unique situation of the clients, the health care agency, and the services provided in the individual areas where clients may be seeking medical attention, contribute to positive and negative Allied Health care outcomes. Some barriers faced by clients can include individual characteristics or simply be the result of where the service was received, as well as the systemic barriers that can appear to be of an enormous burden to clients.

INDIVIDUAL BARRIERS

Individual characteristics of the client can be defined as client-based factors that may impact access to services. These are individual barriers. Individual characteristics are described as financial, socioeconomic, sexual orientation, and race. These characteristics may limit a client's access to services and negatively affect the quality of services received. More pointedly stated, the negative perception of individuals characteristics (e.g., race) can lead to counterproductive outcomes. The following paragraphs address how each of these factors (e.g., financial, socio-economic, sexual orientation, and race) affect barriers faced by clients in the Allied Health case management system.

FINANCIAL. Financial barriers may impact access to resources for clients. Having access to healthcare insurance is one area of concern for clients. The playing field is not level when it comes to financial access to healthcare services, because the uninsured client will undoubtedly face significant barriers when trying to access healthcare services. Having insurance requires paying a deductible, which is the amount the client must pay upfront before the insurance company pays the remaining amount. Being able to afford health care can be a challenge for clients who are not able to pay the deductible. Although a client may have insurance, there is no guarantee that services will be affordable or the quality of care equal. Understanding the client from a holistic view, rather than just one individual factor, can help Allied Health case managers and healthcare providers recognize how the lack of finances is a barrier to services. It is important to note that there is a correlation between financial resources and gender and race, for example.

SOCIOECONOMIC STATUS. Education and employment are key components of the client's socioeconomic status. The client's socioeconomic status, which is connected to the affordability of services, can have an impact on access to and the quality of health care services for low-income communities. Similarly, clients with low or no education at all may have similar experiences. Individuals from low socioeconomic backgrounds may find that there is a lack of access to healthcare resources due to their inability to pay. Another barrier is the nature of an individual's employment. For example, a person who works with an organization that does not provide health insurance or incentives may face barriers to accessing healthcare services. Simply stated, these individuals may work full time but have little money to afford a particular kind of health care services. In short, a client's socio-economic status can and have determined the quality of services they may have access to.

SEXUAL ORIENTATION. Sexual orientation is often ignored when providing Allied Health case management. Individuals who identify as members of the Lesbian, Gay, Bisexual Transgendered (LGBT) are often afraid of being stigmatized, shamed, and negatively categorized. Often overlooked, individuals who belong to the LGBT community experience marginalization, and homophobic attitudes that prevent adequate access to healthcare and increase psychological health issues.[4] Health care providers working with people from the LGBT community should preserve a culturally sensitive approach that includes respect, dignity, empowerment, validation, and acceptance as a measure to improve service outcomes. Thus, client's sexual orientation can be a barrier to access health care services, but Allied health case managers can work proactively to ensure that they are advocates for facilitating access and adequate health care for all clients.

RACE. African Americans, along with other racial and ethnic groups, have historically been misdiagnosed by white mental health professionals.[4]

Misdiagnosing racial and ethnic minorities is a barrier for clients in obtaining services by obstructing the client from receiving appropriate and high-quality treatment (e.g., misdiagnosing mental health disorders). The diagnosis of a mental health disorder may be high among specific groups resulting in an impact on case management. Wang, Demler, and Kessler[16] discovered that specific factors, such as being young and African American, were predictors in not receiving adequate mental health treatment services.[16] As noted by their research, race can act as a barrier and thus have an impact on the experience of receiving quality treatment.

Allied health professionals provide services to clients from diverse cultures and backgrounds. Clients from diverse cultures are often ambivalent about seeking help and support services because of past negative experiences with health care systems. Reaching out for help may not be supported in many communities where underrepresented groups reside. In many underrepresented groups, the client's culture may require religious or other forms of help when seeking assistance to facilitate personal or family problems.[12] In fact, seeking help (e.g., mental health, substance abuse) from outside the community can be stigmatizing and seen as a weakness in many underrepresented communities. For example, according to Han and Pong, expressing and acknowledging psychiatric problems is often impacted by culture.[5] For this reason, it is imperative that the case management process embody a multicultural approach that promotes and encourages competence and sensitivity to the unique characteristics of all clients seeking services.

SYSTEMIC BARRIERS

Systemic barriers are the obstacles that are caused by policies and procedures, resulting in lack of access to resources and services. Systemic barriers exist in accessing health care, particularly for marginalized clients, including people of color, people with disabilities, and women.[3] Racism in health care is systemic and has multidimensional effects.[3] The attitudes toward marginalized communities can impact and serve as a barrier to receiving adequate services. The presence of implicit bias (a bias that we are not aware of) resulting in a provider's preference for white over black clients, can serve as a systemic barrier.[3] Furthermore, inequality in the delivery of health care services presents a barrier when a health care provider is biased based on the race or gender of a client. For instance, a survey by the Seattle and King County Department of Public Health revealed that African Americans and Native Americans were 3 to 4 times more likely to experience discrimination in health care when compared to European Americans.[3] Additionally, Holtgrave et al. indicated that black men, who have sex with men, are the group most disproportionately affected by HIV with unmet service needs.[6] It is clear from the evidence that experiences of discrimination can deter clients of color from returning to services, impacting the client's' overall service outcome, when compared to European American clients. Again, it is vital that case managers proactively address the aforementioned systemic barriers to ensure a positive outcome for all clients.

HIV + CLIENT'S INTERACTION WITH AN ALLIED HEALTH PROFESSIONAL: CASE STUDY JOSH

Josh is a 26-year-old Latino male who has been referred by his health care physician to the Washington Behavioral health center to receive counseling services. After an intake with a behavioral health RN, Josh is assigned to receive one-on-one counseling with one of the counselors at the center. Josh has been living with HIV for 2 years and he is on medication that has helped to maintain his symptoms. With new advances in medication, he can live a productive and good quality of life. Putting his dating life on hold for many years, Josh is now ready to be in an intimate long-term relationship. He has had some trouble regulating his emotions and has felt alone in the process. He has not kept regular counseling sessions after he was diagnosed. Although he has a loving and supportive family, he often feels sad and lonely. His primary concern for coming to the facility is to find ways to diffuse his depressive thoughts. Additionally, he wants to be prepared for any health concerns when entering a relationship.

CASE STUDY DISCUSSION QUESTIONS

1. What are some systemic barriers that Josh may encounter in the process of receiving Allied Healthcare?

2. How can case managers optimize the service outcome for Josh?

3. What are some considerations for other Allied Healthcare professionals working with Josh?

4. As a case manager, what are some considerations when working with Josh?

5. What are some other ways to engage all the health care providers working with Josh?

QUALITY AND PROCESS OF HEALTHCARE DELIVERY

The location where clients receive services (e.g., inpatient, outpatient, or home health care) may present a barrier to healthcare delivery. The characteristics of healthcare facilities and the delivery of services can impact the service outcomes for clients. Factors impacting a client's service outcomes may include a) delivery of services at the facility, b) management of services, c) implementation of prevention services, and d) incorporation of a trauma informed approach.[8] Healthcare providers and case managers can evaluate the quality of healthcare delivery and ensure easy access to health care services thereby implementing positive service outcomes for clients.

The way healthcare is delivered may not always be in the client's best interest. If healthcare is focused only on one area, other concerns may not be addressed. For example, if a client has a medical diagnosis for arthritis but is also dealing with depression, the client' depression can go unnoticed in a facility that primarily focuses on the medical complaint (arthritis). An integrated model, addressing both physical and behavioral health, can be a useful approach. Treating the client's depression and arthritis in an integrated manner can result in overall improvement in outcomes, satisfaction in care, and a better quality of life.[11] Evaluating healthcare delivery modalities may be an important consideration in assessing client outcomes.

The management of healthcare systems, hospitals, and private agencies can also impact the clients' outcome. Sometimes, the case manager may feel overwhelmed or overworked which may impact the delivery of services to clients. Reallocation of workload can help unload the burden experienced by case managers and result in positive client outcomes.[11]

CONCLUSION

The discipline of Allied Health consists of diverse professionals working together to provide efficient client care. While the practice of Allied Health professionals varies in terms of setting, the overall goal of working from an interdisciplinary perspective expands services and resources for the client. Unlike traditional case management, Allied Health case management utilizes a holistic perspective as it considers the overall needs of the client to ensure specific services and treatment needs.

The diversity of Allied Health professionals helps improve, expand, and effectively manage the client's quality of life. Utilized in various settings such as home health, outpatient and inpatient facilities, Allied Health case management looks at a variety of paths to healthcare, solicits the most appropriate plan, and coordinates the support and expertise of other professionals, agencies, vendors, and family members. As outlined in the chapter, case management is an endorsed practice that is utilized with diverse populations in the healthcare delivery system. Allied Health case management adheres to a model of providing care from a client centered perspective. Each client presents with unique needs and potential barriers. It is equally important for Allied Health case managers to work individually and collectively to address potential barriers that may impact service outcomes. Allied Health case managers are uniquely positioned to address the complex needs of the client. The collective power of the Allied Healthcare team creates a system of care that ensures a positive outcome and better quality of life for the clients and their family.

REFERENCES

[1]About the Ryan White HIV/AIDS Program. (2016, October 01). Retrieved October 06, 2017, from https://hab.hrsa.gov/about-ryan-white-hivaids program/about-ryan-white-hivaids-program

[2]Durbin, A., Durbin, J., Hensel, J., Deber, R., & Hensel, J. M. (2016). Barriers and enablers to integrating mental health into primary care: A policy analysis. *Journal of Behavioral Health Services & Research, 43*(1), 127-139.

[3]Feagin, J., & Bennefield, Z. (2014). Systemic racism and U.S. health care. *Social Science & Medicine, 103*(2), 7-14.

[4]Freedberg, P. (2006). Health care barriers and same-sex intimate partner violence: A review of the literature. *Journal of Forensic Nursing, 2*(1), 15-24.

[5] Han, M., & Pong, H. (2015). Mental health help-seeking behaviors among Asian American community college students: The effect of stigma, cultural barriers, and acculturation. *Journal of College Student Development, 56*(1), 1-14.

[6]Holtgrave, D. R., Kim, J. J., Adkins, C., Maulsby, C., Lindsey, K. D., Johnson, Montoya, D.C., Kelley, R. T. (2014). Unmet HIV service needs among black men who have sex with men in the United States. *AIDS and Behavior, 18*(1), 36-40.

[7]Lamb, G. S. (1992). Conceptual and methodological issues in nurse case management research. *Advances in Nursing Science, 15*(2), 16-24.

[8]Lee. H Y., Yang. B. M., & Kang, M. (2016). Control of corruption, democratic accountability, and effectiveness of HIV/AIDS official development assistance. *Global Health Action, 9,*1-10.

[9] Markle, A. (2004). The economic impact of case management. *The Case Manager, 15*(4), 54-58.

[10] Moxely, D. P. (1989). *The practice of case management*. Newberry Park, CA: Sage

[11] Simmons, N., & Kuys, S. (2011). Trial of an allied health workload allocation model. *Australian Health Review, 35*(2), 168-175.

[12] Solomon, D., Graves, N., & Catherwood, J. (2015). Allied health growth: What we do not measure we cannot manage. *Human Resources for Health, 13*(1), 1-6.

[13] Sosin, M. R., & Durkin, E. (2007). Perceptions about services and dropout from a substance abuse case management program. *Journal of Community Psychology, 35*(5), 583-602.

[14] Summers, N. (2016). *Fundamentals of case management practice: Skills for the human services.* 5th ed. Boston, MA: Cengage Learning.

[15] U.S. Bureau of Labor Statistics. (n.d.). Retrieved October 09, 2017, from https://www.bls.gov/

[16] Wang, P., Demler, O., & Kessler, R. (2002). Adequacy of treatment for serious mental illness in the United States. *American Journal of Public Health, 92*(1), 92-98.

[17] What is Allied Health? [webpage]. Association of Schools of Allied Health Professions. Available from: http://www.asahp. org/about-us/what-is-Allied-Health/. Accessed September 27, 2017.

[18] Wu, L., & Li, X. (2013). Community-based HIV/AIDS interventions to promote psychosocial well-being among people living with HIV/AIDS: a literature review. *Health Psychology and Behavioral Medicine, 1*(1), 31 - 46.

CHAPTER 15

CASE MANAGEMENT IN FORENSIC ENVIRONMENTS

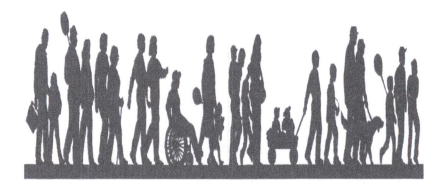

TYRA TURNER WHITTAKER

SHAKEERRAH LAWRENCE

JENNIFER DASHIELL-SHOFFNER

ABSTRACT

Case management in forensic environments involves an exploration of the unique role and function of case managers working in legal settings which include expert testimony, workers compensation, personal injury, disability management, life care planning, and criminal case management. Forensic interviewing in child sexual abuse cases, along with knowledge of the importance of diversity and cultural competency in case managers, is also addressed. Case studies and discussion questions are provided to enhance the reader's critical thinking skills and practical application of concepts learned. Through the examination and analysis of case managers in various roles and functions, the reader is presented with a multifaceted and holistic look into the world of case managers in forensic settings.

CHAPTER HIGHLIGHTS

➢ Role and Function of Case Managers in Forensic Environments.

➢ A Brief Overview of Forensic Environments in Human Services.

➢ The Impact of Diversity in Forensic Case Management.

LEARNING OBJECTIVES

➢ Understand the role and function of case managers working in forensic environments;

➢ Identify the diverse types of forensic environments including expert testimony, workers compensation, personal injury, disability management, life care planning, criminal case management, and forensic interviewing in child sexual abuse cases;

➢ Apply case management concepts using case studies.

ROLE AND FUNCTION OF CASE MANAGERS IN FORENSIC ENVIRONMENTS

Case management is a core function of most human service professionals. Case management is a dynamic process which involves the key functions of individual assessment, case and service coordination; client advocacy, evaluation, planning, and exhaustive documentation. These vital functions are undertaken and coordinated by a case manager. Case managers seek to assess the overall medical, psychological, social, emotional, and financial needs of the individual and family. A case manager's findings from the assessment process are included in a treatment plan that is tailored to the individual. The case manager is the "glue" that connects the three key contributors to the case management process-the case manager, the client, and members of a multidisciplinary treatment team. Under certain circumstances the relationship between the case manager and the client may be ushered into a legal setting. When client-case worker relationship enters a legal setting the strength of the partnership becomes more visible.

Occasionally, case managers interface with the law and legal system. The legal climate is referred to as a forensic setting or environment. Case management services provided to the court or legal system varies and is based upon the expertise of the professional. In forensic settings, there are several types of helping professionals who may be called upon to render their expertise, such as social workers, psychologists, nurses, and rehabilitation counselors.

Forensic social workers may serve as child advocates, or be involved in and assist with child custody disputes; child support, child abuse and criminal misconduct cases.[1] Forensic psychologists may conduct a battery of assessments to determine if an individual is competent enough to stand trial. Likewise, forensic psychologists may also assist attorneys during the jury selection process.[3] Forensic or rehabilitation nurses draw connections and inferences between law and medicine by providing medical testimony in cases of sexual assault, trauma, domestic violence, and neglect.[7] Similar to forensic social workers, psychologists, and nurses, rehabilitation counselors are often summoned to provide expert testimony to determine if a person can return to work after sustaining an injury or illness. If the individual can return to work; rehabilitation counselors provide a list of suitable jobs for the client as well as suggest any supportive treatment or assistive technology that may be needed. Case managers come in a variety of professions, such as social workers, psychologists, rehabilitation nurses, and rehabilitation counselors. When serving in forensic environments, case managers represent the diversity of the human service profession. Although the human services fields may be distinct, the services offered are not mutually exclusive in all cases.

The reader may notice that a significant degree of overlap exists between the case manager's professional roles and the type of case management services provided. For example, forensic social workers and rehabilitation counselors use a range of skills to provide community-based services to an inmate upon release from a correctional institution. The range of skills includes ongoing assessment of needs, coordination of services, linkage, advocacy, outreach, housing placement, and skill development. Law firms and insurance companies may solicit the services of a rehabilitation or nurse case manager to evaluate the impact of an injury or illness upon the individual. Forensic social workers and psychologists may determine if an individual is responsible for his or her actions and is competent to stand trial. As can be seen, forensic case managers are uniquely positioned to make "high stake" decisions about the client's competence which has great implications in legal environments.

The case manager's role becomes even more significant when interacting with the legal system. Consequently, it is important for the case manager to remain abreast of relevant laws, ordinances, and their profession's code of ethics. Equally important is knowing how to handle situations in which the law contradicts the case manager's professional code of ethics. In short, case managers utilize their evidence-based competencies to facilitate the client's continuum of care. Facilitating the continuum of care is described as developing a "roadmap" that outlines the health care a client needs over a period of time. (*see Chapter 12, Case Management, Mental Health, and Substance Abuse. Chapter 12 provides a more detailed description of continuum of care.*) Even when case managers maintain their knowledge of applicable laws, and adhere to their professional code of ethics, their client's roadmap can be altered significantly when there are legal issues to consider. When human services and forensic environments intersect, the impact on the individual can be truly significant, and once again, the role of the case manager takes center stage. The following sections explore a variety of forensic environments where case managers can employ their unique skills and expertise.

FORENSIC ENVIRONMENTS IN HUMAN SERVICES

EXPERT TESTIMONY

Case management has broadened its framework to include components related to forensic environments, including legal terminology, court procedures, and expert witness, also called expert testimony. Case managers are often called upon to render expert testimony. Expert testimony involves testimony made by a qualified person due to their professional expertise, knowledge, or training in a specialized field. Participation in expert testimony is highly structured with limited flexibility, specifically during litigation cases (lawsuits).

When working in a structured legal setting, the testimony provided should remain impartial and objective, based only on facts presented in the case. Regardless of specialty area, case managers should rely on their expertise in making the most effective decisions. Case managers should also strive to use less complex language when testifying. Doing so provides greater understanding for attorneys, judges, and members of the jury, specifically when providing clarity for specialty-specific terms. Expert testimony can be provided by case managers of various specialties within the human services field, including psychology, social work, psychiatry, and counseling. Case managers, when working in forensic environments, must be aware that their testimony has legal and financial implications for the individual involved, especially when working in criminal settings

Forensic psychologists maintain an integral role in forensic environments, especially in criminal settings, jails, and prisons. Forensic psychologist case managers may provide expert testimony in the way of psychological assessment and evaluation of offenders, specifically explaining mental health diagnoses and treatment. Case managers, with a specialization in social work, focus their expert testimony on cases that deal with inner workings of the family unit. For example, forensic social worker case managers may provide testimony regarding proper custody of a child who has been neglected based on facts presented in the case. In addition to child custody cases, forensic social workers may also provide testimony regarding parental rights, juveniles, and proper placement of a child. Case managers with a focus in psychiatry, also called forensic psychiatric case managers, may use their knowledge and expertise to determine mental competency of offenders who are to stand trial. Through assessments and evaluations, these case managers further appraise if an offender will be able to testify, or if the offender has significant mental, cognitive, or intellectual limitations to prevent him or her from testifying. As with all areas of case management, case managers need excellent critical thinking, problem solving, and communication skills due to interactions with judges, juries, and attorneys.

Like social work and psychology, counselors, specifically mental health and rehabilitation counselors, are also employed in forensic environments. Counselor case managers may provide testimony regarding an offender's current mental health status or suitable treatment options. Expert testimony is further used by case managers with a vocational lens. Vocational experts, also called VEs, are knowledgeable in labor market information, job availability, and functional components of jobs. VEs are highly used in disability hearings with the Social Security Administration. In most cases, the impartial opinion of the VE can help determine if a person will be awarded disability. With the VE being responsible for determining past work and current work capability, the case manager can be used to further support expert testimony given during disability hearings. Additionally, a medical evaluation can also be used to help determine suitable work environments based on a person's functional limitations. Due to the nature of the cross-examination process by attorneys, case managers testifying must remain calm and focused, particularly when asked a series of questions aimed at discrediting their testimony. Case management in forensic environments encompasses multiple areas within the human services profession, including psychology, social work, counseling, and psychiatry. The vocational lens of case management also extends to workers compensation.

WORKERS COMPENSATION

Workers compensation is considered by some to be the oldest Social Security insurance program in the country.[12] Workers compensation is a form of insurance, and has three primary goals:

➢ provide medical assistance for those injured on the job;

➢ provide financial assistance to replace lost wages for those injured on the job and consequently are unable to work;

➢ protect the employer from legal ramifications, such as lawsuits and court cases, that the employee may consider because of work-related injuries and lost wages.

Workers compensation plans vary depending on the state and area of jurisdiction. A person can receive weekly payments, past and future compensation, reimbursement for medical expenses, or payable benefits to family members if the injury resulted in death. Individuals with workers compensation claims can also benefit from the assistance of case managers. For example, if a person sustains an injury on the job that leads to a psychological diagnosis, such as anxiety, a case manager with a focus in psychology or counseling can assist him or her with coordinating services to receive proper care. A case manager with a vocational focus can help determine if the injured person is best suited for sedentary work, such as a secretary, due to extensive review of the treatment plan. Effective communication is also needed as the case manager consults with employers for work availability and insurance companies to determine negotiated payoff amounts, specifically if these payoff amounts are determined by the injured person's employer.

When determining negotiated payoff amounts, case managers in forensic environments are aware that workers compensation exists at the state level and the state determines monetary amounts given, requirements, and additional benefits applicable to awardees. Each state also has a governing board that specifically develops guidelines that specify as to how workers compensation benefits will be dispersed to those who qualify. Workers compensation programs not only vary by state and jurisdiction level, but also by groups and organizations. For example, the Veterans Administration (VA) has its own set of regulations dictating how workers compensation will be awarded to those within the VA system. Information on impairments that are covered under workers compensation has changed throughout the past few decades. Several types of occupational related illnesses and psychological disorders have also been added to the list of impairments, including skin disorders (e.g., eczema), hearing loss, heat stroke, lead poisoning, social anxiety, and panic disorder. As laws continue to evolve, clients may consider additional options regarding their specific needs. Workers compensation, although a useful program, may not meet the needs of every individual. In such cases other avenues, such as filing a personal injury claim for example, may need to be explored.

PERSONAL INJURY

Personal injury is defined as an injury that occurs physically, cognitively, emotionally, or in combination, that causes significant injury to the mind, body, and emotions of that individual. Personal injury cases are usually filed by the injured person. As with workers compensation cases, laws regarding how personal injury cases are handled vary from state to state. Three types of personal injury cases include those that cause physical injury (e.g., automobile accidents), medical malpractice (e.g., faulty medical equipment) and product liability (e.g., injury caused by machinery malfunctioning).[12] Case managers involved in personal injury cases are usually heavily involved with the intake process. Medical records and financial documentation of lost wages are two examples of background information needed by a case manager during the intake process. Despite the uniqueness of each case, the case manager is usually tasked with reviewing the individual's background to better determine severity of injury. Nurse case managers provide a critical service to those requiring assistance with the management of chronic conditions, often seen in severe personal injury cases.

Managing chronic conditions require case managers to track the client's individual's case, specifically answering questions of changes that occur throughout the process, such as settlement amounts. Examples of how personal injury can occur include the following: motor vehicle accidents, work-related accidents, occupational-related diseases (e.g., asbestos related diseases), and repetitive strain diseases or disorders (e.g., carpal tunnel syndrome). Medical malpractice claims can result from faulty medical equipment or a medical procedure that resulted in a debilitating injury. For example, a doctor may leave an object inside of a patient during surgery, resulting in internal damage or permanent disability. Product liability, another type of personal injury, usually occurs due to equipment malfunction. A personal injury case of this type can involve more than one person at fault, especially if the person filing the personal injury claim decides to sue either his or her employer and manufacturer of the product. While personal injury claims can arise from various circumstances, specific requirements should be in place to ensure compensation is awarded and received.

For a person to receive monetary compensation from a personal injury case, the injured person must prove that neglect occurred at the fault of another person or company. The injured person must also prove that the injury caused financial hardship in his or her life. The amount of money awarded in a personal injury case depends on the severity of the injury. The most common type of personal injury involves motor vehicle accidents. For a claim to be supported in these cases, as with all personal injury cases, medical evidence is essential. For example, if a person is diagnosed with a traumatic brain injury

(TBI) because of a motor vehicle accident, they will need to provide substantial medical evidence for verification. Documents that can be used for verification in this case include magnetic resonance imaging (MRI) or computed tomography (CT) scans, both integral in the process of capturing detailed, computerized images of physiological injuries. This information can also help determine how much financial compensation a person will receive.[12] Financial compensation can also be a factor in helping to restore a portion of the individual's quality of life, or general overall physical, mental, and emotional well-being, which encompasses their overall satisfaction with life. With issues involving workers compensation or personal injury, one of the overarching concerns is helping the individual to transition back to work as quickly as possible. One of the programs developed specifically to assist individuals with their return-to-work transition is known as disability management.

DISABILITY MANAGEMENT

Disability management is a workplace program that provides a safe return to work for employees who have been diagnosed with a chronic illness, a disability, or both. Disability management programs may also focus on improving the overall safety of the workplace. According to the Certification of Disability Management Specialists (DMS), Disability Management Specialists' work roles are divided into four distinct domains:

> ➤ Disability and Work Interruption Case Management;

> ➤ Workplace Intervention for Disability Prevention;

> ➤ Program Development, Management, and Evaluation, and

> ➤ Employment Leaves and Benefits Administration.[2]

When providing disability and work interruption case management, DMS gather relevant information regarding the individual's case in an effort to develop an individualized case management plan, which is extremely helpful with implementing recommendations.

DMS provide specific recommendations to employers to mitigate the occurrence of workplace injuries. Additionally, DMS also ensure that job descriptions accurately reflect essential job functions to reduce the likelihood of disability and maximize productivity in the workplace.[9] Essential job functions are work tasks that are required to perform a specific job without accommodations. DMS provide programming to employees to enhance their education about disability in the workplace and collaborate with key staff and human resource specialists to assist in managing the disability management program. DMS also assist with managing health-related employment leaves.[2, 10] Workers compensation is not provided with all employment opportunities; not all employers provide this benefit. For workers who are hurt in work-related instances, if the individual can receive assistance through workers compensation or by filing a personal injury case, the individual can often get the needed assistance. Work-related injuries come in various levels of severity. Some injuries are minor while others are catastrophic. Work-related injuries that are considered catastrophic usually benefit from life care planning services.

LIFE CARE PLANNING

Life care planning has emerged as one of the most popular forms of case management due to its focus on catastrophic injuries and illness, as well as the associated long-term consequences. Case managers also find that life care planners are well-paid which adds to the popularity of this type of case management. Life care planning is best described as a comprehensive systematic process of case management that involves the development of a dynamic document that addresses medical and non-medical needs and projects the current and future costs of needed services over the persons estimated life span.[8,15] This document, otherwise known as a life care plan, is a dynamic document that describes the diverse needs of a person with a disability from the point of injury throughout the remainder of their life. A case manager in this environment is called a life care planner. Rehabilitation counselors and rehabilitation nurses are active in life care planning due to their educational background and the medical and psychological impact of disability. Despite their professional background, the goal of a life care planner is to maximize the overall function and quality of life for a person with a catastrophic injury or illness. A life care plan may include a range of components from projected evaluations needed (e.g., speech therapy, occupational therapy, physical therapy) to architectural renovations (e.g., ramp in the home, bars in the hallway). The components addressed in the life care plan depend on the type and impact of the disability. Life care planners utilize a multidisciplinary team approach when developing the life care plan to maximize the individual's quality of life. A life care planner may consult and coordinate services with many individuals including physicians, rehabilitation nurses, neuropsychologists, physical therapists, occupational therapists, speech-language pathologists, rehabilitation counselors, social workers, and therapeutic recreation specialists. Life care planners consult with those multidisciplinary team members who can inform the client's quality of care. The growth and popularity of life care planning provides case managers with a unique opportunity to not only gain substantial income, but also work alongside others to improve the quality of life for individuals who require the greatest need.

Up to this point, we have discussed forensic case management as it relates to employment and livelihood. We have discussed forensic case management as related to work-related injuries and workers compensation; forensic case management as related to personal injury cases, forensic case management as related to disability management, and forensic case management as related to life care planning. What happens when helping professionals are required to perform case management in instances involving crimes of criminal activity?

Next, we'll examine criminal case management and then examine forensic interviewing for sex crimes against children.

CRIMINAL CASE MANAGEMENT

Individuals enter the criminal system because of being charged with committing an illegal act or offense. The person who commits a crime or infringes upon the civil liberties of another individual is known as an offender. It is important to establish a mutual understanding of the types and levels of crime before discussing the role of the case manager in this environment. Criminal offenses can be divided into four distinct categories- personal crimes, property crimes, inchoate crimes, and statutory crimes. Personal crimes are offenses against the individual and can include negligence, robbery, rape, homicide, battery, or any other type of personal assault. An offense against an individual's property or belongings is referred to as a property crime. Property crimes include, but are not limited to, burglary, theft, embezzlement, and stealing cars. Inchoate crimes describe attempts to commit a crime or failing to follow through with a crime. A classic example of an inchoate or "incomplete" crime is attempted rape. One of the authors is familiar with a case involving a teenager who was taken home by her uncle who was abusing alcohol. Thinking that her uncle had left the property, she locked the doors of the home. She was unaware that her uncle was hiding in a room in the back of the house. Her uncle began to fondle her with the intent of molesting her. However, she could escape the situation and the uncle was unable to complete the crime. Statutory crimes involve breaking a federal or state law. Examples of statutory crimes include traffic offenses, driving under the influence, and drug possession. Along with the four distinct types of criminal offenses described, the following two additional subcategories are mentioned to distinguish the level of severity.

Criminal offenses can be categorized as a misdemeanor which is a minor violation that does not carry a stiff penalty and may or may not involve jail time. A more serious crime is often categorized as a felony which often results in a prison sentence of at least one year. Upon completing the time sentenced, the individual leaving incarceration becomes an ex-offender or a re-entering adult that has a criminal record or history. The authors use the term ex-offender to refer to those who were incarcerated in a federal or state prison or a local jail. Usually because of good behavior, an ex-offender may be discharged to complete his or her sentence in the community under supervision (i.e., parole). It is during this transition back into the community that the case manager becomes an integral support in the life of the ex-offender.

Case managers assume a critical role in assisting the ex-offender to re-enter the community. Criminal case managers develop a service plan for an ex-offender. Case managers assist ex-offenders in securing resources that will contribute to their overall recovery and successful transition into the community post-incarceration.[14] In this setting, the case manager may refer the ex-offender to a halfway house which is a residential facility that helps ex-offenders reintegrate into society.[14] Case managers must develop strategic relationships with the community and local employers to ensure that the ex-offender successfully transitions into the community and ultimately acquires gainful employment.[5] The case manager may be required to provide specific services as a condition of deferred sentencing or probation.[14] Securing employment is often a condition of supervised prison release. The criminal case manager may secure job development and placement services to increase the ex-offender's employability. The individual may need specific assistance with resume writing and completing job applications. According to the Center for Substance Abuse Treatment (2012),[14] case management benefits the criminal justice system by:

➢ Increasing supervision through drug testing;

➢ Reducing drug use and criminal behavior;

➢ Broadening the range of sanctions available to the criminal justice system;

➢ Providing systems of graduated interventions;

➢ Offering treatment in lieu of or in combination with punishment;

➢ Providing information to the criminal justice system;

➢ Providing a basis for judicial decision-making;

➢ Extending the power of the court to influence drug-using behavior.[p.60]

The reintegration of ex-offenders necessitates a comprehensive and holistic approach to reentry. Ex-offender's basic survival needs including food, clothing, and shelter must be addressed. Additionally, the case manager in this capacity must consider issues related to any disability the ex-offender's may have, as well as the severity of the disability, criminal offense and history, and ex-offender status (e.g., parole, completion of sentence).[5] While case managers are essential with the reintegration of ex-offenders transitioning back into the community, they are also utilized in child sexual abuse cases, specifically during forensic interviewing.

FORENSIC INTERVIEWING IN CHILD SEXUAL ABUSE CASES
Child Sexual Abuse (CSA) is any sexual act involving a child and includes both physical (e.g. touching a child's genitals) and non-physical (e.g. showing pornography to a child). Often the abuse occurs in secret and the abuser denies any wrongdoing. Sexual abuse has a long-term psychological impact on the child. Often, children are abused by someone they know. In most cases, the abuser is either a family member or a family acquaintance that has purposely befriended the child.[4]

When CSA occurs, case management services require the assistance of several professionals with specific knowledge about various aspects of CSA. These professionals come together to form a multidisciplinary team, each providing case management services based on their specific area of expertise. For example, a social worker typically has the most contact with the abused child via the hospital emergency room or child protection agencies.[17] As the case manager of record, service provision may include assisting medical staff by clarifying the medical processes that will occur, crisis intervention, and referral and follow-up services such as coordinating visits from child welfare and law enforcement, linking the family with associated child abuse programs, and serving as the liaison between the family and the prosecuting attorney.[16]

Although social workers may serve in other roles, their main priority is to ensure that the child is safe from further harm. The social worker may be required to investigate the family's history, ensure that the child's (and the family's) mental health and emotional needs are addressed, and in general, be available to attend to any needs that arise as the case is being resolved.[17] If the CSA victim resides in the same home as the abuser, the case manager must make decisions about the future safety of the child which may involve removing the child from the home. Social workers in this arena also help families understand and navigate the procedures of the criminal justice system.[17] Additional aid for the family may include crisis intervention services, expert testimony, and preventative community activities. For example, if the court recommends that a CSA victim be evaluated, the social worker can help clarify the purpose of the evaluation and explain how it is separate from ongoing treatment.[11] Social workers are a crucial part of the case management process as they serve as the cornerstone of the team, and are vital to the organization of the team's recommendations as the case moves forward.[16]

A forensically trained nurse may also be a part of the case management process. Registered nurses who have completed a Sexual Assault Forensic Examiner (SAFE) course are considered experts in forensic evidence collection and appropriate medical management.[7] SAFE courses generally do not include pediatric training; therefore, forensic nurses who serve as a member of a CSA team must have some additional training in pediatric normal anatomy, physiology, developmental milestones, and child protective issues prior to working with CSA victims.[7]

Social workers and psychologists often serve as forensic interviewers and are essential members of the CSA multidisciplinary treatment team. A forensic interview, by definition, is a developmentally sensitive and legally sound method of gathering factual information regarding allegations of abuse or exposure to violence. The goal of the forensic interview is to obtain accurate and complete information to determine the validity of the allegations of abuse. The forensic interviewer meets with the child and directs other aspects of the investigation.[6] The interviewer must proceed cautiously and ensure that the interview and resulting report are free of bias. It is important to note that any professional receiving forensic interviewing training can conduct forensic interviews. The American Professional Society on the Abuse of Children, the National Child Advocacy Center, and Child First offer forensic interviewing training to a range of professionals.

THE IMPACT OF DIVERSITY IN FORENSIC CASE MANAGEMENT

The changing cultural landscape of the United States requires health and human service professionals to become culturally competent. Being culturally competent means that the case manager makes efforts to increase the level of awareness of his or her own personal assumptions, biases, and beliefs and actively address these areas through consultation. Case managers must also increase their awareness and knowledge of the cultural beliefs, practices, and the impact of cultural oppression on their clients. Finally, cultural competence mandates that case managers acquire and apply the needed skills to work with diverse cultural groups. Case managers must commit themselves fully to the idea and practice of cultural competence to effectively manage cases for clients different from themselves. Case managers must understand that cultural competence is not attained but rather maintained.[13] In essence, case managers can't just *be* culturally competent, but rather they must *work* at being culturally competent with all clients at all times. Cultural competence is a *process* of change that occurs over time as case managers encounter clients from diverse populations.

Highlighting the process of becoming culturally competent comes with a few warnings for the forensic case manager. The authors caution case managers working in forensic environments to avoid feeling culturally competent just because they (i.e., case managers) completed a multicultural counseling course or training. If one is culturally competent due to completing a course or having friends from a specific cultural group can negatively impact the case manager-client relationship and impact the nature and quality of services received. In fact, there is ample research showing that people of color experience patterns of inequity and lower acceptance rates for vocational rehabilitation services.[18] When accepted for services, European American case managers have low expectations of clients of color, especially African-American clients.[9] In some instances, case managers "forget" to inform clients about services that enhance the client's wellness and development and instead reserve (intentionally or unintentionally) those recommendations for the clients with whom they "connect."

Any discussion regarding patterns of inequity must include the impact of language barriers on the case management process. When working with clients who speak English as their Second Language (ESL), culturally competent case managers consider the impact (i.e., formal documents that require a signature) of the language barrier on the case management process. The impact of not addressing linguistic barriers is evident when a case manager providing expert testimony presents a biased statement due to not fully understanding what the client was communicating during the individual assessment process. Culturally competent case managers respect the client's language and enlist the services of additional individuals (e.g., interpreters, family members), with the client's permission, to maximize the quality of the services provided.

Not only does a culturally competent case manager value linguistic differences, the client's sexual orientation is also respected. Lesbian, Gay, Bisexual, Transgender (LGBT) clients also have a right to be treated with dignity and respect when receiving case management services. Culturally competent case managers are fully aware of their own values and beliefs about sexuality. Unresolved bias may manifest as open hostility towards the client that results in premature termination of the case manager-client relationship and ultimately, harm to the client. For example, a forensic case manager working with a transgendered sexually abused teenager may not fully advocate for the teenager to the same degree as an individual who is not transgendered. The forensic case manager's lack of advocacy is likely due to deeply held beliefs about individuals identifying with a gender that is opposite of their sex at birth. The same culturally insensitive case manager may believe that the sexual abuse was a result of failure to create a safe environment for the client (not the counselor) promotes ineffective and inappropriate service delivery with little consideration of the client's needs.

Receiving culturally competent services is a client's right and not a privilege. Case managers working in a forensic environment must provide culturally competent services that result in better client outcomes and effective service delivery. The following case studies further explore the effect cultural competency has while working as a case manager within forensic environments.

CASE STUDY
CARLA

Carla is a 35-year old Hispanic wife and mother of two children who was recently employed as a front-desk manager at the Plaza hotel. The Plaza is a part of a large hotel chain which generates $4 million annually. Carla earns a net salary of $50,000 per year. Carla was working one day when several members of the housekeeping staff were unable to come to work due to a contagious illness. Carla was very concerned about the staff shortage as she realized it was going to take longer to clean the rooms. She also remembered that a large group was checking into the hotel at 3:00pm that day. In her desire to ensure high quality services for her arriving guests, Carla asked the assistant front-desk manager to cover the desk, so she could assist the staff with housekeeping. While this is not something she would normally do, she *felt it was necessary to avoid future complaints about the service at the Plaza. Carla thought she was simply going above and beyond her normal duties.*

While she was making the bed in one of the rooms, she began to feel pain in her lower back. Thinking the pain was related to her sudden increase in physical activity from cleaning, she brushed it aside and kept working. The pain persisted throughout her shift, but Carla was convinced she would feel better once she went home, took some Tylenol, and rested. As such, she did not report the pain to her immediate supervisor or staff. The next morning, Carla struggled to get out of bed and could barely walk. She had no choice but to call in sick and see a doctor. Upon examination, her doctor shared that she had strained her back and would need to stay out of work for at least six weeks and begin physical therapy immediately. Carla informed the Plaza of her diagnosis and subsequently filed a worker's compensation claim so she could continue to receive monetary compensation while she was out of work. To Carla's surprise, her claim was denied. The Plaza contended that cleaning the rooms for one day could not have caused her to strain her back and remain out of work for such a prolonged period. Their position was that she likely injured herself at some other time and was simply trying to gain benefits from the Plaza so she could collect a check while sitting at home. Carla was angered by the Plaza's response, and immediately began researching her options. She hired an attorney who in turn sought the services of a vocational expert.

Carla shared her story with her attorney and the vocational expert, both of whom vowed to help Carla win her case. The attorney informed Carla that she would seek the assistance of a vocational expert in the field who was knowledgeable with Carla's type of injury and had previously served as an expert during many cases such as this one. The attorney told Carla that she has worked with this expert many times on several cases so there was no need to worry. Upon hearing this information, Carla felt confident that between her attorney and the vocational expert, she would win her case.

Although the attorney had prior experience working with the vocational expert, she did not tell Carla that there were rumors that the vocational expert did not have the appropriate credentials to serve as an expert in the field. In fact, the attorney never questioned the expert about her credentials. When the attorney and the vocational expert met to discuss the case, the attorney told the expert that Carla was an ESL client and so there was no need to interview her because she would have to use technical jargon that Carla probably wouldn't understand anyway. The vocational expert did not meet Carla until the day she testified in court.

During the court proceedings, the opposing attorney discredited the vocational expert by exposing her lack of credentials and her lack of knowledge about the nature of Carla's injury. Furthermore, he enlightened the court to the fact that the vocational expert had never met Carla before that day. Carla was fearful of the outcome of her case because she knew this information was damaging. After four days of court proceedings, to the shock and surprise of many, the jury found in favor of Carla. However, her reward was reduced from $100,000 to $20,000 because of the damaging testimony.

CASE STUDY
DISCUSSION QUESTIONS

1. What were your initial feelings upon reading the above case study?

2. Describe the concerns that Carla may have about her present and future.

3. Discuss how receiving workers' compensation will benefit Carla.

4. Was the vocational expert culturally competent? Explain.

CASE STUDY
JOHN

John is a 19-year-old African-American male who was charged with child sexual abuse (CSA) and is currently completing a two-year prison sentence. John was sexually abused by a neighbor at five years old. He has an extensive criminal history that began when he was 14 years old when he was arrested for prostitution to help his mother pay the bills. He was arrested multiple times for petty crimes including possession of marijuana, theft, auto theft, breaking and entering, and simple assault. John lives with his mother and father, aunt, and 10-year-old cousin. His family continually tried to help him but to no avail. John was assigned a criminal case manager to coordinate and facilitate his successful reentry into the community.

Dave, the criminal case manager/counselor, is a 37-year-old Caucasian male and has been working with John in prison to address his negative behaviors and attitude. Dave believes there is hope for John if he can just address the root of the anger that John is feeling which causes him to behave negatively. For the past two years, Dave and John met weekly to discuss his behavior. Dave suggested on more than one occasion that John has a poor view of, and poor relationship with, his parents and that he should work on improving this relation-

ship as well as learning to control his anger. Dave also worked with John on his vocational goals and plans. Dave has been working hard with John to reintegrate him into the work environment in a setting where John can thrive by assisting with interviewing skills.

John's behavior seemed to improve. However, when Dave heard about John's recent conversion to the Nation of Islam (a religious organization that supports the African-American empowerment), he was shocked and dismayed. Dave began to slowly distance himself from John. Previously whenever John was having a rough day or a meltdown, he would request a meeting with Dave and receive an immediate response. Since John joined the Nation of Islam, Dave rarely meets with him. If Dave happened to be in the building when John requested a meeting, he would tell John that he was busy. When John scheduled an appointment, Dave would cancel the appointment and not offer an immediate date to reschedule his appointment. One of John's inmates shared that he overheard Dave expressing disgust toward John and his decision to join the Nation of Islam. When John was eventually able to meet with Dave to discuss the information he received and confirm his release date, Dave denied making any comments about his client.

John knew inwardly that Dave was not telling the truth which caused him to become angry and frustrated. John told Dave that he did not believe him. Dave confessed that he made the comments but did not know that someone overheard him. Dave further expressed that he never expected John to be like "one of them." Dave then told John that he is uncomfortable being around him and felt that he could no longer provide services to him. John was hurt by Dave's words and lashed out at him as he exited the room. Dave silently expressed relief that John departed his office, and does not plan to contact John again.

CASE STUDY
DISCUSSION QUESTIONS

1. What role does the systematic oppression of African-American males play in the case of John?

2. How should Dave have approached his work with John?

3. What are the implications of Dave's actions? What are the possible outcomes?

4. Now that Dave is not working with John, how will receiving criminal case management services from his new case manager help him?

CONCLUSION

The roles and responsibilities of case managers have significantly evolved over the years. Once considered integral in healthcare and nursing settings, the need for case management advanced to other areas, including mental health and the legal system. The need for case managers in forensic environments offers them the opportunity to further enhance their knowledge, skills, and expertise in a variety of areas, including expert testimony and life care planning. While case managers are utilized from different backgrounds (e.g., social work, nursing, and psychology), their role remains unique within forensic settings, whether assisting with coordination of care in life care planning to aiding offenders during the criminal case management process as they readjust to life outside of prison. While case studies are helpful tools to help apply practice knowledge to real-life scenarios, hands-on training and experience foster continued growth and development for case managers seeking to make a difference in the lives of those in need. The use of hands on training is especially helpful working with individuals from diverse backgrounds. Culture and diversity continue to make an impact across various fields, with case management and forensic environments being no exception. The need for cultural competency is necessary for every profession due to the nation's ever-changing diverse climate. Regardless of gender, race, ethnicity, or sexual orientation, case managers must remain diligent and mindful, showing respect to others despite differences. Along with showing respect, case managers may also seek to understand their own personal biases to develop greater awareness about themselves and others. Greater awareness of self and others and knowledge of evidence-based practices are vital components to success as a culturally competent case manager working in forensic environments.

REFERENCES

[1]Barker, R., & Branson, D. (2000). *Forensic social work: Legal aspects of professional practice* (2nd ed.). New York: Haworth Press. International Association of Forensic Nurses (2017). What is forensic nursing? Retrieved at http://www.forensicnurses.org/?page=whatisfn

[2] Certified Disability Management Specialists (2017). Retrieved from http://www.cdms.org/index.php/About/Content/scope-of-practice.html.

[3]Franklin, K. (2014). Forensic psychology: Is it the career for me? Retrieved from https://www.psychologytoday.com/blog/witness/201409/forensic-psychology-is-it-the-career-me.

[4]Glaser, D., & Wiseman, M. (2000). Child sexual abuse. *Principles of Medical Biology*, *14*, 357-378. http://ncat.idm.oclc.org/login?url=https://search-proquest   com.ncat.idm.oclc.org/docview/1645135726?accountid=12711

[5] Harley, D. A., Cabe, B., Woolums, R., & Turner-Whittaker, T. (2014). Vulnerability and marginalization of adult ex-offenders with disabilities in community and employment reintegration. *Journal of Applied Rehabilitation Counseling, 45*(4), 4-14.

[6] Hershkowitz, I., Orbach, Y., Lamb, M. E., Sternberg, K. J., & Horowitz, D. (2006). Dynamics of forensic interviews with suspected abuse victims who do not disclose abuse. *Child Abuse & Neglect, 30*(7), 753-769.

[7] International Association of Forensic Nurses (2017). What is forensic nursing? Retrieved at http://www.forensicnurses.org/?page=whatisfn.

[8] Reid, C., & Grisham, S.R. (2015). The importance of work or productive activity in life care planning and case management. *Neurorehabilitation, 36*(3), 267-274. doi:10.3233/NRE-151215

[9] Rosenthal, D.A. (2004). Effects of client race on clinical judgment of practicing European American vocational rehabilitation counselors. *Rehabilitation Counseling Bulletin, 47*, 131-141.

[10] Rosenthal, D.A., Hursh, N., Isom, R., Sasson, J., & Lui, J. (2007). A survey of current disability management practice: Emerging trends and implications for certification. *Rehabilitation Counseling Bulletin, 50*(2), 76-124.

[11] Strand, V. C. (1994). Clinical social work and the family court: A new role in child sexual abuse cases. *Child & Adolescent Social Work Journal, 11*(2), 107-122.

[12] Strauser, D. (2014). Private practice in vocational rehabilitation. In N. Ditchman, M. Wu, F. Chan, S. Fitzgerald, C. Lin & W. Tu. (Eds.), *Career development, employment, and disability in rehabilitation: From theory to practice.* (pp. 361-388). New York, NY: Springer.

[13] Substance Abuse and Mental Health Services Administration. (2006). *Substance Abuse: Administrative Issues in Outpatient Treatment.* (DHHS Publication No. SMA 06-4151). Rockville, MD.

[14] Substance Abuse and Mental Health Services Administration. (2012). *Comprehensive case management for substance abuse treatment.* (DHHS Publication No. SMA 12-4215). Rockville, MD.

[15] Turner, T. N., Taylor, D. W., Rubin, S.E., & May, R. V. (2000). Job functions associated with the development of life care plans. *Journal of Legal Nurse Consulting, 11*(3), 3-7.

[16] Van Pelt, J. (2013). Multidisciplinary child protection teams-The social worker's role. *Social Work Today, 13*(2), 26. Retrieved from http://www.socialworktoday.com/archive/031513p26.shtml.

[17] Wagner, W. G. (1987). Child sexual abuse: A multidisciplinary approach to case management. *Journal of Counseling & Development, 65*(8), 435-439.

[19] Wilson, K. B., & Senices, J. (2005). Exploring the vocational rehabilitation acceptance rates for Hispanics versus Non-Hispanics in the United States. *Journal of Counseling & Development, 83*(1), 86-96.